Genetic Testing:
Defining Your Path to a Personalized Health Plan

AN INTEGRATIVE APPROACH
TO OPTIMIZING HEALTH

CHRISTY L. SUTTON, D.C.

Genetic Testing: Defining Your Path to a Personalized Health Plan

Disclaimer: The information in this book has been obtained from authentic and reliable sources. Although great care has been taken to ensure accuracy of the information presented, the author and publisher cannot assume responsibility for the validity of all materials or the consequences of their use. You should consult with your doctor before starting any regimen of vitamins or supplements. The nutritional supplementation and genetic information in this book is not intended to diagnose, treat, cure or prevent disease. This report is not a diagnostic test. Do not use the information in it to make any decisions about your health without consulting with your healthcare provider. The purpose of this book is to educate and is not intended as a substitute for professional health care advice. The author and publisher are not liable for misperception or misuse of the material provided. The author and publisher are not liable nor do they assume any liability for any information contained within this book. The reader should consult with their health care provider for the diagnosis and treatment of any health care problems. This information has not been evaluated or approved by the FDA and is not necessarily based on scientific evidence from any source. These products are intended to support general well-being and are not intended to treat, diagnose, mitigate, prevent, or cure any condition or disease. The information in this book is not a substitute for obtaining professional medical advice. You should always consult your physician or other healthcare provider before changing your diet or starting an exercise program. This book is not intended to diagnose, treat, cure, or prevent disease.

Intended Use Statement

The content of this book is intended for information purposes only. The medical information in this book is intended as a general information only and should not be used in any way to diagnose, treat, cure, or prevent any disease, and is not intended to be medical advice. The goal of this book is to present and highlight environmentally and nutritionally significant information and offer suggestions for environmental and nutritional support, and health maintenance. It is the sole responsibility of the user of this information to comply with all local and federal laws regarding the use of such information, as it relates to the scope and type of practice.

"23andMe" is a registered trademark of 23andMe®, Inc. Christy Sutton, D.C. and DC&K, PLLC are not affiliated with 23andMe®

Infographic: Produced by Em-press Design, Inc; and Designed by Christy L. Sutton, D.C.

ISBN: 978-0-692-95067-8

Library of Congress number: 2017914711

Cover photo copy writes: Iaroslav Neliubov and everythingpossible

Genetic Testing:
Defining Your Path to a Personalized Health Plan

AN INTEGRATIVE APPROACH
TO OPTIMIZING HEALTH

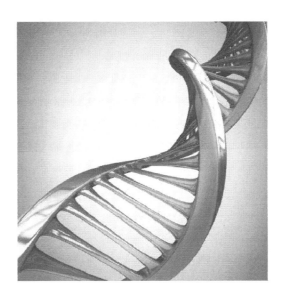

CHRISTY L. SUTTON, D.C.

For my daughter, Madison—You are perfect, even though you have my genes.

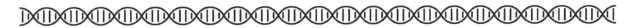

"A person's health isn't generally a reflection of genes, but how their environment is influencing them. Genes are the direct cause of less than 1% of diseases: 99% is how we respond to the world."

—Bruce Lipton

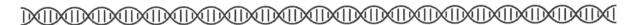

CONTENTS

Christy L. Sutton D.C.

Who is this book for?

This book is for a diverse readership. This book is for the person who wants to make informed decisions about their health and desires to have a better understanding of what they can talk to their doctor about doing to possibly improve their health, and possibly prevent future problems. This book is for the mother-to-be who wants to be as healthy as possible before becoming pregnant. It's for the children who want to be healthier than their parents, and the parents who want their child to grow up to be healthier than themselves. This book is for the grandparents who want to be able to dance at their grandchild's wedding. This book is for the layperson, medical practitioners, students of health and health care providers. This book can be used by many different people for many different reasons. The information in this book can act as a guide to help you work with your doctor to create a personalized health plan.

How should this book be used?

1.) Get genetic testing done through "23andMe"

Simply order a test kit online from www.23andMe.com and complete the test with a small sample of saliva. Once you've completed the genetic testing and your DNA has been sequenced, you can search the "23andMe" website to discover your genotype. "23andMe" will provide ancestry and genetic information to you. This book, and the corresponding genetic report from http:geneticdetoxification.com, is designed to be and expansion upon what "23andMe" gives you. There are many things in this book, and the corresponding GeneticDetoxification report, that are not included on "23andMe". Similarly there are many things that "23andMe" give you information about that I do not include in this book or the corresponding GeneticDetoxification report.

2.) Learn all about your specific genes and order report to go along with this book at http://geneticdetoxification.com.

"23andme" will provide you with some health reports. This book focuses on additional genetic information that isn't covered in the health reports that "23andMe" provides. Once "23andMe" has finished sequencing your DNA, you can use the genetic information they collected to learn what health problems you might be at risk for developing, and what you can talk to you doctor about doing to potentially decrease health risks.

Christy L. Sutton D.C.

Have a customized genetic report created based on the genetic information within this book—If you want a customized report that will provide your genetic information within the context of this book, go to **www.geneticdetoxification.com** Here you'll find directions on how to order a customized report based on your "23andMe" results and all the information within this book.

What makes this book and report stand out is that I've tried to aim for transparency, quality and accuracy within the book and coinciding report.

3.) Work with your doctor to create a personalized health plan.

We don't know everything about genes, but we know enough to potentially make a significant difference in your health

While we can learn a lot from looking at our genes, it's important to remember that we *do not* know everything about our genes. However, we know enough to potentially make a positive and significant difference in your health.

You may think that your genes predetermine your fate, but this isn't necessarily true. Think of your genes as more of a road map that can guide you in your health care journey.

There are many different paths you can take to arrive at each destination in life. If health is your destination of choice, then make the best life choices that will get you there. With the proper understanding, you can make choices that will help you avoid the hazards that your genes may present along your path to health.

We live in an exciting and challenging time in science, medicine and nutrition, with access to more personalized information about our physiological and genetic states than ever before. But the continually changing environment presents new challenges to our health. Throughout this book you'll learn what you can do to better navigate your environment by creating an individualized plan guided by your genes.

Genetic analysis, lab testing and symptoms are all part of the big picture, and must be considered in an integrative manner to better understand potential problems and solutions. Use this book, and the coinciding genetic report, to work with your doctor to help you create a personalized health plan.

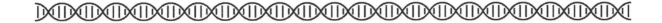

<u>Introduction</u>

"Waiting until you are sick to get healthy is like digging a well when you are thirsty."
— Chinese proverb

Why your environment may be more important than your genes:

Epigenetics—The study of how genes are affected by the environment. This could also be called the science of preventing disease rather than just treating disease.

Epigenetics is the reason you should choose salad over donuts, exercise versus sitting on the couch, getting a good night's sleep instead of partying the night away, and becoming a yogi versus a lawyer. We can't always do what we know is best for our health, but we can support our health to minimize damage from the wear and tear of daily life.

We know that our environment can turn genes on and off, but we have much to learn about what type of environment is best for each individual's genetic makeup. This book is about using the environment to smartly and effectively tip the scale toward health— despite how strongly our genes might be trying to tip the scale toward disease.

What you can do to suppress "bad" genes and promote health:

1. **Exercise, exercise, exercise**—Exercise is the best preventive drug[1]. It's been shown to prevent cancer genes from being turned on while also slowing the aging process. If you have a history of heart problems, stroke or diabetes,

Christy L. Sutton D.C.

exercise is proven to be as effective as many drugs in preventing these problems from recurring[2]. Similar findings exist for arthritis, cancer, respiratory illnesses and some other chronic conditions[3-9]. Moderate exercise, such as walking for 450 minutes weekly (just over an hour a day), has the best effect for promoting longevity[10-11].

2. **Reduce exposure to chemicals and toxins**—Reducing exposure to chemicals in your normal environment will eliminate many toxic triggers that turn on "bad" genes, thus decreasing your risk of cancer, autoimmune diseases and other chronic conditions. Toxins are everywhere, but you can minimize your exposure.

   Common toxic triggers to avoid include:

   - Using cleaning supplies with toxic ingredients
   - Using lawn care treatments
   - Eating non-organic foods
   - Eating foods canned in BPA-lined cans
   - Using artificial sweeteners and ingredients
   - Eating highly processed foods
   - Drinking out of plastic bottles
   - Using cosmetics and lotions with toxic ingredients
   - Getting mercury dental fillings
   - Eating foods with nitrates, including bacon, sausage, and anything with celery seed
   - Using nicotine, alcohol or drugs
   - Consuming excess caffeine

3. **Promote healthy detox and metabolic pathways**—Promoting detox pathways is closely related to avoiding toxins. Because we can't avoid toxins entirely, we must promote detoxification to remove the toxins that we inevitably come in contact with—thus preventing toxins from accumulating in the body. Being able to detoxify and neutralize toxins in your environment is *essential* for health. Unfortunately, certain genetic variations prevent some people from being able to properly detoxify. Promoting healthy detoxification pathways based on your specific genetic defects is covered throughout this book, particularly in part I chapters 1-4 (pg. 19-140).

4. **Ensure a healthy gut**—One way your body eliminates toxins is through your bowels, making it essential to have at least one bowel movement daily. A healthy digestive lining protects your body from infections, prevents allergies and

autoimmune disease, and promotes nutrient absorption for health and longevity. Maintaining a healthy digestive system by eating a diet high in fresh fruits and vegetables while also supplementing with probiotics goes a long way toward influencing what genes get turned on, or expressed, in your body. Certain genetic predispositions are more likely to experience digestive problems. Promoting a healthy digestive system based on your specific genetic variants is covered throughout this book, particularly in part 4 chapter 9 (pg. 269).

5. **Stress less**—Stress (particularly chronic stress) is a killer. Stress-relieving techniques are an essential part of maintaining good health. It's easy to know when you're stressed, but calming yourself down is another matter! Science has proven that stress-relieving activities like meditation, praying, yoga and light exercise can alter your DNA to promote health and longevity. Certain genes can predispose you to enter a stress response more quickly, while others decrease your ability to decompress from a stressful situation. Throughout this book you'll find specific details to enable you to better handle stressful situations, as well as how to calm down more easily when you do become overly stressed (chapter 7 pg. 179-224).

6. **Strive for a more stable blood sugar level**—A blood sugar level that's too high or too low is very stressful on your body. Eating five small meals daily that are high in protein, fat and fiber is a great way to promote a normal blood sugar level throughout the day.

7. **Get adequate sleep**—Sleep is the time when your body heals and recovers from the day's stress. Sleep affects everything in your body, including blood pressure, memory and metabolism. Inadequate sleep can raise the risk of a car crash, diabetes, heart disease, stroke and Alzheimer's disease[12]. Research shows that within two weeks, a young, healthy, fit individual can be transformed into a pre-diabetic state if put on an *irregular* sleep schedule[12]. People who aren't getting enough sleep are also 200-300 times more likely to get a cold when exposed to a cold-causing virus[12]. Two additional things to keep in mind regarding sleep:

   • *Poor sleep will make your brain and body toxic*—Sleep is when your body clears out many of the toxins that build up in your brain and body while you're awake. This book details some of the genes associated with poor sleep and what may help to improve sleep (chapter 7, pg 179-224).

   • *Both sleep quantity and quality are essential for health*—Many people experience low-quality sleep due to waking often through the night or having sleep apnea. Sleep apnea is a serious health problem where breathing repeatedly stops and starts throughout the night. Maintaining an ideal weight, avoiding alcohol and smoking, and getting adequate sleep can decrease sleep apnea.

8. **Decrease inflammation levels**—Inflammation is not only a symptom of an underlying health problem, but it's also a trigger for future medical problems. Monitoring and decreasing inflammation is essential for health. Certain genetic variations can predispose you to have inflammation problems. This book details some of the genes associated with higher inflammation levels and what can be done to naturally decrease them (chapters 9-10, pg 269-318).

9. **Schedule regular lab testing**—Ignorance is *not* bliss. Get routine and thorough lab work and testing to analyze how the environment is affecting your genes.

The body's 20,000 genes manifest as 2,500 metabolites throughout the body. Measuring and monitoring certain metabolites through various lab tests can provide valuable insight into how your genes are reacting in your body.

Certain blood analysis markers serve as red flags, telling us that we need to pay attention and make some changes to our environment. Throughout this book are recommendations for specific testing that should be considered for each genetic variation.

It is important to work with an experienced doctor to help you analyze and understand the labs that you are having performed.

References:

1.) Baulkman, Jaleesa. University Herald. Exercise is the best preventative drug against many health problems. (2013. Dec 30th) Retrieved from: http://www.universityherald.com/articles/6505/20131230/exercise-is-the-best-preventive-drug-against-many-health-problems.htm#ixzz3ZqlVXsnd

2.) Huseyin Naci. Comparative effectiveness of exercise and drug interventions on mortality outcomes: metaepidemiological study. British Medical Journal 2013;347:f5577.

3.) Fong DYT, Ho JWC, Hui BPH, Lee AM, Macfarlane DJ, et al. Physical activity for cancer survivors: meta-analysis of randomised controlled trials. BMJ2012;344:e70.

4.) Sigal RJ, Kenny GP, Wasserman DH, et al. Physical activity/exercise and type 2 diabetes: a consensus statement from the American Diabetes Association. Diabetes Care2006;29:1433-8.

5.) Fletcher GF, Balady G, Blair SN, et al. Statement on exercise: benefits and recommendations for physical activity programs for all americans: a statement for health professionals by the Committee on Exercise and Cardiac Rehabilitation of the Council on Clinical Cardiology, American Heart A Association. Circulation1996;94:857-62.

6.) Garcia-Aymerich J, Lange P, Benet M, et al. Regular physical activity reduces hospital admission and mortality in chronic obstructive pulmonary disease: a population based cohort study. Thorax2006;61:772-8.

7.) Kujala UM. Evidence for exercise therapy in the treatment of chronic disease based on at least three randomized controlled trials—summary of published systematic reviews. Scand J Med Sci Sports2004;14:339-45.

8.) Kujala UM. Evidence on the effects of exercise therapy in the treatment of chronic disease. Br J Sports Med2009;43:550-5.

9.) Byberg L, Melhus H, Gedeborg R, et al. Total mortality after changes in leisure time physical activity in 50 year old men: 35 year follow-up of population based cohort. BMJ2009;338:b688.

10.) Reynolds, Gretchen. New York Times April 15, 2015.The Right Dose of Exercise for a Longer Life. Retrieved from: http://well.blogs.nytimes.com/2015/04/15/the-right-dose-of-exercise-for-a-longer-life/?_r=0

11.) NCI news notes. JAMA Internal Medicine April 6, 2015. Retrieved from: http://www.cancer.gov/news-events/press-releases/2015/peak-longevity-physical-activity

12.) Hamilton, John. Snooze Alert: A Sleep Disorder May Be Harming Your Body And Brain. (2015. Aug 24th). Retrieved from: http://www.npr.org/sections/health-shots/2015/08/24/432764792/snooze-alert-a-sleep-disorder-may-be-harming-your-body-and-brain

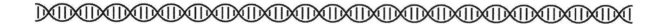

Genes and Your Environment

"It isn't the hand of cards you're dealt, but how you play the hand you're dealt." ### *—Randy Pausch*

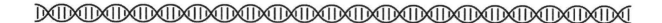

Everyone is dealt a certain "genetic hand" when they're born—something that is, of course, completely out of our control. Some people are dealt a better hand of genes than others. You don't have control over the genes you inherit. But you *do* have control over how wisely you play the hand you're dealt.

For example, some people expose themselves to more environmental triggers, while others modify their environment in ways that limit potential health problems—despite their genes. Understanding your genetic make-up enables you to take certain actions to "bypass" or protect yourself against the genes that predispose you to certain health conditions.

Having a genetic predisposition to a disease doesn't necessarily mean you'll get that disease. On the flip side, not having a genetic predisposition to a disease doesn't mean that you'll never get that disease.

While genes are important, your environment is one of the most important determining factors for your health. You may have inherited great genes with very few genetic predispositions to ill health. But if you're exposed to an unhealthy environment, then you may experience more health problems than someone with less fortunate genes who lives in a healthier environment.

Multiple factors determine if and when a "bad" gene will actually manifest into a disease—including your exposure to toxins and heavy metals, previous bacteria or viral infections, dietary choices, antioxidant intake, exercise habits, mental and physical stress, and sleep habits.

Part 1
Detoxification Genes

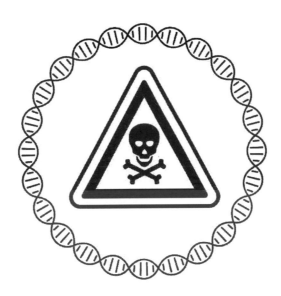

Detoxification genes are critical to allow your body to remove the toxins you are exposed to through daily living. However, some people are genetically hindered in their ability to detoxify. Before genetic testing, "poor detoxifiers" were much harder to identify. "Poor detoxifiers" need to protect their bodies from toxicity and support their detox pathways, just as light-skinned people need to protect their skin when they're at the beach.

Having certain genetic variations can hinder your ability to detoxify everything from caffeine to hormones to pesticides. Knowing your genetic make-up and specific detoxification issues can shed light on where you're most vulnerable. This section will help you identify if you're a "poor detoxifier," where your genes make you most vulnerable, and how to protect yourself from your genetic vulnerabilities.

Christy L. Sutton D.C.

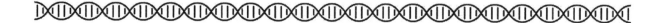

Chapter 1
Phase I Detoxification Genes

PHASE I DETOXIFICATION GENES

Toxin ingested

Phase I
Detox Pathway and Genes

Intermediate highly toxic stage

Phase II
Detox Pathway and Genes

Toxin removed from the body

Phase I detox pathways are an entry point for your body to detoxify drugs, hormones, toxins, caffeine and many more chemicals found in the environment. There are some genetic variations that can compromise the body's ability to detoxify using the Phase I detox pathways. Some of the health problems associated with inheriting genes that compromise Phase I detox pathways include cancer, neurological issues, heart attack, stroke, pregnancy-related issues, birth defects, autism and autoimmune disease.

In this chapter you'll learn if you've potentially inherited genes that negatively affect your ability to perform Phase I detoxification, what specific health problems you're predisposed to develop based on your specific genetic make-up, how to protect yourself from developing those health problems, and how to monitor your health for problems that can result from inheriting genes that compromise your body's ability to perform Phase I detoxification.

All genes that begin with "CYP" are cytochrome P450 Phase I detoxification genes.

Christy L. Sutton D.C.

CYP1A1 gene
Cytochrome P450 1A1 - Phase I detoxification gene

Names of CYP1A1 genetic variants (SNP identification)	rsnumber	Risk allele
CYP1A1*2C A4889G	rs1048943	Risk allele is C
CYP1A1 C2453A	rs1799814	Risk allele is T
CYP1A1	rs2606345	Risk allele is A

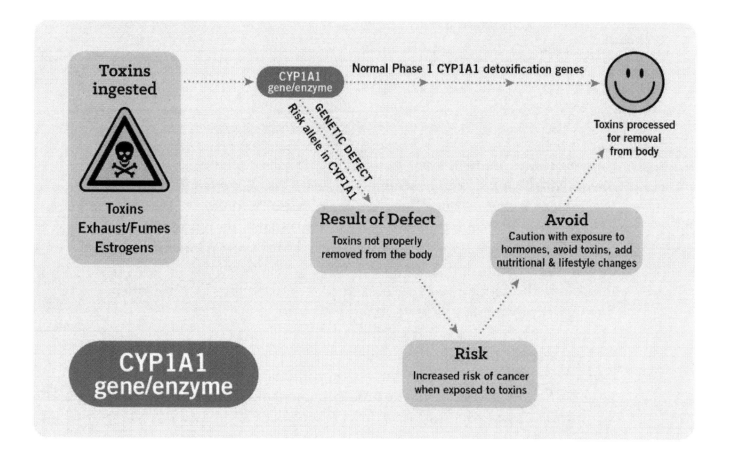

What does the CYP1A1 gene do?

The CYP1A1 gene is essential for Phase I detoxification, the body's initial detoxification step. The CYP1A1 enzyme that is made from the CYP1A1 gene is responsible for the 2-hydroxylation of estrogen.

The CYP1A1 gene helps detoxify:

- *Polycyclic Aromatic Hydrocarbons (PAH)*—The CYP1A1 gene detoxifies PAH, found in exhaust, fumes and cigarettes. PAH also results from cooking meat at a high temperature over an open flame. Having the risk alleles for the CYP1A1 gene carries an increased cancer risk, particularly if you smoke.

- *Estrogen*—Because the CYP1A1 gene metabolizes and removes excess estrogen from the body, having the risk allele carries a decreased ability to metabolize and remove estrogen from the body—a risk factor for cancer. The CYP1A1 gene is responsible for the 2-hydroxylation of estrogen, which is necessary to metabolize and remove estrone from the body.

What health problems are associated with the CYP1A1 risk allele?

- *Estrogen dominance*—This is due to CYP1A1 not detoxifying and removing estrogen as efficiently as it should. Uterine fibroids and fibrocystic breast cancer can also occur with high levels of estrogen build-up. Estrogen dominance can increase your cancer risk. If you have a CYP1A1 risk allele, you're at an increased risk for having high levels of estrogen in the forms called estrone and estradiol. Estrone and estradiol are the most proliferative forms of estrogen, and are the forms most strongly linked to cancer risk.

- *Increased cancer risk*—This particularly applies when you're exposed to high levels of estrogen and PAH from exhaust, fumes and cigarettes.

I have one or more CYP1A1 risk alleles. What should I talk to my doctor about doing so that I can reduce my health risks?

- *Avoid excessive estrogen exposure*—Estrogen can be given as a hormone in birth control and hormone replacement therapy. However, many chemicals in our environment act like estrogen in the body (i.e. soy, BPA plastics, pesticides, nail polish, nail polish remover, stearalkonium chloride, and certain creams and cosmetics with parabens).

- *Exercise regularly*—One of the best ways to prevent cancer is to make time for regular exercise. Just 30 minutes of walking daily can reduce your breast cancer risk by 30 to 40 percent.

Christy L. Sutton D.C.

- ***Keep your waist-to-hip ratio around 0.8 (women) and 1.0 (men) or lower***—Being overweight can lead to extra estrogen production. You can determine this ratio by measuring your waist in the narrowest area and your hips in the widest area. Then divide your waist measurement by your hip measurement.

- ***Ensure sufficient vitamin B-12 (methylcobalmain) and vitamin B-9 (folate) levels***—Both are important for the body's ability to eliminate excess estrogen.

- ***Increase your body's ability to detoxify estrogen***—CYP1A1 detoxification genes are important for the body's ability to eliminate extra hormones, especially estrogen. Things that can help the body detoxify excess estrogen include:

  - ➤ ***Cruciferous vegetables***—Broccoli, cabbage, cauliflower, Brussel sprouts and watercress. Cruciferous vegetables are high in substances that detoxify estrogen and can reduce cancer risk.

  - ➤ ***DIM in supplemental form***—Diindolylmethane (DIM) is naturally occurring in cruciferous vegetables, but can also be taken in a supplemental form to help remove extra estrogen and reduce cancer risk.

  - ➤ ***Fish oil***—Fish oil helps the body metabolize and detoxify estrogen.

  - ➤ ***Calcium D-glucarate***

  - ➤ ***High-fiber diet***

- ***Avoid eating large amounts of food cooked over an open flame at a high temperature***.

- ***Don't smoke.***

- ***Avoid air pollution and exhaust whenever possible.***

- ***Consider supplementing with a high-quality B-complex***—Ensure that it contains the activated form of all B vitamins, which are required for the CYP1A1 detoxification pathways to function properly.

- ***Correct any iron-deficient anemia***—Iron is necessary for CYP1A1 enzymes to work correctly.

- ***Ensure a sufficient vitamin D level***—Vitamin D helps activate CYP1A1 enzymes. A level of 70 to 100 is considered healthy. A low vitamin D level can increase your risk of developing osteoporosis, cancer and autoimmune disease.

- ***Eat more foods that stimulate CYP1A1-Phase I detoxification***—Berries, garlic, onions, green tea, basil, turmeric, cumin and black pepper help support healthy Phase I detox pathways.

- ***Avoid acid-reducing drugs***—These suppress the CYP1A1 phase I detoxification process.

- ***Sweat regularly***—Sweating allows your body to bypass many detox pathways, including Phase I detoxification performed by the CYP genes. Taking niacin (vitamin B3) right before sweating can provide an added detoxification boost by increasing circulation, decreasing toxicity and potentially decreasing cholesterol levels. However, high niacin levels can cause an increased heart rate, so it should only be taken under a doctor's supervision. Also, you should consume additional electrolytes, minerals and water to offset those lost as you sweat.

- ***Increase your antioxidant intake***—Although Phase I detoxification is essential for health and detoxification, it does produce many cancer-causing free-radicals in the body. The best way to protect yourself from dangerous free radicals is to increase your antioxidant intake, including vitamin A, vitamin C, vitamin E, glutathione and alpha-lipoic acid. It's important to eat fresh fruits and vegetables to increase antioxidant levels.

Aging is bad for your ability to detoxify

There is a predictable age-related decline of about 30 percent in the Phase I detox enzymes. This means that even if you have perfect Phase I detox genes, your body's ability to process toxins through Phase I detox pathways will still become 30 percent less efficient due to aging. Thus, whatever Phase I detox genetic vulnerabilities you inherited will become more pronounced as you age. Unfortunately, bodies, like cars, work less efficiently as they age, thus requiring more maintenance.

As we age our overall toxic load tends to increase due to a lifetime of accumulative toxin exposure. That's why it's important to be *proactive and thoughtful* about your toxicity exposure and levels as you age.

Christy L. Sutton D.C.

I have one or more CYP1A1 risk alleles. What labs/testing should I consider to continually monitor my health?

✓ **Routine cancer screenings**—All applicable tests should be performed regularly: colonoscopy, EGD (upper endoscopy of the stomach), skin exam, thyroid exam, prostate exam, Pap smear, breast exam and routine blood work.

✓ **Comprehensive hormonal testing**—Hormone imbalances can be early predictors for breast cancer, adrenal issues, osteoporosis and prostate cancer. Hormone testing can reveal if you're estrogen-dominant, meaning you have either too much estrogen or not enough progesterone.

> ➤ **Essential-estrogen by Genova Diagnostics**—This is an excellent way to find out if you aren't detoxifying estrogen as well as you need to be to prevent high estrogen levels, estrogen dominance, and cancer.

✓ **Toxicity testing**—These tests provides information about your toxicity levels, as well as how quickly you're accumulating toxins in your body.

✓ **Labs to ensure you're not anemic (blood work)**—CBC, hemoglobin, hematocrit, serum iron and ferritin are all necessary labs to ensure you're not anemic.

✓ **Vitamin D (blood test)**— I prefer to see vitamin D level around 70 to 100 on lab work. A low vitamin D level can increase your risk of developing osteoporosis, cancer and autoimmune disease.

Why acid-reducing drugs can make you highly toxic

Acid-reducing drugs suppress all Phase I detoxification pathways. This means that even if you have perfect Phase I detox genes, you can still experience serious detoxification problems from simply taking an acid-reducing drug.

What your body is exposed to from the environment can be much more significant to your health than the genes that you inherit from our parents. Our genes aren't our whole story.

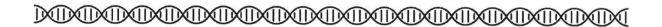

CYP1A2 gene

Cytochrome P450 1A2 - Phase I detoxification gene

Names of CYP1A2 genetic variants (SNP identification)	rsnumber	Risk allele
CYP1A2*1F C164A	rs762551	Risk allele is C
CYP1A2*1F	rs2472304	Risk allele is A

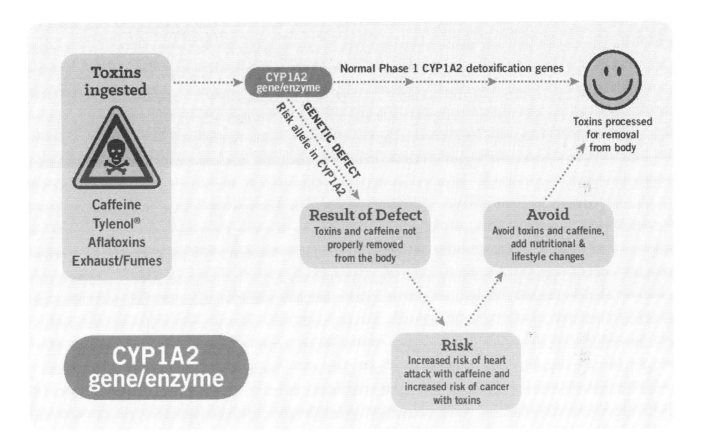

What does the CYP1A2 gene do?

The CYP1A2 gene plays an important role in initiating Phase I detoxification (the first step in detoxification) and in the detoxification of many environmental toxins.

The CYP1A2 gene helps detoxify:

- *Caffeine*—The CYP1A2 (rs762551) gene is important for the body to metabolize caffeine properly. Having one or two C risk alleles for CYP1A2 can cause you to be a "slow caffeine metabolizer." Therefore, drinking caffeine can have a more

Christy L. Sutton D.C.

stimulatory effect because caffeine is metabolized out of your body at a slower pace. Drinking caffeinated beverages such as coffee, tea and sodas could also increase your cancer risk.

- **Acetaminophen/Tylenol**—The CYP1A2 gene is important for detoxifying Tylenol/ acetaminophen.

- **Aflatoxin B1**—The CYP1A2 gene is important for detoxifying aflatoxin B1, which is arguably the most potent cancer-causing substance known. You're exposed to aflatoxin when you eat peanuts, cottonseed meal, corn and other grains[2]. The toxin is produced by a fungus that grows on these foods.

- **Polycyclic Aromatic Hydrocarbons (PAH)**—The CYP1A2 gene detoxifies PAH, found in exhaust, fumes and cigarettes. PAH also results from cooking meat at a high temperature over an open flame. Having the risk alleles for the CYP1A2 gene carries an increased cancer risk, particularly if you smoke.

What health problems are associated with the CYP1A2 risk allele?

- **Increased heart attack risk**—An increased heart attack risk is a concern for anyone who drinks large quantities of caffeine and has one or more CYP1A2 risk alleles. The largest risk for having a heart attack comes from drinking caffeine while having the risk allele for CYP1A2*1F C164A (rs762551):

  - **People with two risk alleles, (or the C/C genotype), for CYP1A2*1F C164A (rs762551) genetic variant**—These people are 36 percent more likely to have a heart attack if they drink two to three cups of coffee a day, and 64 percent more likely if they drink more than three cups a day[1]. This increased heart attack risk was highest in women[1].

- **Increased cancer risk**—The increased cancer risk is from a decreased ability to detoxify and remove toxins such as caffeine, Tylenol, aflatoxin B1 and PAH.

I have one or more CYP1A2 risk alleles. What should I talk to my doctor about doing so that I can reduce my health risks?

- **Avoid excessive caffeine consumption**

- **Avoid Tylenol**

- *Avoid eating foods high in Aflatoxin B1*—This includes peanuts, cottonseed meal, corn and other grains.

- *Exercise regularly*—Exercise is an excellent way to reduce your risk of developing cancer.

- *Avoid eating foods exposed to very high temperatures over an open flame, such as grilling.*

- *Don't smoke.*

- *Avoid air pollution and exhaust whenever possible.*

- *Consider Supplementing with a high-quality B-complex*—Ensure that it contains the activated form of all B vitamins, which are required for the CYP1A2 detoxification pathways to function.

- *Correct any iron-deficient anemia*—Iron is necessary for CYP1A2 enzymes to work properly.

- *Ensure a sufficient vitamin D level*—Vitamin D helps activate CYP1A1 enzymes. I prefer to see vitamin D level around 70 to 100 on lab work. A low vitamin D level can increase your risk of developing osteoporosis, cancer and autoimmune disease.

- *Eat more foods that stimulate CYP1A2 Phase I detoxification*—Berries, garlic, onions, green tea, basil, turmeric, cumin and black pepper help support healthy Phase I detox pathways.

- *Avoid acid-reducing drugs*—These suppress the CYP1A2 phase I detoxification process.

- *Sweat regularly*—Sweating allows your body to bypass many detox pathways, including Phase I detoxification performed by the CYP genes. Taking niacin (vitamin B3) right before sweating can provide an added detoxification boost by increasing circulation, decreasing toxicity and potentially decreasing cholesterol levels. However, high niacin levels can cause an increased heart rate, so it should only be taken under a doctor's supervision. Also, you should consume additional electrolytes, minerals and water to offset those lost as you sweat.

Christy L. Sutton D.C.

- ***Increase your antioxidant intake***—Although Phase I detoxification is essential for health and detoxification, it does produce many cancer-causing free-radicals in the body. The best way to protect yourself from dangerous free radicals is to increase your antioxidant intake, including vitamin A, vitamin C, vitamin E, glutathione, alpha-lipoic acid and superoxide. It's important to eat fresh fruits and vegetables to increase antioxidant levels.

I have one or more CYP1A2 risk alleles. What labs/testing should I consider to continually monitor my health?

- ✓ ***Monitor heart health***—This includes continually monitoring your blood pressure, having regular cardiac stress tests and undergoing routine follow-ups with a physician who is licensed and trained to diagnose heart problems.

- ✓ ***Routine cancer screenings***—All applicable tests should be performed regularly: colonoscopy, EGD (upper endoscopy of the stomach), skin exam, thyroid exam, prostate exam, Pap smear, breast exam and routine blood work.

- ✓ ***Toxicity testing***—This test provides information about your toxicity levels and how quickly you're accumulating toxins in your body.

- ✓ ***Labs to ensure you're not anemic (blood work)***—CBC, hemoglobin, hematocrit, serum iron and ferritin are all necessary labs to ensure you're not anemic.

- ✓ ***Caffeine challenge test***—The caffeine challenge test provides a more accurate representation of how well the CYP1A2 detoxification pathways are clearing caffeine from your body.

- ✓ ***Vitamin D (blood test)***— I prefer to see vitamin D level around 70 to 100 on lab work. A low vitamin D level can increase your risk of developing osteoporosis, cancer and autoimmune disease.

References:

1.) Marilyn C. Cornelis, BSc; Ahmed El-Sohemy, PhD; Edmond K. Kabagambe. Coffee, CYP1A2 Genotype, and Risk of Myocardial Infarction. JAMA. 2006;295(10):1135-1141.

2.) Galvano F., Ritieni A., Piva G., Pietri A. Mycotoxins in the human food chain. In: Diaz D.E., editor. The Mycotoxin Blue Book. Nottingham University Press; Nottingham, UK: 2005. pp. 187–224.

CYP1B1 gene

Cytochrome P450 1B1 - Phase I detoxification gene

Names of CYP1B1 genetic variants (SNP identification)	rsnumber	Risk allele
CYP1B1 L432V	rs1056836	Risk allele is C
CYP1B1 N453S	rs1800440	Risk allele is T
CYP1B1 R48G	rs10012	Risk allele is C

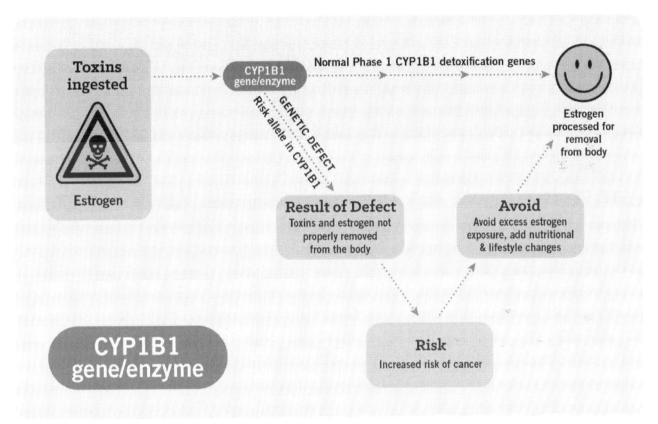

What does the CYP1B1 gene do?

The CYP1B1 gene helps detoxify estrogen from the body. The CYP1B1 enzyme that is made from the CYP1B1 gene is responsible for the 4-hydroxylation of estrogen.

What health problems are associated with the CYP1B1 risk allele?

- **Increased cancer risk**—Having CYP1B1 risk alleles can lead to a decreased ability to properly detoxify estrogen, increasing your risk for developing estrogen dominance and cancer. This risk is exacerbated when you're exposed to

Christy L. Sutton D.C.

excessive hormones and xenobiotics. Xenobiotics are foreign chemicals found in the body that aren't normally present (i.e. drugs, antibiotics, dioxin, pesticides and other toxins). The CYP1B1 gene is responsible for the 4-hydroxylation of estrogen, which is necessary to metabolize and remove estrone from the body.

- **Estrogen dominance**—This condition occurs when the ratio of estrogen is too high, and can also occur due to having inherited CYP1B1 risk alleles that cause Phase I detoxification to be hindered in its ability to detoxify estrogen as efficiently as it should. Uterine fibroids and fibrocystic breast can also occur with high levels of estrogen build-up. Estrogen dominance can increase your cancer risk. If you have a CYP1B1 risk allele, then you're at an increased risk for having high levels of estrogen in the forms called estrone and estradiol. Estrone and estradiol are the most proliferative forms of estrogen, and are the forms that are most strongly linked to cancer risks.

I have one or more CYP1B1 risk alleles. What should I talk to my doctor about doing so that I can reduce my health risks?

- *Avoid radiation*—If you have the CYP1B1 L432V (rs1056836) risk allele, there is some evidence that you may be more sensitive to radiation exposure. Your risk of developing breast cancer may also be significantly increased with radiation exposure[1] from sources such as X-rays and mammograms. If you have the CYP1B1 L432V (rs1056836) risk allele, you should be particularly careful about radiation exposure, especially to your breast tissue.

- *Avoid excessive estrogen exposure*—Estrogen can be given as a hormone in birth control and hormone replacement therapy. However, many chemicals in our environment act like estrogen in the body (i.e. soy, BPA plastics, pesticides, nail polish, nail polish remover, stearalkonium chloride, and certain creams and cosmetics with parabens).

- *Increase your body's ability to detoxify estrogen*—CYP1B1 detoxification genes are important for the body's ability to eliminate extra hormones, especially estrogen. Things that help your body detoxify excess estrogen include:

  - ➤ *Cruciferous vegetables*—Broccoli, cabbage, cauliflower, Brussel sprouts and watercress are high in substances that detoxify estrogen and reduce cancer risk.

- ➤ ***DIM in supplemental form***—Diindolylmethane (DIM) is naturally occurring in cruciferous vegetables, but can also be taken in a supplemental form to help your body remove extra estrogen and reduce cancer risk.

- ➤ ***Fish oil***—Fish oil helps the body metabolize and detoxify estrogen.

- ➤ ***Calcium D-glucarate***

- ➤ ***High-fiber diet***

- ***Exercise regularly***—One of the best ways to prevent cancer is to make time for regular exercise. Just 30 minutes of walking daily can reduce your breast cancer risk by 30-40 percent.

- ***Keep your waist-to-hip ratio around 0.8 (women) and 1.0 (men) or lower***—Being overweight can lead to extra estrogen production. You can determine this ratio by measuring your waist in the narrowest area and your hips in the widest area. Then divide your waist measurement by your hip measurement.

- ***Ensure sufficient vitamin B-12 (methylcobalamin) and vitamin B-9 (folate) levels***—Both are important for the body's ability to eliminate excess estrogen.

- ***Consider supplementing with a high-quality B-complex***—Ensure that it contains the activated form of all B vitamins, which are required for the CYP1B1 detoxification pathways to function properly.

- ***Correct any iron-deficient anemia***—Iron is necessary for CYP1B1 enzymes to work properly.

- ***Ensure a sufficient vitamin D level***—Vitamin D helps activate CYP1B1 enzymes. I prefer to see vitamin D level around 70 to 100 on lab work. A low vitamin D level can increase your risk of developing osteoporosis, cancer and autoimmune disease.

- ***Eat foods that stimulate CYP1B1 Phase I detox pathways***—Berries, garlic, onions, green tea, basil, turmeric, cumin and black pepper support healthy Phase I detox pathways.

Christy L. Sutton D.C.

- *Avoid acid-reducing drugs*—These suppress the CYP1B1 phase I detoxification process

- *Sweat regularly*—Sweating allows your body to bypass many detox pathways, including Phase I detoxification performed by the CYP genes. Taking niacin (vitamin B3) right before sweating can provide an added detoxification boost by increasing circulation, decreasing toxicity and potentially decreasing cholesterol levels. However, high niacin levels can cause an increased heart rate, so it should only be taken under a doctor's supervision. Also, you should consume additional electrolytes, minerals and water to offset those lost as you sweat.

- *Increase your antioxidant intake*—Phase I detoxification is essential for health and detoxification, but can produce many cancer-causing free-radicals in the body. The best way to protect yourself from dangerous free radicals is to increase your antioxidant intake, including vitamin A, vitamin C, vitamin E, glutathione, alpha-lipoic acid and superoxide. It's important to eat fresh fruits and vegetables to increase antioxidant levels.

I have at least one risk allele for the CYP1B1 gene. What labs/testing should I considered to continually monitor my health?

- ✓ *Routine cancer screenings*—All applicable tests should be performed regularly: colonoscopy, EGD (upper endoscopy of the stomach), skin exam, thyroid exam, prostate exam, Pap smear, breast exam and routine blood work.

- ✓ *Comprehensive hormonal testing*—Hormone imbalances can be early predictors for breast cancer, adrenal issues, osteoporosis and prostate cancer. Hormone testing can reveal if you are estrogen-dominant, meaning you have either too much estrogen or not enough progesterone

  - ➤ *Essential-estrogen by Genova Diagnostics*—This is an excellent way to find out if you aren't detoxifying estrogen as well as you need to be to prevent high estrogen levels, estrogen dominance, and cancer.

- ✓ *Labs to ensure you aren't anemic (blood work)*—CBC, hemoglobin, hematocrit, serum iron and ferritin are all necessary labs to ensure you aren't anemic.

✓ **Vitamin D (blood test)**— I prefer to see vitamin D level around 70 to 100 on lab work. A low vitamin D level can increase your risk of developing osteoporosis, cancer and autoimmune disease.

References:

1.) Sigurdson AJ1, Bhatti P, et al. Polymorphisms in estrogen biosynthesis and metabolism-related genes, ionizing radiation exposure, and risk of breast cancer among US radiologic technologists. Breast Cancer Res Treat. 2009 Nov;118(1):177-84.

2.) Retrieved from: https://www.mygenefood.com/cyp1b1-gene-estrogen-metabolism-cancer-risk/

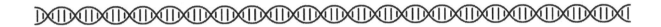

CYP2A6 gene

Cytochrome P450 2A6 - Phase I detoxification gene

Names of C2P2A6 genetic variants (SNP identification)	rsnumber	Risk allele
CYP2A6*2 1799T>A	rs1801272	Risk allele is T

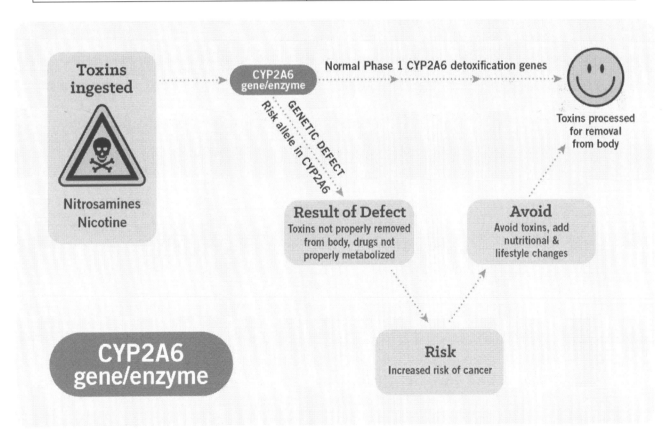

Christy L. Sutton D.C.

What does the CYP2A6 gene do?

The CYP2A6 gene is important for nitrosamine and nicotine detoxification. When you eat processed meats containing nitrates, your body converts the nitrates to nitrosamines; thus, a good reason to avoid processed meats containing nitrates. nitrosamines can be found in beer, pesticides, some cosmetics, most rubber products and e-cigarette vapor. Nicotine is found in tobacco products.

What health problems are associated with the CYP2A6 risk allele?

Increased cancer risk—Having the CYP2A6 risk allele brings an increased cancer risk, particularly lung cancer. Caffeine and smoking are problematic for people with a CYP2A6 risk allele. Avoiding smoking and caffeine may help decrease your cancer risk.

I have the CYP2A6 risk allele. What should I talk to my doctor about doing so that I can reduce my health risks?

- *Avoid cancer-causing nitrates in food*—These are found in bacon, sausage, processed meats and celery powder.

- *Avoid nicotine, smoking and caffeine*.

- *Avoid nitrosamines*—These are found in beer, pesticides, some cosmetics, most rubber products and e-cigarette vapor.

- *Exercise regularly*—One of the best ways to prevent cancer is to make time for regular exercise. Just 30 minutes of walking daily can reduce your breast cancer risk by 30 to 40 percent.

- *Consider supplementing with a high-quality B-complex*—Ensure that it contains the activated form of all B vitamins, which are required for the CYP2A6 detoxification pathways to function.

- *Correct any iron-deficient anemia*—Iron is necessary for CYP2A6 detoxification pathways to work properly.

- *Ensure a sufficient vitamin D level*—Vitamin D helps activate the CYP2A6 detoxification pathways. I prefer to see vitamin D level around 70 to 100 on lab work. A low vitamin D level can increase your risk of developing osteoporosis, cancer and autoimmune disease.

- *Increase your antioxidant intake*—A high antioxidant intake from fruits, vegetables and nutritional supplements will prevent the overwhelming of detox pathways.

- *Eat foods that stimulate the CYP2A6 Phase I detox pathways*—Berries, garlic, onions, green tea, basil, turmeric, cumin and black pepper will support healthy CYP2A6 Phase I detox pathways.

- *Avoid acid-reducing drugs*—These suppress the CYP2A6 phase I detoxification process.

- *Sweat regularly*—Sweating allows your body to bypass many detox pathways, including Phase I detoxification performed by the CYP genes. Taking niacin (vitamin B3) right before sweating can provide an added detoxification boost by increasing circulation, decreasing toxicity and potentially decreasing cholesterol levels. However, high niacin levels can cause an increased heart rate, so it should only be taken under a doctor's supervision. Also, you should consume additional electrolytes, minerals and water to offset those lost as you sweat.

- *Increase your antioxidant intake*—Although Phase I detoxification is essential for health and detoxification, it does produce many cancer-causing free-radicals in the body. The best way to protect yourself from dangerous free radicals is to increase your antioxidant intake, including vitamin A, vitamin C, vitamin E, glutathione, alpha-lipoic acid and superoxide. It's important to eat fresh fruits and vegetables to increase antioxidant levels.

I have the CYP2A6 risk allele. What labs/testing should I consider to continually monitor my health?

- ✓ *Routine cancer screenings*—All appropriate tests should be performed regularly: colonoscopy, EGD (upper endoscopy of the stomach), skin exam, thyroid exam, prostate exam, Pap smear, breast exam and routine blood work should be performed regularly.

- ✓ *Vitamin D (blood test)*— I prefer to see vitamin D level around 70 to 100 on lab work. A low vitamin D level can increase your risk of developing osteoporosis, cancer and autoimmune disease.

Christy L. Sutton D.C.

✓ ***Toxicity testing (blood and urine tests)***—These tests provides information about your toxicity levels and how quickly you're accumulating toxins in your body.

✓ ***Labs to ensure you're not anemic (blood work)***—CBC, hemoglobin, hematocrit, serum iron and ferritin are all necessary labs to ensure you're not anemic.

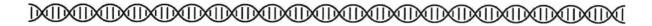

CYP2C9 gene

Cytochrome P450 2C9 - Phase I detoxification gene

Names of CY22C9 genetic variants (SNP identification)	rsnumber	Risk allele
CYP2C9*2 C430T	rs1799853	Risk allele is T
CYP2C9*3 A1075C	rs1057910	Risk allele is C

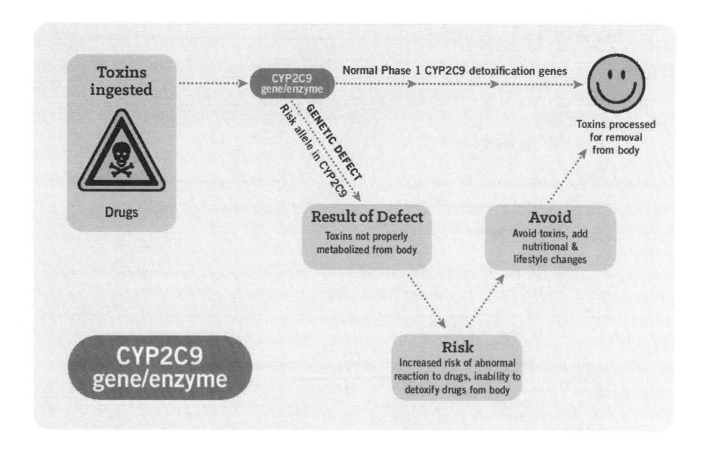

Personalized genetic report found at http://geneticdetoxification.com

What does the CYP2C9 gene do?

The CYP2C9 gene enables the body to detoxify recreational, over-the-counter and pharmaceutical drugs.

What types of health problems are associated with having the CYP2C9 gene risk allele(s)?

Having the risk allele(s) for the CYP2C9 gene can lead to abnormal drug reactions and an increased risk for certain drug side effects.

- *Abnormal drug reactions for CYP2C9*3 A1075C rs1057910. Risk allele is C*—People with the C risk allele may experience stronger side effects when taking certain drugs because they metabolize drugs at a slower rate. Therefore, drugs will remain in the body for a longer time and have a stronger effect.

- *Bleeding ulcers*—Having a risk allele for CYP2C9 can increase your risk of developing a bleeding ulcer from taking NSAIDS such as aspirin (Bayer, Bufferin, Excedrin), ibuprofen (Advil, Motrin IB), and naproxen (Aleve).

*Contact your prescribing doctor before changing or stopping any medications.

I have the CYP2C9 gene risk allele(s). What should I talk to my doctor about doing so that I can reduce my health risks?

- *If you're taking NSAIDs, consider taking L-glutamine*—Bleeding stomach ulcers are a common and potentially life-threatening side effect of taking NSAIDs. Supplementing with L-glutamine will help to maintain a healthy digestive lining and protect you from developing a bleeding ulcer. If you're taking NSAIDs and are experiencing stomach pain, talk to your doctor.

- *Consider supplementing with a high-quality B-complex*—Ensure that it contains the activated form of all B vitamins, which are required for the CYP2C9 detoxification pathways to function.

- *Correct any iron-deficient anemia*—Iron is necessary for CYP2C9 enzymes to work properly.

Christy L. Sutton D.C.

- ***Ensure a sufficient vitamin D level***—Vitamin D helps activate the CYP2C9 detoxification pathways. I prefer to see vitamin D level around 70 to 100 on lab work. A low vitamin D level can increase your risk of developing osteoporosis, cancer and autoimmune disease.

- ***Eat foods that stimulate Phase I detox pathways***—Berries, garlic, onions, green tea, basil, turmeric, cumin and black pepper will support healthy Phase I detox pathways.

- ***Avoid acid-reducing drugs***—These drugs suppress the CYP2C9 phase I detoxification process.

- ***Sweat regularly***—Sweating allows your body to bypass many detox pathways, including Phase I detoxification performed by the CYP genes. Taking niacin (vitamin B3) right before sweating can provide an added detoxification boost by increasing circulation, decreasing toxicity and potentially decreasing cholesterol levels. However, high niacin levels can cause an increased heart rate, so it should only be taken under a doctor's supervision. Also, you should consume additional electrolytes, minerals and water to offset those lost as you sweat.

- ***Increase your antioxidant intake***—Although Phase I detoxification is essential for health and detoxification, it does produce many cancer-causing free-radicals in the body. The best way to protect yourself from dangerous free radicals is to increase your antioxidant intake, including vitamin A, vitamin C, vitamin E, glutathione, alpha-lipoic acid and superoxide. It's important to eat fresh fruits and vegetables to increase antioxidant levels.

I have a CYP2C9 risk allele. What labs/testing should I consider to continually monitor my health?

- ✓ ***Vitamin D (blood test)***— I prefer to see vitamin D level around 70 to 100 on lab work. A low vitamin D level can increase your risk of developing osteoporosis, cancer and autoimmune disease.

- ✓ ***Labs to ensure you're not anemic (blood work)***—CBC, hemoglobin, hematocrit, serum iron and ferritin are all necessary labs to ensure you're not anemic.

Drugs known to be metabolized by CYP2C9

You may be at an increased risk for developing side effects or having abnormal reactions from taking these drugs if you have the risk allele for CYP2C9:

- **Tolbutamide**—Used to treat diabetes
- **Glipizide (sulfonylurea)**—Used to treat diabetes
- **Phenytoin**—Used to treat epilepsy
- **Coumadin (warfarin)**—Used to treat clotting disorders
- **NSAIDs**—Used for pain and inflammation
  - ➤ **Celebrex**
  - ➤ **Aspirin (Bayer, Bufferin, Excedrin)**
  - ➤ **ibuprofen (Advil, Motrin IB)**
  - ➤ **Naproxen (Aleve)**

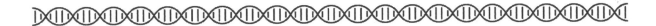

CYP2C19*17

Cytochrome P450 2C19*17 - Phase I detoxification gene

Names of CYP2C19*17 genetic variants (SNP identification)	rsnumber	Risk allele
CYP2C19*17	rs12248560	Risk allele is T

What does the CYP2C19*17 gene do?

The CYP2C19 gene detoxifies drugs like proton pump inhibitors (such as Prilosec), many anticonvulsant drugs (such as valium), and antidepressants.

What types of health problems are associated with having a risk allele for the CYP2C19*17 gene?

- *Your body may break down certain drugs faster*—Having this risk allele is associated with *an increased rate of breaking down drugs.* Therefore, people with this risk allele may require larger drug doses to achieve the desired effect.

Christy L. Sutton D.C.

- ***You may be more likely to benefit from tamoxifen***—Cancer patients with the risk allele for CYP2C19*17 are more likely to benefit from tamoxifen treatment as a part of their breast cancer prevention regimen[1].

Contact your prescribing doctor before changing or stopping any medications.

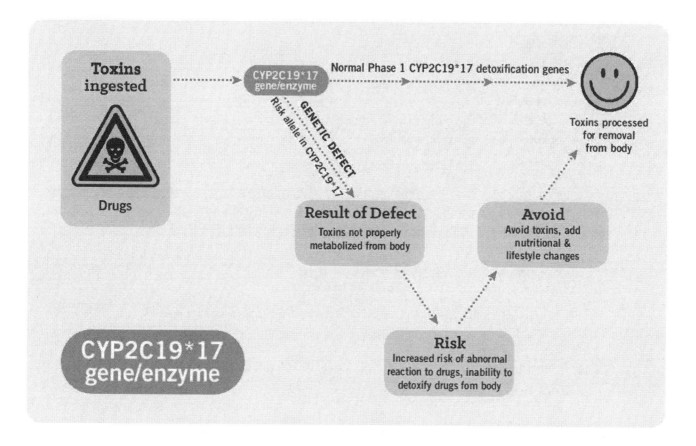

I have the CYP2C19*17 (rs12248560) T risk allele. What should I talk to my doctor about doing so that I can reduce my health risks?

- ***Consider supplementing with a high-quality B-complex***—Ensure that it contains the activated form of all B vitamins, which are required for the CYP2C19*17 detoxification pathways to function properly.

- ***Correct any iron-deficient anemia***—Iron is necessary for CYP2C19*17 enzymes to work correctly.

- ***Maintain an adequate vitamin D level***—Vitamin D helps activate the CYP2C19*17 detoxification pathways. I prefer to see vitamin D level around 70 to 100 on lab work. A low vitamin D level can increase your risk of developing osteoporosis, cancer and autoimmune disease.

- ***Avoid acid-reducing drugs***—Acid-reducing drugs will suppress the CYP2C19*17 phase I detoxification process.

- ***Sweat regularly***—Sweating allows your body to bypass many detox pathways, including Phase I detoxification performed by the CYP genes. Taking niacin (vitamin B3) right before sweating can provide an added detoxification boost by increasing circulation, decreasing toxicity and potentially decreasing cholesterol levels. However, high niacin levels can cause an increased heart rate, so it should only be taken under a doctor's supervision. Also, you should consume additional electrolytes, minerals and water to offset those lost as you sweat.

- ***Increase your antioxidant intake***—Although Phase I detoxification is essential for health and detoxification, it does produce many cancer-causing free-radicals in the body. The best way to protect yourself from dangerous free radicals is to increase your antioxidant intake, including vitamin A, vitamin C, vitamin E, glutathione, alpha-lipoic acid and superoxide. It's important to eat fresh fruits and vegetables to increase antioxidant levels.

I have the CYP2C19*17 risk allele. What labs/testing should I consider to continually monitor my health?

- ✓ ***Vitamin D (blood test)***— I prefer to see vitamin D level around 70 to 100 on lab work. A low vitamin D level can increase your risk of developing osteoporosis, cancer and autoimmune disease.

- ✓ ***Labs to ensure you're not anemic (blood work)***—CBC, hemoglobin, hematocrit, serum iron and ferritin are all necessary labs to ensure you're not anemic.

References:

1.) Schroth W1, Antoniadou L, Fritz P, et al. "Breast cancer treatment outcome with adjuvant tamoxifen relative to patient CYP2D6 and CYP2C19 genotypes." J Clin Oncol. 2007 Nov 20;25(33):5187-93.

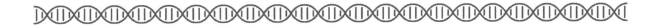

Christy L. Sutton D.C.

CYP2D6 gene

Cytochrome P450 2D6 - Phase I detoxification gene

Names of C2P2D6 genetic variants (SNP identification)	rsnumber	Risk allele
CYP2D6 100C>T	rs1065852	Risk allele is A
CYP2D6 2850C>T	rs16947	Risk allele is G

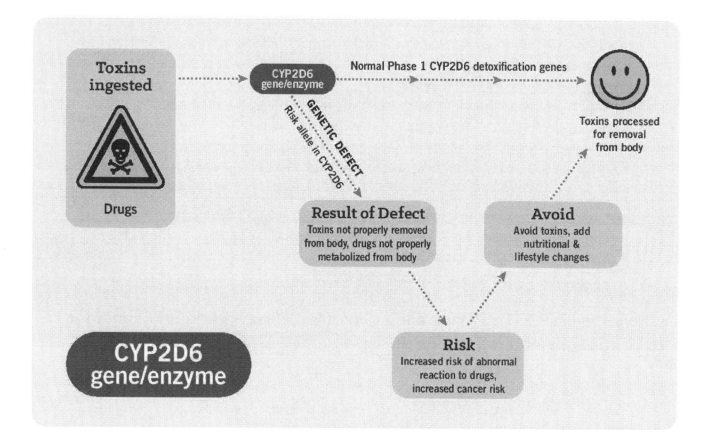

What does the CYP2D6 gene do?

The CYP2D6 gene detoxifies approximately 20 percent of all prescription drugs, including tricyclics, monoamine oxidase inhibitors (MAOIs), selective serotonin re-uptake inhibitors (SSRIs), opiates, antiarrhythmics, beta blockers and Cimetidine.

What types of health problems are associated with having the risk alleles for the CYP2D6 gene?

- *Abnormal processing and possible side effects to certain drugs:*

  - **CYP2D6 100C>T (rs1065852); risk allele is A**—Having the A risk allele for CYP2D6 (rs1065852) can cause your body to break down certain drugs more slowly, including debrisoquine, Dextromethorphan, Sparteine, nortriptyline, atomoxetine and codeine. Therefore, people with the A risk allele may require a smaller dose, or have more side effects, when taking these drugs.

  - **CYP2D6 2850C>T (rs16947); risk allele is G**—Having the G risk allele for CYP2D6 (rs16947) can cause your body to break down *certain drugs and toxins faster* than normal. This means that the drugs and toxins are removed from your body more quickly than normal. While having the G risk allele may increase your ability to detoxify faster, it can also create other problems, including overwhelming phase II detoxification. Anyone with the G risk allele must vigilantly support Phase II detox pathways through diet, lifestyle and nutrition. There is more information about how to specifically support Phase II detox pathways in chapter 2 (pg. 55)

- *Increased prostate cancer risk*—There is an increased risk of prostate cancer associated with having the risk alleles for CYP2D6[1].

Contact your prescribing doctor before changing or stopping any medications.

I have the CYP2D6 risk allele(s). What should I talk to my doctor about doing so that I can reduce my health risks?

- *Consider supplementing with a high-quality B-complex*—Ensure that it contains the activated form of all B vitamins, which are required for CYP2D6 detoxification pathways to function properly.

- *Correct any iron-deficient anemia*—Iron is necessary for CYP2D6 enzymes to work properly.

- *Maintain an adequate vitamin D level*—Vitamin D helps activate the CYP2D6 detoxification pathways. I prefer to see vitamin D level around 70 to 100 on lab work. A low vitamin D level can increase your risk of developing osteoporosis, cancer and autoimmune disease.

- *Eat more foods that stimulate CYP2D6-Phase I detoxification*—Berries, garlic, onions, green tea, basil, turmeric, cumin and black pepper help support healthy Phase I detox pathways.

- *Avoid acid-reducing drugs*—Acid-reducing drugs suppress the CYP2D6 phase I detoxification process.

- *Sweat regularly*—Sweating allows your body to bypass many detox pathways, including Phase I detoxification performed by the CYP genes. Taking niacin (vitamin B3) right before sweating can provide an added detoxification boost by increasing circulation, decreasing toxicity and potentially decreasing cholesterol levels. However, high niacin levels can cause an increased heart rate, so it should only be taken under a doctor's supervision. Also, you should consume additional electrolytes, minerals and water to offset those lost as you sweat.

- *Increase your antioxidant intake*—Although Phase I detoxification is essential for health and detoxification, it does produce many cancer-causing free radicals in the body. The best way to protect yourself from dangerous free radicals is to increase your antioxidant intake, including vitamin A, vitamin C, vitamin E, glutathione, alpha-lipoic acid and superoxide. It's important to eat fresh fruits and vegetables to increase antioxidant levels.

I have one or more CYP2D6 risk allele(s). What I labs/testing should I consider to continually monitor my health?

- ✓ *Routine cancer screenings*—All appropriate tests should be performed regularly: colonoscopy, EGD (upper endoscopy of the stomach), skin exam, thyroid exam, prostate exam, Pap smear, breast exam and routine blood work.

- ✓ *Vitamin D (blood test)*— I prefer to see vitamin D level around 70 to 100 on lab work. A low vitamin D level can increase your risk of developing osteoporosis, cancer and autoimmune disease.

- ✓ *Labs to ensure you're not anemic (blood work)*—CBC, hemoglobin, hematocrit, serum iron and ferritin are all necessary labs to ensure you're not anemic.

References:

1.) Febbo PG1, Kantoff PW, Giovannucci E, et al. "Debrisoquine hydroxylase (CYP2D6) and prostate cancer. Cancer Epidemiol Biomarkers Prev..1998 Dec;7(12):1075-

CYP2E1 gene

Cytochrome P450 2E1 - Phase I detoxification gene

Names of C2P2E1 genetic variants (SNP identification)	rsnumber	Risk allele
CYP2E1 A46G	rs2480256	Risk allele is A
CYP2E1 T8845C	rs8192772	Risk allele is C
CYP2E1	rs1329149	Risk allele is T
CYP2E1	rs2070676	Risk allele is G
CYP2E1	rs6413419	Risk allele is A

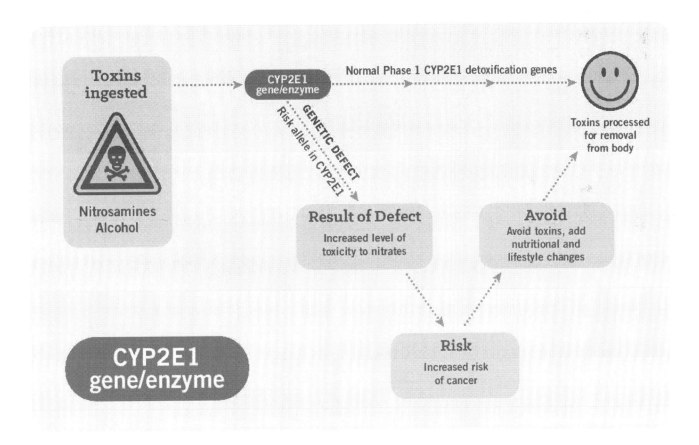

Christy L. Sutton D.C.

What does the CYP2E1 gene do?

The CYP2E1 gene detoxifies and metabolizes chemicals found in the environment, drugs, nitrosamines and ethanol (present in alcohol).

What health problems are associated with having the risk allele for CYP2E1 genes?

There is an increased cancer risk associated with having the risk allele(s) for CYP2E1 genes. Specifically, this includes an increased risk for developing:

- *Colon cancer*—Having a CYP2E1 risk allele has also been linked to an increased colorectal cancer risk[1]. Your risk for developing cancer is increased if you consume nitrates, nitrosamines and/or alcohol.

- *Head and neck cancer*—If you have a CYP2E1 risk allele, you're at an increased risk for developing cancer of the head and neck, especially if you consume alcohol and tobacco. Concurrent drinking and smoking are specifically known to increase the risk of esophageal and laryngeal cancer[7].

I have one or more CYP2E1 risk allele(s). What should I talk to my doctor about doing so that I can reduce my health risks?

- *Avoid exposure to things that the CYP2E1 gene detoxifies, including*:

  - *Alcohol*—The CYP2E1 gene plays a role in detoxifying alcohol.

  - *Smoking*—The CYP2E1 gene converts some of the cancer-causing chemicals from smoking into even more toxic substances.

  - *Nitrates*—Nitrates can increase the risk for cancers of the digestive system and are found in processed meats, bacon, sausage and celery powder.

  - *Nitrosamines*—Nitrosamines can be found in beer, latex, pesticides, some cosmetics, most rubber products and e-cigarette vapor.

- **Avoid acid-reducing drugs**—Acid-reducing drugs suppress the CYP2E1 phase I detoxification process.

- **Consider supplementing with a high-quality B-complex**—Ensure that it contains the activated form of all B vitamins, which are required for CYP2E1 detoxification pathways to function properly.

- **Correct any iron-deficient anemia**—Iron is necessary for CYP2E1 enzymes to work properly.

- **Ensure a sufficient vitamin D level**—Vitamin D helps activate CYP2E1 enzymes in both the liver and intestines. I prefer to see vitamin D level around 70 to 100 on lab work. A low vitamin D level can increase your risk of developing osteoporosis, cancer and autoimmune disease.

- **Increase intake of foods that stimulate CYP2E1 Phase I detoxification**—Berries, garlic, onions, green tea, basil, turmeric, cumin and black pepper help support healthy Phase I detox pathways.

- **Sweat regularly**—Sweating allows your body to bypass many detox pathways, including Phase I detoxification performed by the CYP genes. Taking niacin (vitamin B3) right before sweating can provide an added detoxification boost by increasing circulation, decreasing toxicity and potentially decreasing cholesterol levels. However, high niacin levels can cause an increased heart rate, so it should only be taken under a doctor's supervision. Also, you should consume additional electrolytes, minerals and water to offset those lost as you sweat.

- **Increase your antioxidant intake**—Phase I detox performed by the CYP2E1 enzyme increases cancer-causing free-radicals. The best way to protect your body from dangerous free radicals is to increase your intake of antioxidants such as vitamin C, vitamin E, vitamin A, glutathione, alpha-lipoic acid and superoxide dismutase (SOD). Increased consumption of fresh fruits and vegetables is also a great way to increase your antioxidant level.

 Christy L. Sutton D.C.

I have one or more CYP2E1 risk allele(s). What labs/testing should I consider to continually monitor my health?

✓ **_Routine cancer screenings_**—All appropriate tests should be performed regularly: colonoscopy, EGD (upper endoscopy of the stomach), skin exam, thyroid exam, prostate exam, Pap smear, breast exam and routine blood work.

✓ **_Vitamin D (blood test)_**— I prefer to see vitamin D level around 70 to 100 on lab work. A low vitamin D level can increase your risk of developing osteoporosis, cancer and autoimmune disease.

✓ **_Toxicity testing (blood and urine)_**—These tests provides information about your toxicity levels and how quickly you're accumulating toxins in your body.

✓ **_Labs to ensure you're not anemic (blood work)_**—CBC, hemoglobin, hematocrit, serum iron and ferritin are all necessary labs to ensure you're not anemic.

References:

1.) Yang H, Zhou Y, Zhou Z, et al. (2009) A novel polymorphism rs1329149 of CYP2E1 and a known polymorphism rs671 of ALDH2 of alcohol metabolizing enzymes are associated with colorectal cancer in a southwestern Chinese population. Cancer Epidemiol Biomarkers Prev 18: 2522–2527.

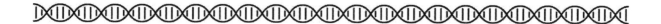

CYP3A4*1B

Cytochrome P450 3A4*1B - Phase I detoxification gene

Names of CYP3A4*1B genetic variants (SNP identification)	rsnumber	Risk allele
CYP3A4*1B	rs2740574	Risk allele is T

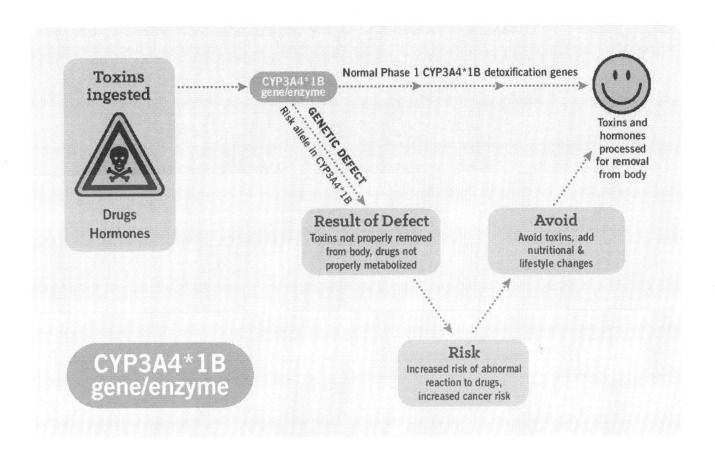

What does the CYP3A4*1B gene do?

The CYP3A4 gene detoxifies more than 50 percent of all prescription medications, as well as most steroid hormones, including corticosteroids, prednisone, estrogen, testosterone, cortisol, progesterone and dehydroepiandrosterone (DHEA). The CYP3A4 enzyme that is made from the CYP3A4 gene is responsible for the 16-hydroxylation of estrogen.

Christy L. Sutton D.C.

What health problems are associated with having the risk allele for CYP3A4*1B?

- *Increased cancer risk, especially prostate* cancer—Your cancer risk is increased if you have the CYP3A4 risk allele. Having the (T,T) genotype is associated with approximately a tenfold higher risk of aggressive prostate cancer in African-American males[1]. There is a 2.5-2.8x increased risk of ovarian cancer for women with the (T, T) genotype[2]. This enzyme is important in metabolizing estrogen, which is probably why it's linked to various cancers.

- *Estrogen dominance*—This is due to CYP3A4 not detoxifying and removing estrogen as efficiently as it should. Uterine fibroids and fibrocystic breast can also occur with high levels of estrogen build-up. Estrogen dominance can increase your cancer risk. If you have a CYP3A4 risk allele, you're at an increased risk of having high estrogen levels in the estrone and estradiol forms. Estrone and estradiol are the most proliferative forms of estrogen, and are the forms most strongly linked to cancer risks

I've inherited one or more CYP3A4*1B risk allele(s). What should I talk to my doctor about doing so that I can reduce my health risks?

- *Increase fiber intake*—Fiber is important for removing toxins and extra hormones from the body. Examples of fiber include vegetables, grapefruit, avocado, oatmeal, fruits, apples and psyllium husk.

- *Increase your body's ability to detoxify estrogen*—The CYP3A4*1B gene is important for the body's ability to eliminate extra hormones, especially estrogen. Things that help the body detoxify estrogen include:

  - ➢ *Cruciferous vegetables*—Broccoli, cabbage, cauliflower, Brussel sprouts and watercress are high in substances that detoxify estrogen and can reduce cancer risk.

  - ➢ *DIM in supplemental form*—Diindolylmethane (DIM) is naturally occurring in cruciferous vegetables, but can also be taken in a supplemental form to help your body remove extra estrogen and reduce cancer risk.

  - ➢ *Fish oil*—Fish oil helps the body metabolize and detoxify estrogen.

  - ➢ *Calcium D-glucarate*

> *   *High-fiber diet*

*   *Increase your antioxidant intake*—Phase I detox performed by the CYP3A4*1B enzyme increases cancer-causing free-radicals. The best way to protect your body from dangerous free radicals is to increase intake of antioxidants such as vitamin C, vitamin E, vitamin A, glutathione, alpha-lipoic acid and SOD. You can also eat more fresh fruits and vegetables to increase antioxidant levels.

*   *Avoid acid-reducing drugs*—These suppress the CYP3A4 phase I detoxification process.

*   *Consider supplementing with a high-quality B-complex*— Ensure that it contains the activated form of all B vitamins, which are required for the CYP3A4*1B detoxification pathways to function properly.

*   *Correct any iron-deficient anemia*—Iron is necessary for CYP3A4*1B enzymes to work properly.

*   *Ensure a sufficient vitamin D level*—Vitamin D helps activate CYP3A4*1B enzymes in both the liver and intestines. I prefer to see vitamin D level around 70 to 100 on lab work. A low vitamin D level can increase your risk of developing osteoporosis, cancer and autoimmune disease.

*   *Increase your intake of foods that stimulate CYP3A4*1B Phase I detoxification*—Berries, garlic, onions, green tea, basil, turmeric, cumin and black pepper support healthy Phase I detox pathways.

*   *Sweat regularly*—Sweating allows your body to bypass many detox pathways, including Phase I detoxification performed by the CYP3A4*1B genes. Taking niacin (vitamin B3) right before sweating can provide an added detoxification boost by increasing circulation, decreasing toxicity and potentially decreasing cholesterol levels. However, high niacin levels can cause an increased heart rate, so it should only be taken under a doctor's supervision. Also, you should consume additional electrolytes, minerals and water to offset those lost as you sweat.

I've inherited one or more risk allele(s) for the CYP3A4*1B gene. What labs/testing should I consider to continually monitor my health?

✓ **Routine cancer screenings**—All appropriate tests should be performed regularly: colonoscopy, EGD (upper endoscopy of the stomach), skin exam, thyroid exam, prostate exam, Pap smear, breast exam and routine blood work.

✓ **Comprehensive hormonal testing**—Hormone imbalances can be early predictors for breast cancer, adrenal issues, osteoporosis and prostate cancer. Hormone testing can reveal if you're estrogen-dominant, meaning you have either too much estrogen or not enough progesterone.

> ➢ **Essential-estrogen by Genova Diagnostics**—This is an excellent way to find out if you're not detoxifying estrogen as well as you need to be to prevent high estrogen levels, estrogen dominance, and cancer.

✓ **Labs to ensure you're not anemic (blood work)**—CBC, hemoglobin, hematocrit, serum iron and ferritin are all necessary labs to ensure you're not anemic.

✓ **Vitamin D (blood test)**— I prefer to see vitamin D level around 70 to 100 on lab work. A low vitamin D level can increase your risk of developing osteoporosis, cancer and autoimmune disease.

References:

1.) Bangsi D1, Zhou J, Sun Y, Patel NP, et al. "Impact of a genetic variant in CYP3A4 on risk and clinical presentation of prostate cancer among white and African-American men."

2.) Pearce CL, Near AM, Van Den Berg DJ, et al. Validating genetic risk associations for ovarian cancer through the international Ovarian Cancer Association Consortium. Br J Cancer. 2009 Jan 27;100(2):412-20.

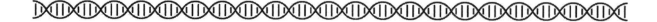

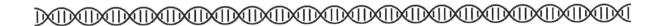

<u>Chapter 2</u>
Phase II Detoxification Genes

Christy L. Sutton D.C.

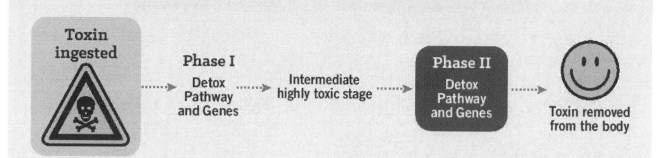

Phase II detox pathways are an essential part of metabolizing and removing toxins from the body. Some genetic variations can compromise the body's ability to detoxify using the Phase II detox pathways. Some of the health problems associated with having inherited genes that compromise Phase II detox pathways include cancer, neurological issues, heart attack, stroke, pregnancy-related issues, birth defects, autism and autoimmune disease.

In this chapter you'll learn if you've potentially inherited genes that negatively affect your ability to perform Phase II detoxification, any specific health problems you're predisposed to develop based on your specific genetic make-up, how to protect yourself from developing those health problems, and how to monitor your health for issues resulting from inherited genes that compromise your ability to perform Phase II detoxification.

Phase II Detoxification Genes
Glutathione Genes

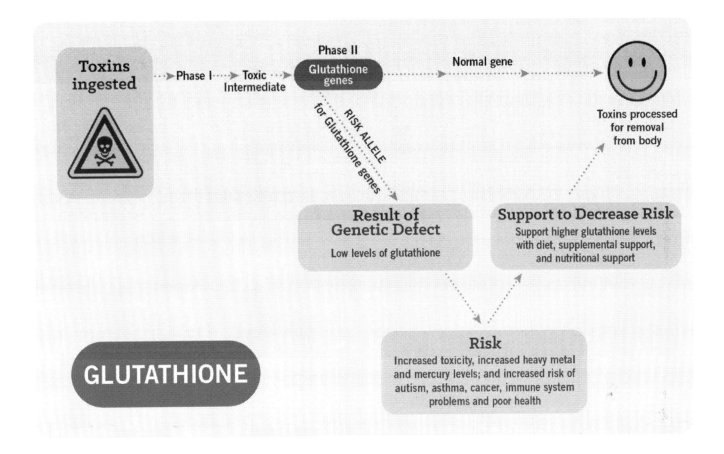

One of the body's most significant detoxification pathways is the glutathione pathway. Glutathione is one of the body's most important antioxidants. Some people have a genetic predisposition that causes them to produce low levels of glutathione. If you have low glutathione levels, you're at an increased risk of developing cancer, autoimmune disease or even autism.

This section provides valuable insight to help you understand if you're genetically predisposed to low glutathione levels and how you can protect yourself from the potential health risks associated with a genetic predisposition toward low glutathione levels.

Christy L. Sutton D.C.

Glutathione genetic variants
Glutathione-Disulfide Reductase (GSR)
Glutathione Synthetase (GSS)
Glutathione S-Transferase Mu 1 (GSTM1)
Glutathione S-Transferase Mu 3 (GSTM3)
Glutathione S-Transferase Pi 1 (GSPT1)

Names of glutathione genetic variants (SNP identification)	rsnumber	Risk allele
GSR	rs2551715	Risk allele is C
GSS G11705T	rs6060124	Risk allele is A
GSTM1 7730C>T	rs1056806	Risk allele is T
GSTM3 V224I	rs7483	Risk allele is T
GSTP1 A114V	rs1138272	Risk allele is T
GSTP1 I105V	rs1695	Risk allele is G

ANTIOXIDANTS

- Vitamin C, A, E
- Alpha Lipoic Acid
- Glutathione
- Super Oxide Dismutase (SOD)
- Catalase (CAT)

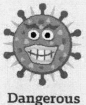
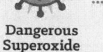

Dangerous Superoxide Free Radical

SOD2 gene/enzyme

Hydrogen Peroxide
(Dangerous Free Radical)

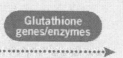
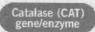

Glutathione genes/enzymes

Catalase (CAT) gene/enzyme

Water + Oxygen
(Free Radical Eliminated)

What do the glutathione genes do?

The glutathione genes provide instructions for your body to metabolize and maintain adequate glutathione levels. Having a risk allele in the glutathione genes can lead to low glutathione levels, which is bad for your health because it can lead to a buildup of toxins and an increased rate of degeneration of the entire body, including the brain.

In general, glutathione genes help your body to:

- ***Detoxify chemicals and heavy metals***—Glutathione detoxification genes are essential for detoxifying chemicals and heavy metals such as mercury.

- ***Prevent cancer***—Glutathione, a powerful antioxidant, protects the body from free radicals, which can damage DNA and lead to cancer. It acts much like a bulletproof vest against DNA damage.

- ***Prevent immune problems, including autoimmune disease***—Glutathione is an immune modulator that helps support healthy immune function. Other immune modulators include vitamin D, probiotics, and fish oil.

What type of health problems are associated with having the risk allele(s) in the glutathione genes?

Some health problems associated with low levels of glutathione and having risk allele(s) in the glutathione genes include:

- Cancer[1,2]
- Autoimmune disease
- Asthma
- Heavy metal toxicity, especially mercury toxicity
- General poor health
- Viral infections[2]
- Immune dysfunction[2]
- Autism spectrum disorder[3]
- Macular degeneration
- Chemical sensitivity

Christy L. Sutton D.C.

The glutathione and autism connection

Blood glutathione levels are significantly lower in children with autism spectrum disorder[3]. Low glutathione levels increase your child's risk for developing toxicity and immune system issues—both of which are common problems for individuals diagnosed with autism.

Some pediatricians will determine if a child should delay exposure to toxins found in vaccines based on the child's low glutathione levels. Vaccines are a controversial subject. However, the idea that a child with low glutathione levels has a higher risk of serious health problems is not a controversial subject, and can provide an objective measuring stick for some pediatricians.

I have one or more risk allele(s) for the glutathione genes. What should I talk to my doctor about doing so that I can reduce my health risks?

- *Consider avoiding the following because they deplete glutathione levels:*

  - *Alcohol*

  - *Acetaminophen (Tylenol)*—Tylenol depletes glutathione levels rapidly and could cause your child to get asthma. *Having high glutathione levels is very important for lung health.* Children who take Tylenol are at a higher risk of developing asthma because it depletes the body's glutathione levels. Anyone with lung problems should closely examine their glutathione genes and levels and work to get their glutathione levels as high as possible.

  - *Smoking*—Smoking puts a lot of pressure on the glutathione pathways, especially with GSTP1 risk alleles.

  - *Smog*

  - *Heavy metals, especially mercury*—Mercury exposure can result from eating fish, having mercury amalgam fillings in the mouth and being exposed to coal power plants.

  - *Exposure to pesticides, herbicides and toxic cleaning chemicals*

- **Work to increase glutathione levels**—Some ways to increase glutathione levels include:

  - ➤ **Consider supplementing with NAC (n-acetylcysteine)**—NAC is a precursor to glutathione and can be taken in supplemental form to help increase glutathione levels. If you go to the hospital for Tylenol-induced liver failure, the emergency room will give you an I.V. of NAC to reduce your body's absorption of Tylenol and help you produce more glutathione to detoxify the Tylenol.

  - ➤ **Ensure you have adequate levels of selenium**—Selenium is needed for the body to make glutathione naturally.

  - ➤ **Consider supplementing with a high-quality B-complex consisting of vitamins in the activated form**—B vitamins are necessary for the body to make glutathione naturally.

  - ➤ **Consume sulfur rich foods**—This includes vegetables such as garlic, cabbage, cauliflower, broccoli, and onions. Sulfur is necessary for glutathione production. Supplementing with MSM is another way to boost sulfur levels.

  - ➤ **Ensure adequate levels of protein, specifically foods high in the amino acids that make up glutathione**—These amino acids include cysteine, glycine and glutamic acid. Foods naturally high in these amino acids include gelatin, lamb, turkey, chicken, beef, bison, fish, poultry, yogurt, egg yolks, red pepper, garlic, onions, broccoli, Brussel sprouts, oats and wheat germ.

  - ➤ **Consider supplementing with milk thistle**—Milk thistle is a herb that can help increase glutathione levels by supporting a healthy liver cells and liver function.

  - ➤ **Apply topical glutathione cream**—Glutathione in its topical form can quickly increase glutathione levels because the glutathione absorbs through the skin.

  - ➤ **Glutathione nebulizer**—This is an effective way to increase glutathione levels when all else fails.

  - ➤ **Oral glutathione supplementation**—Glutathione tends to be poorly absorbed in the digestive system. However, oral glutathione supplementation

Christy L. Sutton D.C.

in the form called liposomal glutathione may be more absorbable, and therefore help increase glutathione levels.

➢ **Ensure adequate levels of vitamins C and E**—These are essential for keeping glutathione levels elevated.

➢ **Consider supplementing with glucoraphanin**—This promotes phase II detox pathways. Glucoraphanin converts into Sulforaphane, which is found to be an effective long-acting indirect antioxidant and significant inducer of phase II detoxification enzymes. The anti-oxidant effects of glucoraphanin are significantly longer lasting than vitamins C, E, and A. Because they assist in maintaining health throughout adult life, phytonutrients, such as glucoraphanin, are considered "lifespan essentials." Glucoraphanin is believed to play an important role in maintaining healthy gastrointestinal flora; healthy cellular life cycles; immune, eye, and cardiovascular health; and a normal response to inflammation.

Breast cancer prevention can mean eating your broccoli

Some research shows that women with the GSTP1 rs1695 risk allele are significantly more likely to get breast cancer, particularly postmenopausal women[1]. However, it's also been found that increasing intake of cruciferous vegetables may reduce that risk. Cruciferous vegetables include cabbage, cauliflower, broccoli and Brussel sprouts.

Talk to your doctor about possibly supplementing with Glucoraphanin or diindolylmethane (DIM), which are compounds isolated from cruciferous vegetables that's been shown to decrease breast cancer by helping the body metabolize estrogen and estrogenic-like chemicals found in the environment.

I have one or more risk allele(s) for the glutathione genes. What labs/testing should I consider to continually monitor my health?

✓ ***Monitor liver health with ALT, AST, and GGT (blood test)***—Liver enzymes, especially GGT, monitor liver health. Low glutathione levels can lead to liver damage and high liver enzymes. GGT should ideally be below 25 on blood work.

✓ ***Blood glutathione level (blood test)***—It's highly advisable for anyone with the risk alleles for the glutathione genes to measure their glutathione levels through a blood test.

> ➤ ***Nutreval by Genova Diagnostics (blood and urine)***—This lab test measures glutathione, vitamins, minerals, amino acids, fatty acids, antioxidants, heavy metals and some chemical toxicity levels. This test measures for nutrient deficiencies that may lead to low glutathione levels.
> ➤ ***Oxidative Stress Profile by Dunwoody Labs***—This lab measures total glutathione and reduced glutathione. The reduced glutathione is what the body needs to repair and prevent tissue damage.

✓ ***Acetaminophen challenge (blood test)***—Acetaminophen is the active ingredient in Tylenol that depletes glutathione levels. This test consists of ingesting a small amount of acetaminophen and then measuring how well it's cleared out of the body. If the acetaminophen is not cleared efficiently, that suggests that the glutathione pathways aren't operating at an adequate level.

✓ ***Oxidative stress test (blood test)***—This test measures the levels of oxidative stress (degeneration) and antioxidant reserves that protect you from oxidative stress. Antioxidants like glutathione neutralize free radicals that cause oxidative stress/DNA damage. High oxidative stress/free radicals, low levels of antioxidants and high levels of DNA damage *increase your risk of developing cancer*.

References:

1. Lee SA1, Fowke JH, Lu W, Ye C, et al. "Cruciferous vegetables, the GSTP1 Ile105Val genetic polymorphism, and breast cancer risk." Am J Clin Nutr. 2008 Mar;87(3):753-60.

2.) Fraternale A, Paoletti MF, et al. "Antiviral and immunomodulatory properties of new pro-glutathione (GSH) molecules." Curr Med Chem. 2006;13(15):1749-55.

3.) James B Adams, et al. "Nutritional and metabolic status of children with autism vs. neurotypical children, and the association with autism severity". Nutr Metab (Lond). 2011; 8: 34. 2011 June 8.

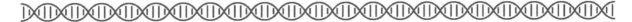

Christy L. Sutton D.C.

CTH gene
Cystathionine Gamma-lyase

Names of CTH genetic variants (SNP identification)	rsnumber	Risk allele
CTH S4031I	rs1021737	Risk allele is T
CTH T16147C	rs12723350	Risk allele is C

What does the CTH gene do?

The CTH gene provides the body's instructions to produce the enzyme cystathionine gamma-lyase (CTH), which is necessary to create glutathione. Specifically, CTH helps convert cystathionine into cysteine. Cysteine is an amino acid required to make glutathione. Therefore, having the risk allele for CTH can decrease the body's ability to make glutathione naturally.

What health problems are associated with having the risk allele for CTH?

- *High homocysteine levels*—Having the risk allele for CTH S4031I (rs1021737) is associated with *significantly* higher levels of homocysteine in the blood. High homocysteine levels increase your risk of developing Alzheimer's disease, cardiovascular disease, heart attack, stroke and cancer.

- *Low glutathione levels*—Low glutathione levels can increase your risk for cancer, autoimmune disease, degenerative disease, autism, toxicity issues and other chronic conditions. Read more about low glutathione levels on page 57.

I have one or more risk allele(s) for the CTH gene. What should I talk to my doctor about doing so that I can reduce my health risks?

- *Maintain adequate vitamin-B6 (P-5-P)*—The activated form of vitamin B-6 (p-5-p) is required for the CTH enzyme to work effectively. Being deficient in vitamin B-6 can exacerbate health problems associated with a CTH risk allele.

- *Increase cysteine intake*—Cysteine is an amino acid found in protein that's required to produce glutathione. Having a risk allele in the CTH gene can lead to low levels of cysteine, and to subsequent low levels of glutathione. Foods high in cysteine include pork, poultry, eggs, dairy, garlic, onions, broccoli, Brussel sprouts, oats and lentils.

- **Increase glutathione levels**—Some ways to increase glutathione levels include supplementing with a high-quality B-complex (consisting of vitamins in the activated form), NAC (n-acetylcysteine), selenium, milk thistle, topical glutathione cream, glutathione nebulizer and a glutathione I.V.

I have one or more risk allele(s) in the CTH gene. What labs/testing should I consider to continually monitor my health?

✓ **Monitor liver health with ALT, AST, and GGT (blood test)**—Liver enzymes, especially GGT, monitor liver health. Low glutathione levels can lead to liver damage and high liver enzymes. GGT should ideally be below 25 on blood work.

✓ **Measure cysteine, cystathionine, and glutathione levels**

➤ **Nutreval by Genova Diagnostics (blood and urine)**—This test measures your levels of cysteine, cystathionine and glutathione. Having the risk allele for the CTH gene can make you low in the amino acid cysteine due to an inability to covert cystathionine into cysteine. A low cysteine level can lead to a low glutathione level.

➤ **Oxidative Stress Profile by Dunwoody Labs**—This lab measures total glutathione, reduced glutathione, and two other markers of oxidative stress. Reduced glutathione is what the body needs to repair and prevent tissue damage.

✓ **Homocysteine level (blood test)**—Having a risk allele in the CTH gene can lead to a high homocysteine level. I prefer to see homocysteine below 8 on blood work.

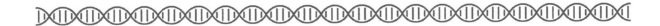

Christy L. Sutton D.C.

Phase II Detoxification Genes
Acetylation Genes

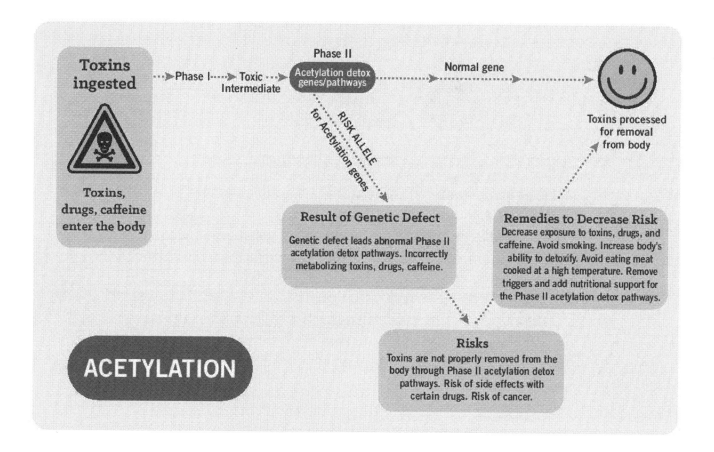

The acetylation detox pathways are also essential detoxification pathways. Some people are genetically hindered in their ability to have healthy acetylation detox pathways because of the genes they inherited from their parents. These people can be at an increased risk of developing cancer, having abnormal drug reactions, and experiencing chemical sensitivities.

This section provides valuable insight to help you discover if you're possibly genetically predisposed to detoxification problems with the acetylation detox pathways, and what you can do to help protect yourself from potential health risks.

NAT1 and NAT2 genes
N-acetyltransferase 1 and 2 genes

Names of NAT1 and NAT2 acetylation Phase II detox genetic variants (SNP identification)	rsnumber	Risk allele
NAT1 R187Q—*slow* detoxifier / *metabolizer*	rs4986782	Risk allele is A
NAT2 C282T—generally *fast* detoxifier / *metabolizer*	rs1041983	Risk allele is T
NAT2 C481T—generally *fast* detoxifier / *metabolizer*	rs1799929	Risk allele is T
NAT2 G191A—generally *fast* detoxifier / *metabolizer*	rs1801279	Risk allele is A
NAT2 G286E—generally *fast* detoxifier / *metabolizer*	rs1799931	Risk allele is A
NAT2 I114T—generally *fast* detoxifier / *metabolizer*	rs1801280	Risk allele is C
NAT2 K268R—generally *fast* detoxifier / *metabolizer*	rs1208	Risk allele is A
NAT2 R197Q—generally *fast* detoxifier / *metabolizer*	rs1799930	Risk allele is A
NAT2- *slow detoxifier / metabolizer*	rs1495741	Risk allele is A

What do the NAT1 and NAT2 genes do?

The NAT1 and NAT2 genes provide the body's instructions to make important detoxification enzymes called N-acetyltransferase (NAT) during Phase II detoxification. These genes are essential for detoxifying carcinogens, drugs and caffeine by facilitating the Phase II acetylation detox pathways. The detox pathways associated with the NAT1 and NAT2 genes are necessary for the body to convert toxic chemicals into a form that's easier for the body to excrete. NAT1 is more active in the liver, whereas NAT2 is active in both the liver and intestines.

What health problems are associated with having the risk alleles for NAT1 and NAT2 genes?

Having the risk alleles for the NAT1 and NAT2 genes can cause either an increase or decrease in the speed of the Phase II acetylation detoxification pathways. Both faster *and* slower detoxification pathways can have negative consequences. Slower detoxifiers lead to toxin build-up because the body cannot remove them efficiently. Fast detoxifiers tend to make detoxification mistakes that covert ingested toxins into even more toxic chemicals once in the body.

Some specific health problems associated with having a risk allele in the NAT1 or NAT2 genes include:

- *A higher cancer risk*—The increased risk of cancer from having a risk allele for NAT1 or NAT2 genes is especially concerning when you're exposed to cancer-

Christy L. Sutton D.C.

causing actions or substances in the environment such as smoking, pesticides, herbicides or eating a large amount of meat cooked at a high temperature. The types of cancer for which you're at an increased risk largely depend on whether your NAT1 or NAT2 risk allele makes you a slow or fast detoxifier.

> ### Slow detoxifiers/metabolizers

  - Urinary, bladder and lung cancer are most strongly associated with having the risk alleles that make Phase II acetylation detox pathways *slower* than normal. The risk for lung cancer is highest when someone both smokes and has a risk allele for NAT1 R187Q (rs4986782). Having the risk allele for rs1495741 is associated with an increased risk for developing bladder cancer.

> ### Fast detoxifiers/metabolizers

  - Colon and bladder cancer are most strongly associated with having the risk alleles that make Phase II acetylation detox pathways *faster* than normal. Other cancers associated with these risk alleles include lung, head and neck cancers, and non-Hodgkin's lymphoma. If you have the risk allele(s) that causes your Phase II acetylation pathways to be faster than normal, you're at risk of making the toxins you ingest even more toxic. That's why it's important to minimize your overall toxin exposure if you have these risk allele(s). The risk of developing cancer increases if you consume large amounts of meat, especially if the meats are roasted or cooked at a high temperature.

- **Higher risk for drug toxicity due to a decreased ability to properly remove certain drugs from the body**

- **Problems with sulfa drugs**—This is due to a decreased ability to metabolize and detoxify sulfa drugs once consumed.

- **An overall increased toxicity level**—Having the risk alleles for the NAT1 and NAT2 genes can creates a higher level of toxicity because the Phase II acetylation detox pathways cannot clear toxins out of the body correctly.

I have one or more risk allele(s) in the NAT1 and NAT2 genes. What should I talk to my doctor about doing so that I can reduce my health risks?

- *Don't smoke*—If you have the risk allele for the NAT1 or NAT2 genes and you smoke, you're *significantly* more likely to develop lung cancer.

- *Avoid exposure to toxins as much as possible*—Avoiding exposure to toxins means eating a clean diet with organic foods, eliminating toxic chemicals from household cleaning and lawn care, drinking clean water rather than sodas or alcohol, and avoiding processed foods. In short, avoid caffeine, drugs and carcinogens (pesticides, insecticides, toxic chemicals, smog, smoking, etc.).

- *Consider increasing nutrients necessary for the NAT1 and NAT2 Phase II detox pathways*—This includes vitamin C and a high-quality B-complex that contains the activated form of all B vitamins, but especially vitamins B1, B5 and B6 (P-5-P).

- *Eat your veggies*—Liberal consumption of cruciferous vegetables (broccoli, cauliflower, Brussel sprouts and cabbage) increases the detoxification capabilities of all Phase II detoxification pathways, including NAT1 and NAT2 (acetylation). A diet filled with a both a large variety and quantity of vegetables and fruits is necessary to help prevent cancer.

- *Avoid eating large amounts of meat cooked at a high temperature*—There is an increased cancer risk with consumption of meats cooked at a high temperature, such as with grilling and frying.

- *Detoxify*—Consider doing a 21- or 30-day detox diet, including eating ample amounts of vegetables, adequate clean protein, fruits and healthy fats. I don't recommend doing a one-size-fits-all detox protocol. Any detoxification program needs to be tailored to the individual and monitored by a trained and licensed health care professional.

- *Exercise and sweat daily*—Sweating allows your body to bypass many detox pathways and remove toxins without causing damage. Exercise is an essential and irreparable part of keeping your body healthy and preventing cancer.

- *Drink plenty of water*—Water is necessary to help the body properly detoxify.

Christy L. Sutton D.C.

- ***Consider supplementing with n-acetylcysteine (NAC)***—Supplementing with NAC can help support both the acetylation and the glutathione Phase II detoxification pathways.

- ***Consider supplementing with glucoraphanin***—This promotes phase II detox pathways. Glucoraphanin converts into Sulforaphane, which is found to be an effective long-acting indirect antioxidant and significant inducer of phase II detoxification enzymes. The anti-oxidant effects of glucoraphanin are significantly longer lasting than vitamins C, E, and A. The antioxidant activity can last several days longer than typical antioxidants. Because they assist in maintaining health throughout adult life, phytonutrients, such as glucoraphanin, are considered "lifespan essentials." Glucoraphanin is believed to play an important role in maintaining healthy gastrointestinal flora; healthy cellular life cycles; immune, eye, and cardiovascular health; and a normal response to inflammation.

I have one or more risk allele (s) for the NAT1 or NAT2 genes. What labs/testing should I consider to continually monitor my health?

There are no functional tests specific to the detoxification pathways associated with the NAT1 and NAT2 genes. Anyone with NAT1 or NAT2 risk alleles should consider supporting all detox pathways by supporting their overall ability to detoxify while also limiting toxin exposure. If you want to know your level of toxicity, please see below for more information.

- ✓ ***Toxic Effects Core Profile by Genova Diagnostics (blood and urine)***—The Toxic Effects Core Profile provides more information on your carcinogen and toxin levels. This won't tell you exactly how well you're detoxifying, but it will tell you how many toxins are accumulating in your body, which is an indirect indicator of how well you're detoxifying.

- ✓ ***Routine cancer screenings***—All appropriate tests should be performed regularly: colonoscopy, EGD (upper endoscopy of the stomach), skin exam, thyroid exam, prostate exam, Pap smear, breast exam and blood work.

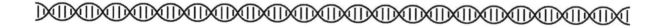

Phase II Detoxification Genes
Glucuronidation Genes

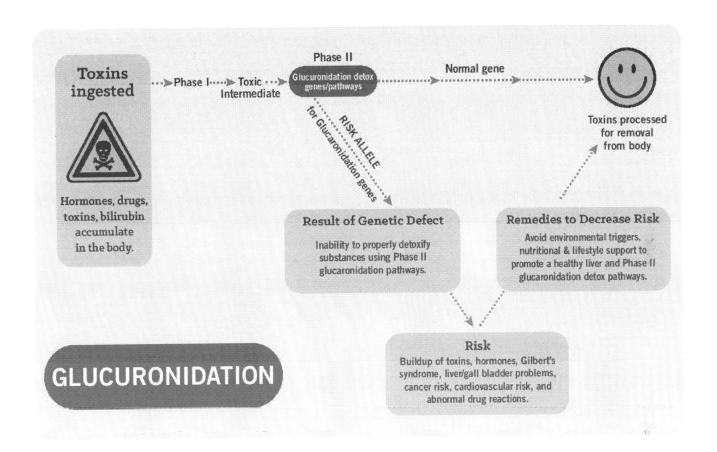

The glucuronidation detox pathways are essential for detoxification. Some people are genetically hindered in their ability to have healthy glucuronidation detox pathways because of the genes they inherited from their parents. These people can be at an increased risk of developing liver problems such as Gilbert's disease, as well as cancer, cardiovascular disease, abnormal drug reactions and chemical sensitivities.

This section provides valuable insight to help you discover if you're possibly genetically predisposed to detoxification issues using the glucuronidation detox pathways, and what you can do to help protect yourself from potential health risks.

Christy L. Sutton D.C.

UGT1A1 and UGT2A1 genes
UDP glucuronosyltransferase gene

Names of UGT1A1 and UGT2A1 glucuronidation Phase II detox genetic variants (SNP identification)	rsnumber	Risk allele
UGT1A1 C175181T	rs887829	Risk allele is T
UGT1A1 C179920T	rs4148325	Risk allele is T
UGT1A1 G179250T	rs6742078	Risk allele is T
UGT1A1 G182349A	rs62625011	Risk allele is A
UGT1A1 G211A	rs4148323	Risk allele is A
UGT1A1 G354A	rs72551351	Risk allele is G
UGT2A2 G308R	rs4148301	Risk allele is T

What do the UGT1A1 and UGT2A2 genes do?

The UGT1A1 and UGT2A2 genes are necessary for your body's ability to detoxify properly through the Phase II glucuronidation pathways. The glucuronidation detox pathways are the most common phase II pathways[1] and are essential for your body to be able to metabolize fat-soluble compounds, such as steroids, bilirubin, hormones and drugs, into water-soluble substances that can be easily excreted[1]. UGT1A1 and UGT2A2 genes provide instructions for the body to make the enzymes that facilitate Phase II glucuronidation detox pathways.

What health problems are associated with having the risk allele for these UGT1A1 and UG2A2 genes?

- *Increased risk of liver problems, such as Gilbert syndrome, and a high bilirubin level*

- *Increased risk for developing gall stones*

- *Increased cardiovascular disease risk*

- *Inability to properly detoxify and remove certain drugs, which can lead to abnormal reactions when taking those drugs*

- *Increased risk for developing cancer*

I have one or more risk allele(s) in the UGT1A1 and UGT2A2 genes. What should I talk to my doctor about doing so that I can reduce my health risks?

- *Promote a healthy gut:*

  - ➢ *Consider supplementing with Saccharomyces boulardii*—This beneficial yeast probiotic prevents toxins from being recirculated in the body and promotes proper excretion through the bowels. It's possible for a toxin to go through the Phase II-glucuronidation detox pathways and then be converted back to its original, more toxic form by bad bacteria in the intestines. *Saccharomyces boulardii* helps reduce the number of problematic intestinal organisms that could inhibit the Phase II-glucuronidation pathway. Having a healthy bacterial flora and intestinal system will promote a healthy Phase II-glucuronidation pathway.

  - ➢ *Eat plenty of fiber to ensure at least daily bowel movements*—Fiber promotes the growth of good bacteria and helps with regular elimination of toxins through the bowels. If you aren't eating enough fiber and/or aren't having regular bowel movements, toxins are not being properly removed and are likely being recirculated in the body.

- *Don't smoke*—Smoking adds extra stress to these glucuronidation detox pathways and increases your cancer risk. If you have a risk allele for the UGT1A1 or UGT2A2 genes, you're particularly vulnerable to smoking-induced cancers.

- *Avoid high levels of hormones, and exercise cautiously when taking hormones (corticosteroids, estrogen, progesterone, testosterone, DHEA, etc.)*—These UGT1A1 and UGT2A2 (glucuronidation) genes help detoxify hormones from the body.

- *Increase intake of foods that promote the glucuronidation detox pathways*—Apples, grapefruit, broccoli, alfalfa, fish, legumes, dairy products, beef, chicken and green leafy vegetables support the Phase II glucuronidation pathway made from the UGT1A1 and UGT2A2 genes[2].

- *Consider nutritional support*—Magnesium, the amino acid glycine and B vitamins (particularly vitamin B3) is needed for Phase II glucuronidation to occur.

Christy L. Sutton D.C.

- **Milk thistle**—Milk thistle can help with healthy liver function and promote Phase II glucuronidation detox pathways.

- **Avoid toxins**—Toxic chemicals are frequently found in cleaning products, cosmetics, non-organic foods, etc.

- **Detoxify**—Consider doing a 21-day detox diet, including eating ample amounts of vegetables, adequate clean protein, fruits and healthy fats. I don't recommend doing a one-size-fits-all detox protocol. Any detoxification program needs to be tailored to the individual and monitored by a trained and licensed health care professional.

- **Exercise and sweat daily**—Sweating allows your body to bypass many detox pathways and remove toxins without causing damage. Exercise is an essential and irreparable part of keeping your body healthy and preventing cancer.

- **Drink plenty of water**—Water is necessary to help the body properly detoxify.

- **Consider supplementing with glucoraphanin**—This promotes phase II detox pathways. Glucoraphanin converts into Sulforaphane, which is found to be an effective long-acting indirect antioxidant and significant inducer of phase II detoxification enzymes. The anti-oxidant effects of glucoraphanin are significantly longer lasting than vitamins C, E, and A. The antioxidant activity can last several days longer than typical antioxidants. Because they assist in maintaining health throughout adult life, phytonutrients, such as glucoraphanin, are considered "lifespan essentials." Glucoraphanin is believed to play an important role in maintaining healthy gastrointestinal flora; healthy cellular life cycles; immune, eye, and cardiovascular health; and a normal response to inflammation

I have one or more risk allele (s) for the UGT1A1 and UGT2A2 genes. What labs/testing should I consider to continually monitor my health?

- ✓ **Hormone testing**—Adrenal and sex hormones should be tested. Having a risk allele in the UGT1A1 and UGT2A1 genes can interfere with the body's ability to metabolize and remove hormones. The only way to know if your hormone levels are too low or high is through testing.

- ✓ **Bilirubin (blood test)**—High bilirubin can indicate a liver problem such as Gilbert's Syndrome.

- ✓ ***Routine cancer screenings***—All appropriate tests should be performed regularly: colonoscopy, EGD (upper endoscopy of the stomach), skin exam, thyroid exam, prostate exam, Pap smear, breast exam and blood work.

References:

1.) Le, Jennifer, PharmD. Merck Manual professional version. Retrieved from: http://www.merckmanuals.com/professional/clinical_pharmacology/pharmacokinetics/drug_metabolism.html

2.) Dwivedi C, Heck WJ, Downie AA, et al. Effect of calcium glucarate on beta-gluconidase activity and glucarate content of certain vegetables and fruits. Biochemical Medicine and Metabolic Biology. 43(2):83-92, 1990.

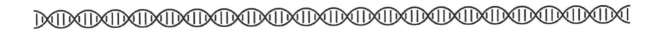

Christy L. Sutton D.C.

Phase II Detoxification Genes
Sulfation Genes

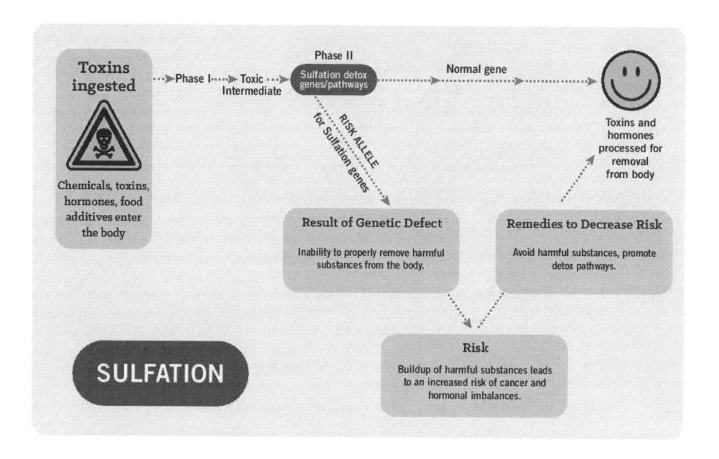

The sulfation detox pathways are essential detoxification pathways. Some people are genetically hindered in their ability to have healthy sulfation detox pathways because of genes inherited from their parents. These people can be at an increased risk of developing cancer and experiencing hormonal imbalances.

This section provides valuable insight into helping you discover if you're genetically predisposed to have detoxification problems with the sulfation detox pathways, and what you can do to help protect yourself from potential health risks.

SULT1A1, SULT1C3 and SULT2A1 genes

Sulfotransferase genes

Names of SULT1A1, SULT1C3, and SULT2A1 sulfation Phase II detox genetic variants (SNP identification)	rsnumber	Risk allele
SULT1A1 C*85G-- Most commonly expressed	rs1042157	Risk allele is A
SULT1C3 C13545841T	rs13392744	Risk allele is T
SULT1C3 G535A	rs2219078	Risk allele is A
SULT2A1 G9598T	rs2547231	Risk allele is A

What do the SULT1A1, SULT1C3 and SULT2A1 (sulfation) genes do?

Phase II SULT genes detoxify carcinogens, drugs and caffeine, as well as harmful chemicals found in the environment such as xenobiotics (chemicals that are foreign to our body), food additives and hormones[1]. While all sulfation genes are important, the SULT1A1 gene is the most commonly used[1]. All genes that begin with the letters "SULT" are Phase II sulfation detox genes.

What health problems are associated with having the risk allele for theSULT1A1, SULT1C3 or SULT2A1 genes?

- *Increased cancer risk*—The SULT genes are essential for proper detoxification; therefore, having a risk allele in these genes can lead to an increased risk of cancer and degenerative diseases, especially with toxin exposure.

- *Hormonal imbalances*—Sulfation detoxification pathways remove excess hormones from the body. Having a risk allele in the Phase II sulfation detox genes can lead to a decreased ability to properly metabolize and remove hormones from the body.

  - *High levels of testosterone and DHEA as seen in polycystic ovarian syndrome (PCOS)*—The SULT2A1 gene may play a role in inherited adrenal androgen excess in women with PCOS[2]. If sulfation detox pathways don't work properly, hormones can build up in the body.

  - *Hot flashes*

Christy L. Sutton D.C.

I have one or more risk allele(s) for the SULT1A1, SULT1C3, or SULT2A1 genes. What should I talk to my doctor about doing so that I can reduce my health risks?

- *Increase your intake of raw fruits and vegetables and avoid cooking at a high temperature*—Sulfation genes help activate harmful substances that result from cooking meat at high temperatures. The best way to prevent this is to be moderate with your amount of fried and grilled foods, as well as foods cooked at very high temperatures. Increased intake of raw food, especially raw vegetables, fruits, and nuts has shown to help reduce cancer risk.

- *Avoid NSAIDs and yellow food dye*—The sulfation detox pathway facilitated by the SULT genes is inhibited by NSAIDS (i.e., aspirin) and yellow food dyes. Therefore, avoiding artificial coloring and NSAIDS could be helpful.

- *Eat a sulfur-rich diet:*

  - *Foods high in sulfur*—Broccoli, cabbage, kale, garlic and onion

  - *High-sulfur supplements to consider*—MSM and glutathione

- *Avoid toxins*—Toxic chemicals are frequently found in cleaning products, cosmetics, non-organic foods, etc.

- *Detoxify*—Consider doing a 21-day detox diet, including eating ample amounts of vegetables, adequate clean protein, fruits and healthy fats. I don't recommend doing a one-size-fits-all detox protocol. Any detoxification program needs to be tailored to the individual and monitored by a trained and licensed health care professional.

- *Exercise and sweat daily*—Sweating allows your body to bypass many detox pathways and remove toxins without causing damage. Exercise is an essential and irreparable part of keeping your body healthy and preventing cancer.

- *Drink plenty of water*—Water is necessary to help the body properly detoxify.

Personalized genetic report found at http://geneticdetoxification.com

- **Consider supplementing with glucoraphanin**—This promotes phase II detox pathways. Glucoraphanin converts into Sulforaphane, which is found to be an effective long-acting indirect antioxidant and significant inducer of phase II detoxification enzymes. The anti-oxidant effects of glucoraphanin are significantly longer lasting than vitamins C, E, and A. The antioxidant activity can last several days longer than typical antioxidants. Because they assist in maintaining health throughout adult life, phytonutrients, such as glucoraphanin, are considered "lifespan essentials." Glucoraphanin is believed to play an important role in maintaining healthy gastrointestinal flora; healthy cellular life cycles; immune, eye, and cardiovascular health; and a normal response to inflammation.

I have one or more risk allele(s) for the SULT1A1, SULT1C3 or SULT2A1 genes. What labs/testing should I consider to continually monitor my health?

There are no functional tests specific to the detoxification pathways associated with the sulfation genes. Anyone with the sulfation gene risk allele(s) should consider supporting all detox pathways by improving their overall ability to detoxify and limiting their toxin exposure. If you want to better understand your toxin level, please see below for more information.

- ✓ **Toxic Effects Core Profile by Genova Diagnostics (blood and urine)**—The Toxic Effects Core Profile provides more information on your carcinogen and toxin levels. This won't tell you exactly how well you're detoxifying, but it will tell you how many toxins are accumulating in your body, which is an indirect indicator of how well you're detoxifying.

- ✓ **Hormone testing**—Adrenal and sex hormones are metabolized by the SULT detox pathways. Having a risk allele in the sulfation genes can interfere with the body's ability to metabolize and remove hormones. The only way to know if your hormone levels are too low or high is through testing.

References:

Christy L. Sutton D.C.

1.) Yu D1, Green B2, Marrone A2, et al.Suppression of CYP2C9 by microRNA hsa-miR-128-3p in human liver cells and association with hepatocellular carcinoma. Sci Rep. 2015 Feb 23;5:8534.

2.) NCBI. SULT2A1. Retrieved from: Entrez Gene: SULT2A1 sulfotransferase family, cytosolic, 2A, dehydroepiandrosterone (DHEA)-preferring, member 1". Also retrieved from: http://www.ncbi.nlm.nih.gov/gene/6822

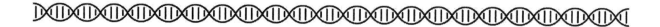

Personalized genetic report found at http://geneticdetoxification.com

Methylation Genes—Phase II Detoxification Genes

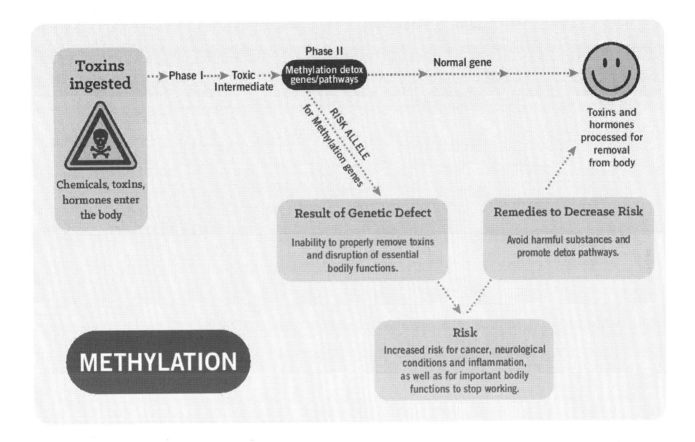

Methylation is a chemical process that turns bodily functions on and off, including promotion or suppression of genes. Some common genetic variations can significantly hinder your body's ability to properly methylate, which can lead to a variety of health conditions, including a decreased ability to detoxify, cardiovascular disease, birth defects, mental illness, Alzheimer's disease, autism, ADHD, and increased pain and inflammation. However, there are some easy and effective ways to prevent genetic predispositions from resulting in actual health problems.

In this section, you'll learn if you have potentially inherited genes that compromise your methylation detox pathways, what having poor methylation genes can mean for your health, and what you can do to protect yourself if you've inherited genes that cause your methylation pathways to perform poorly.

Christy L. Sutton D.C.

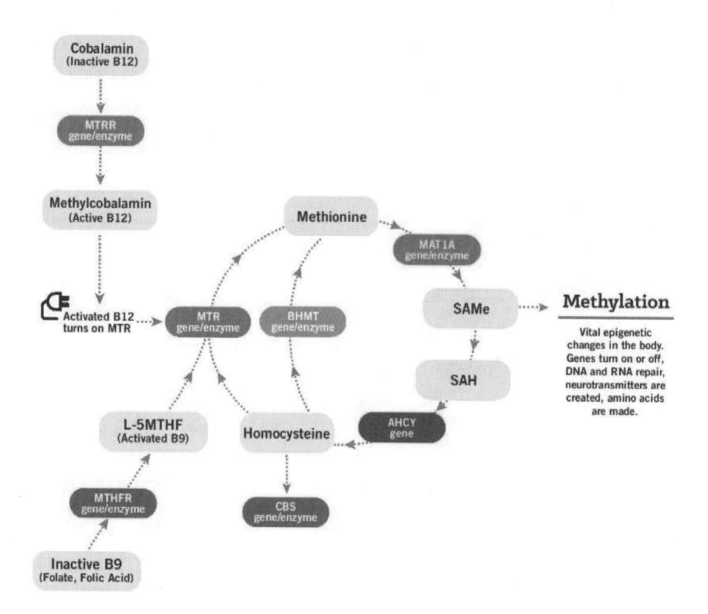

Methylation genetic alterations and autoimmune disease

Having a methylation gene risk allele can increase your risk for developing an autoimmune disease. This is important because the affected tissues of autoimmune patients are often hindered in their ability to perform the methylation process.

For example, in Multiple Sclerosis (MS) patients, the immune system attacks and destroys the myelin sheaths that surround neurons. In studies of MS patients, the myelin sheaths are often shown to have decreased methylation.

In a study of patients with ulcerative colitis (another autoimmune disease), patients were shown to have decreased methylation levels in their immune cells and affected intestinal mucosa of the rectum[1,2].

Having one or more risk alleles in the methylation genes MTHFR, MAT1A, MTRR and BHMT can lead to lower levels of methylation in the tissues, as seen in people with MS and ulcerative colitis. These genetic variants can lower methylation levels in the tissues of people with autoimmune diseases, because they can cause the body to make low levels of SAMe. SAMe is the chemical that ultimately methylates the body's tissues.

Anyone with an increased risk of developing an autoimmune disease should consider having genetic testing to rule out having genetic variants that hinder their ability to methylate, as well as periodic bloodwork to measure how well their methylation pathways are performing.

Many other factors play an important role in developing and managing an autoimmune disease, but diagnosing and properly addressing methylation genetic variants should be part of managing any autoimmune disease.

If you are concerned about having an autoimmune disease, then Cyrex lab's panel 5 can be a valuable test to help determine if you have developed an autoimmune disease. Cyrex panel 5 tests for high levels of multiple antibodies that attack the body's tissues.

References:

1.) Mastroardi, FG, Noor A, Wood DD, et al. Peptidyl argininedeiminase 2 CpG island in multiple sclerosis white matter is hypomethylated. J Neurosci Res. 2007. Jul;85(9):2006-16.

2.) GloriaL, et al. DNA hypomethylation and proliferative activity are increased in the rectal mucosa of patients with long-standing ulcerative colitis. Cancer 78(11): 2300-2306, 1996

Christy L. Sutton D.C.

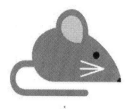

Pregnant Brown Mice

(brown mice are healthier than yellow mice)

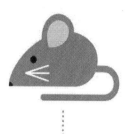

Pregnant brown mice are exposed to BPA to disrupt their methylation detox pathways. These mice **ARE NOT GIVEN nutritional support** to help them promote healthy methylation and compensate for being exposed to toxic chemical BPA.

Pregnant brown mice are exposed to BPA to disrupt their methylation detoxification pathways. These mice **ARE GIVEN nutritional support** that promotes healthy methylation, such as *vitamin B9, vitamin B12, betaine, and choline*. This nutritional support helps them compensate for being exposed to the toxic chemical BPA.

Yellow Offspring

(Unhealthy)

Brown Offspring

(Healthy)

Conclusion

1 BPA is a toxic chemical that can negatively affect the unborn.

2 All females of child bearing years should consider supplementing with nutrients that will help them methylate and protect them from the BPA that they will inevitably be exposed to in the environment.

3 Anyone exposed to BPA from eating or drinking out of plastic containers, eating canned foods, or handling receipt paper should protect themselves with nutrients that will help them methylate.

BPA — Protect yourself through proper nutrition

BPA (bisphenol A) is a dangerous chemical found everywhere in our environment, including in plastic water bottles, on receipts, in dental sealants and lining many canned goods. BPA is an endocrine disruptor that *interferes with methylation detox pathways*, which are essential for the body to detoxify and function properly.

Pregnant mice + BPA exposure = unhealthy offspring
Pregnant mice + BPA exposure + nutrition to promote methylation = healthy offspring

One revealing experiment illustrates how harmful BPA can be to the unborn when mothers are exposed to BPA while pregnant[1]. The experiment exposed healthy, pregnant mice to BPA, causing their offspring to be born yellow and unhealthy[1]. Yellow mice are considered unhealthy and are known to have more health problems than brown mice.

However, the pregnant mice that were also exposed to BPA while simultaneously given a diet high in methylation-promoting nutrition, including vitamin B-9, vitamin B-12, betaine and choline, gave birth to healthy brown mice. These nutrients restored the methylation pathway disrupted by the BPA, thus protecting the unborn mice from the BPA.

Prenatal and childhood exposure to BPA can lead to anxiety and hyperactivity in children

Exposure to BPA while in-utero or as a young child has been shown to increase the risk for boys to develop hyperactivity, anxiety, aggression and depression. It's possible that nutritional support, such as methylated B vitamins, could prevent BPA-associated health problems.

Having a risk allele in methylation genes and BPA can have similar effects on infant health

Genetic variants, or having a risk allele in a pregnant mother's methylation genes is analogous to being exposed to the toxin BPA. This is because both genetic variants and exposure to BPA will interfere with the methylation detox pathways, leading to a decreased ability to detoxify[2]. There are many genetic variants that disrupt the methylation pathways and also make people much more vulnerable to health problems. Fortunately, having genetic variants in the methylation genes can be easily corrected through proper nutrition.

Avoiding BPA and other toxins is essential; unfortunately, we live in a world where complete avoidance is impossible. That's why it's so important to be healthy and practice good nutrition before, during and after pregnancy.

References:

1.) Dolinoy, DC, D Huang and RL Jirtle. 2007. Maternal nutrient supplementation counteracts bisphenol A-induced DNA hypomethylation in early development

2.) Glinda S. Cooper, Kathleen M. Gilbert,Eric L. Greidinger, Judith A. James, et al.Recent Advances and Opportunities in Research on Lupus: Environmental Influences and Mechanisms of Disease. Environ Health Perspect. 2008 June; 116(6): 695–702.

3.) Environmental health news. Prenatal and childhood exposure linked to anxiety hyperactivity in boys. Jul7 25, 2013. Retrieved from: http://www.environmentalhealthnews.org/ehs/newscience/2013/07/boys-bisphenol-a

Christy L. Sutton D.C.

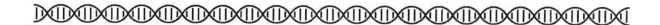

Vitamin B-9 Methylation Genes

The following genes are necessary for your body to correctly methylate (activate) and metabolize vitamin B-9. If you've inherited these "bad" genes, or risk alleles, from your parents, then you might benefit from supplementing with vitamin B-9 in the methyl-activated form. Smartly supplementing with the correct nutrients may help protect you from health problems that might otherwise occur if you inherited the "bad" risk allele for these genes.

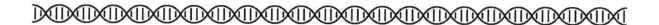

MTHFR gene

Methylenetetrahydrofolate reductase gene

Names of MTHFR genetic variants (SNP identification)	rsnumber	Risk allele
MTHFR C677T	rs1801133	A
MTHFR A1298C	rs1801131	G

MTHFR C677T—Having the risk allele for MTHFR C677T is one of the most significant genetic variations currently known. Thankfully there is a simple solution for anyone who has one or more risk allele(s) for MTHFR C677T.

Who has the MTHFR C677T risk allele(s)?

Ethnic distribution of MTHFR C677T mutations	Homozygous (T, T) genotype
U.S. Africans	0-2%
U.S. Caucasians	10-12%
U.S. Hispanics	20-22%

Table 1 [6,14]

MTHFR A1298C—Having the risk allele for MTHFR A1298C is believed to be less important than MTHFR C677T listed above, but still significant to your health, and still may require nutritional support to protect against this genetic variation. There is a simple solution for anyone who has one or more risk allele(s) for MTHFR A1298C.

What does the MTHFR gene do?

- *The MTHFR gene is important for your ability to activate vitamin B-9*—The MTHFR gene produces an enzyme that is also called MTHFR, which is essential for converting the inactive form of vitamin B-9 into the activated form of vitamin B-9. The methyl-activated form of vitamin B-9 is called Quatrefolic acid or L-5-MTHF, and is what the body needs for normal metabolic functions. Having one or more risk allele(s) in the MTHFR gene simply means that your body can't naturally convert the inactive form of vitamin B-9 into the active form. This means that you won't be able to adequately use the vitamin B-9 from your diet and will require a specific supplemental form of vitamin B-9.

- *MTHFR is important for your ability to detoxify*—Think of MTHFR as a gene that creates a rotating door to remove toxins from the body after they enter

Christy L. Sutton D.C.

through the environment. If you have an MTHFR risk allele, then your rotating door is not working efficiently and you're likely building up toxins. Having the risk allele for MTHFR C677T is much more significant for your health than having the risk allele for MTHFR A1298C. However, having the risk allele for MTHFR A1298C is still an issue that needs to be addressed and properly treated by supplementing with vitamin B-9 in the methyl-activated form called methyl-activated Quatrefolic acid or L-5-MTHF.

- **MTHFR plays an important role in turning genes on and off**—MTHFR plays an extremely important role in the body's ability to methylate, which is essential for turning genes on and off.

What health problems are associated with having a risk allele for the MTHFR gene?

If you have the risk a risk allele for the MTHFR gene, and it's undiagnosed or not treated with proper nutritional supplementation, it can lead to serious health problems. Some of these include:

- Stroke
- Diabetes[4, 7]
- Multiple sclerosis
- Cancer[4, 5, 14]
- Alzheimer's disease
- ALS (amyotrophic lateral sclerosis)
- Depression[2, 3]
- Anxiety disorders[3]
- Atherosclerosis[4]
- Parkinson's disease
- Celiac disease
- Chronic fatigue syndrome
- Fibromyalgia
- Pregnancy complications
- Mitochondrial disease
- Systemic lupus erythematosus
- Neural tube defects (Spina bifida)

- Miscarriages
- Reproductive problems[10, 11]
- Down syndrome
- Bipolar disorder[3]
- Schizophrenia[8, 4]
- Inflammation
- Blood vessel damage
- Thrombosis (blood clots)
- Autism[1,9]
- Autoimmune diseases[12, 13]
- Osteoporosis
- High homocysteine level on blood work—Having a risk allele in the MTHFR gene decreases the body's ability to metabolize homocysteine, resulting in a higher homocysteine level.

MTHFR genetic variants and your child's health

What does having an MTHFR risk allele mean for an unborn child's health?

It's incredibly important for women to be diagnosed and treated for having an MTHFR risk allele before becoming pregnant. If a woman is being treated with proper nutritional supplementation before getting pregnant and while pregnant, her child's chances of developing autism and neural tube defects like spina bifida are dramatically reduced.

Autism and MTHFR risk alleles

There is a *2.79-fold increased risk* for developing autism in children with MTHFR with a risk allele for MTHFR C677T[1]. However, having the risk allele for both MTHFR C677T and A1298C significantly increases the risk of developing autism[1]. There is an *8.11-fold increased risk* of developing autism if someone has all four risk alleles for both MTHFR C677T and MTHFR A1298C[1].

Healthy mommies + healthy pregnancies = healthy babies

All women of child-bearing age, particularly pregnant women, should strongly consider taking a prenatal vitamin with extra vitamin B-9 in the methyl-activated form called Quatrefolic acid or L-5-MTHF. It's particularly important for women with any MTHFR risk alleles to be taking the methyl-activated form of vitamin B-9 before conception, throughout pregnancy and while nursing.

Pregnant women who have one or more MTHFR risk allele(s) are at an increased risk for miscarriage; a more complex, high-risk pregnancy; and developing pre-eclampsia. Even if a pregnant woman doesn't have an MTHFR risk allele, she may still benefit from taking the methyl-activated form of vitamin B-9 called Quatrefolic acid or L-5-MTHF. Her unborn child may also still benefit, particularly if the baby is inheriting a risk-allele paternal MTHFR gene.

One important study showed that women who took at least 400 mcg of vitamin B-9 every day starting at least four weeks before pregnancy, and through eight weeks after the start of their pregnancy, were 40 percent less likely to have a child diagnosed with autism spectrum disorder[13].

An MTHFR risk allele: A big problem or a non-issue?

Thankfully there can be an easy solution to preventing health problems related to having one or more MTHFR risk allele(s). If women are educated about proper nutrition before and during pregnancy, and they ensure that their children get proper nutrition from an early age, their risk for developing MTHFR-related health problems should be a non-issue.

Christy L. Sutton D.C.

I have an MTHFR risk allele. What should I talk to my doctor about doing so that I can reduce my health risks?

While there are many significant health risks related to MTHFR genetic variation, they're easily corrected and bypassed through proper nutritional supplementation.

Nutrition to bypass MTHFR genetic variations:

- *Consider supplementing with the activated form of vitamin B-9 called Quatrefolic acid or L-5-MTHF* —This is an easy and powerful step toward protecting your health and bypassing health problems related to having a risk allele in the MTHFR gene. Having both the knowledge of an MTHFR risk allele and the ability to nutritionally bypass the health problems with a simple nutritional supplement is truly a gift that could add both quality and quantity to your life.

- *Consider supplementing with vitamin B-2*—The MTHFR enzyme requires vitamin B-2 to function properly; therefore, taking a high-quality activated B-complex with the activated forms of both vitamins B-9 and B-2 can be very helpful. The activated form of vitamin B-2 is called riboflavin-5'-phosphate.

- *Avoid high amounts of folic acid*—Folic acid is the inactive, synthetic form of vitamin B-9, which is used to fortify foods and most nutritional supplements. Anyone with one or more MTHFR risk allele(s) should avoid taking the supplemental forms of regular folic acid in large amounts, as it can compete with the activated form of vitamin B-9, causing potential health problems.

- *Eat a diet high in green, leafy vegetables*—Green, leafy vegetables are naturally high in vitamin B-9 (folate) and are essential for health. Eating a diet high in vegetables is important, but diet alone is often not sufficient for people with a risk allele in the MTHFR gene. Only about 50 percent of dietary folate is absorbed from food[13]. For those with a risk allele in the MTHFR gene, only around 30-80 percent of the dietary folate absorbed in the intestines will be converted to the methyl-active form of vitamin B-9 called Quatrefolic acid or L-5-MTHF. And many people are not eating enough green leafy vegetables in the first place. If you have a risk allele for the MTHFR gene, you *need* to take to talk to your doctor about taking a supplemental form of vitamin-B9 in the methyl-activated form called Quatrefolic acid or L-5-MTHF.

- ***Eat a diet high in foods that promote methylation***—These include raw beets; raw, dark, green, leafy vegetables; raw broccoli; egg; chicken; beef; garlic; nuts; pork; fish; broccoli; citrus fruits and beans.

- ***Exercise***—Exercise has been shown to improve methylation in people with a family history of diabetes[7].

I have the risk allele in the MTHFR gene. What type of vitamin B-9 should I consider supplementing with?

You need to consider taking the methyl-activated supplemental form of vitamin B-9 called Quatrefolic acid or L-5-MTHF. These are the naturally occurring, activated form of vitamin B-9. The methyl-activated form of vitamin B-9 is the form of vitamin B-9 that the body needs to function properly, and is the activated form of vitamin B-9 that the body makes using the inactive forms of vitamin B-9 (folic acid or folate). *If you have a risk allele in the MTHFR gene, you won't convert the inactive forms of vitamin B-9 (folate, folic acid) into the active form (Quatrefolic acid or L-5-MTHF).* If you have the risk allele for the MTHFR gene, you should consider including a nutritional supplement that contains the methylated form of vitamin B-9 (Quatrefolic acid or L-5-MTHF).

With the risk allele in the MTHFR gene, what type of vitamin B-9 should I *avoid* supplementing with?

Avoid supplementing with the inactive form of vitamin B-9 called either folic acid or folate. **Folic acid** is a synthetic form of vitamin B-9 in the *inactive* form, found in most nutritional supplements. Vitamin B-9 in the form called folic acid is not sufficient for people with a risk allele in the MTHFR gene. Folic acid is found in fortified foods and most nutritional supplements. Folic acid requires the body to convert it to the methyl-activated form of vitamin B-9 called Quatrefolic acid or L-5-MTHF. This process of converting the folic acid to the activated form doesn't occur efficiently in people with the MTHFR risk allele.

Folate is the inactive form of vitamin B-9 found in food. This form of folate isn't sufficient for people with a risk allele in the MTHFR gene. Folate is a form of vitamin B-9 that is naturally occurring in green leafy vegetables. It requires the body to convert it to the active form of vitamin B-9. The conversion from inactive folate to the active form of vitamin B-9 doesn't occur efficiently in people with the MTHFR risk allele. It's always important to eat a diet high in green, leafy vegetables, but anyone with a risk allele in the MTHFR gene shouldn't depend on diet alone to satisfy their vitamin B-9 requirements.

Talk to your doctor about what type and dosage of B-9 you might need.

Christy L. Sutton D.C.

I have an MTHFR risk allele. What lab/testing should I consider to monitor my health?

✓ *Homocysteine (blood test)*—I prefer to see homocysteine below 8 on blood work. Homocysteine is an excellent test to easily measure how much damage is occurring in the body from having one or more risk allele(s) in MTHFR gene.

✓ *A methylation profile (blood test)*—This should include levels of folate, cystathione, cysteine, homocysteine, methionine, SAMe (S-Adenosyl-L-methionine) and SAH (S-adnosylmethionine).

✓ *Routine cancer screenings*—All appropriate tests should be performed regularly: colonoscopy, EGD (upper endoscopy of the stomach), skin exam, thyroid exam, prostate exam, Pap smear, breast exam and routine blood work

---

Homocysteine: An easy lab test that could save your life

Homocysteine is a lab marker that can tell you a lot about how well your methylation pathways are working. A high homocysteine level can increase your risk for a heart attack, stroke, Alzheimer's disease, cancer and giving birth to a child with birth defects such as spina bifida. It's vital to know your homocysteine level!

What homocysteine level is too high? As a doctor who is highly interested in preventing my patients from developing health problems, when I am reviewing at my patients' lab results, I prefer to see a homocysteine below eight. The *lower* your homocysteine level, the less likely you are to experience hearing loss, macular degeneration, migraines, vascular damage, congestive heart failure, Alzheimer's, dementia, stroke, atherosclerosis, cancer, general inflammation, and pregnancy-related problems such as pre-eclampsia.

What level of homocysteine do most physicians consider too high? Most doctors make their recommendations based on the acceptable lab range for homocysteine; therefore, your doctor will likely not mention your homocysteine level being too high until it is above 15. Unfortunately, most doctors don't include homocysteine in routine lab work they order for their patients.

How can I lower my homocysteine level? If you have a high homocysteine level, then you likely have one or more risk alleles (genetic variants) in your methylation genes. The smartest way to lower your homocysteine level is to get tested to determine your exact genetic variants, then work with your doctor to add the correct nutrition associated with each genetic variant. In general, the active forms of vitamin B-6, vitamin B-9, vitamin B-12, TMG and betaine have shown to help lower homocysteine.

References:

1.) Mohammad et al, Aberrations in folate metabolic pathway and altered susceptibility to autism. Psychiatr Genet 2009 Aug; 19(4):171-6.

2.) Robert J Hedava. Nutrition and Depression: Nutrition, Methylation, and Depression, Part 2 Nutritional support for the methylation cycle plays a critical role. Published on November 22, 2010. http://www.psychologytoday.com/blog/health-matters.

3.) Gilbody S, et al. Methylenetetrahydrofolate Reductase (MTHFR) Genetic Polymorphisms (C677T variant) and Psychiatric Disorders: A HuGE Review. Am J Epidemiol. 2007;165:1-13.

4.) Melas PA, Rogdaki M, Ösby U, et al.Epigenetic aberrations in leukocytes of patients with schizophrenia: association of global DNA methylation with antipsychotic drug treatment and disease onset. FASEB J. 2012, 26:2712–8.

5.) Thillainadesan G, Chitilian JM, et al. TGF-β-dependent active demethylation and expression of the p15ink4b tumor suppressor are impaired by the ZNF217/CoREST complex. Mol Cell. 2012 Jun 8;46(5):636-49.

6.) Siaw-Cheok Liew, Esha Das Gupta. Methylenetetrahydrafolate reductase (MTHFR) C677T polymorphism: epidemiology, metabolism, and the associated diseases.Eur J Med Genet. 2015 Jan;58(1):1-10.

7.) Nitert M. D., Dayeh T., Volkov P., et al.. (2012). Impact of an exercise intervention on DNA methylation in skeletal muscle from first-degree relatives of patients with type 2 diabetes. Diabetes 61, 3322–3332. 10.2337/db11-1653

8.) Rutten BPF, Mill J. Epigenetic mediation of environmental influences in major psychotic disorders. Schizophr Bull. 2009;35(6):1045–56.

9.) Nguyen A., Rauch T. A., Pfeifer G. P., Hu V. W. Global methylation profiling of lymphoblastoid cell lines reveals epigenetic contributions to autism spectrum disorders and a novel autism candidate gene, RORA, whose protein product is reduced in autistic brain. The FASEB Journal.2010;24(8):3036–3051.

10.) Anway MD, et al. Epigenetic Transgenerational Actions of Endocrine Disruptors and Male Fertility Science. 2005 Jun 3,308(5727):1466-9.

11.) Anway MD, et al. Epigenetic transgenerational actions of endocrine disruptors. Endocrinology. 2006 Jun;147(6 Suppl):S43-9

12). Greer, J., P.: The role of epigenetic mechanisms and processes in autoimmune disorders. Biologics. 2012; 6: 307–327. Published online 2012 September 6.

13.) Hamilton, John. Folic Acid for Pregnant Mothers Cuts Kids' Autism Risk. (2013. Feb 12th). Retrieved from: http://www.npr.org/sections/health-shots/2013/02/25/171828067/folic-acid-for-pregnant-mothers-cuts-kids-autism-risk

14.) Thomas, Philip; Fenech, Michael. Methylenetetrahydrofolate reductase, common polymorphisms, and relation to disease. Pg.375-386.

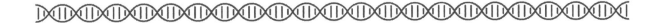

Christy L. Sutton D.C.

MTHFD1L gene
Monofunctional C1-tetrahydrofolate synthase gene

Names of MTHFD1L genetic variants (SNP identification)	rsnumber	Risk allele
MTHFD1L G25264A	rs11754661	Risk allele is A
MTHFD1L G71171A	rs6922269	Risk allele is A
MTHFD1L T31397C	rs17349743	Risk allele is C

What does the MTHFD1L gene do?

The MTHFD1L gene promotes the body's ability to properly methylate through the regeneration of methionine from homocysteine. Having a risk allele in the MTHFD1L gene has been associated with high levels of homocysteine in laboratory testing. Having a high homocysteine level is a sign of inflammation and is associated with many health problems.

What type of health problems are associated with having the risk allele(s) for the MTHFD1L gene?

- *Increased risk of birth defects*—There is an increased risk of neural tube defects, such as spina bifida, associated with MTHFD1L.

- *Increased Alzheimer's risk*—There is an increased risk for Alzheimer's associated for people having both MTHFD1L *and* high homocysteine levels.

- *Increased heart disease risk, particularly coronary artery disease*[1]—An increased risk of cardiovascular disease is a problem for people with one or more risk alleles in MTHFD1L G71171A (rs6922269).

I have a risk allele for the MTHFD1L gene. What should I talk to my doctor about doing so that I can reduce my health risks?

The health problems associated with having a risk allele in the MTHFD1L gene are largely a result of developing a high homocysteine level as a result of having the MTHFD1L risk allele. Therefore, it's very important for anyone with an MTHFD1L risk allele to monitor their homocysteine level through routine blood work. They should also include dietary and nutritional supplementation as part of their everyday routine to promote a lower homocysteine level.

How can I naturally lower my homocysteine level?

- Consider supplementing with the activated form of vitamin B-9 (L- 5-MTHF), the activated form of vitamin-B-12 (methylcobalamin), the activated form of vitamin B-6 (p-5-p), and trimethylglycine (TMG).

- Eat a diet high in green, leafy vegetables and meat for vitamin B-9 and B-12 (vitamin B-12 is only naturally occurring in animal products).

I have a risk allele in the MTHFD1L gene. What labs/testing should I consider to continually monitor my health?

- ✓ *Homocysteine (blood test)*— I prefer to see homocysteine below 8 on blood work.. Homocysteine is an excellent test to easily measure how much damage is occurring in the body due to having one or more risk allele(s) in the methylation genes such as MTHFD1L.

- ✓ *A methylation profile (blood test)*—This should include levels of folate, cystathione, cysteine, homocysteine, methionine, SAMe (S-Adenosyl-L-methionine) and SAH (S-adnosylmethionine).

References:

1.) Wellcome Trust Case Control Consortium. Genome-wide association study of 14,000 cases of seven common diseases and 3,000 shared controls. Nature. 2007; 447:661–678.

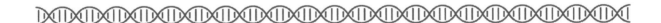

Christy L. Sutton D.C.

MTHFS gene
Methenyltetrahydrofolate synthetase gene

Names of MTHFS genetic variants (SNP identification)	rsnumber	Risk allele
MTHFS – ST20 MTHFS	rs6495446	Risk allele is C
MTHFS – ST20 MTHFS G56057A	rs6495446	Risk allele is T

What does this gene do?

MTHFD1L plays an important role in the body's methylation, and in the pathways that metabolize vitamin B-9.

What health problems are associated with having a risk allele in the MTHFS gene?

- *Chronic kidney disease*—Having the C risk allele for MTHFS (rs6495446), has been associated with chronic kidney disease[1]. Hypertension and diabetes are the two most common causes of chronic kidney disease. If you have both the risk allele for MTHFS and chronic kidney disease, you should consider that hypertension and/or diabetes could be the underlying cause(s) of your kidney problems.

- *Low glutathione levels*—Having the T risk allele for MTHFS (rs2733103) is associated with lower glutathione levels[2]. Glutathione is one of the body's most important antioxidants. Low glutathione is associated with everything from an increased cancer risk to autoimmune disease to autism.

- *Increased rate of depleting vitamin B-9*

I have the MTHFS risk allele. What should I talk to my doctor about doing so that I can reduce my health risks?

- *Avoid dehydration*—Dehydration is very bad for the kidneys.

- *Avoid folinic acid*—Anyone with an MTHFS risk allele should avoid the form of vitamin B-9 called folinic acid, and instead take the methyl activated form of vitamin B-9 called Quatrefolic acid or L-5-MTHF.

- *Ensure adequate magnesium levels*—The MTHFS enzyme requires magnesium to function properly. Foods high in magnesium include green, leafy vegetables; nuts; seeds; fish; beans; whole grains; chocolate and avocados.

- *Increase glutathione levels*—Ways to increase glutathione levels include supplementing with n-acetylcysteine (NAC), selenium, milk thistle and applying a topical glutathione cream. There is more about increasing glutathione levels in the section on glutathione on page 57.

I have a risk allele in the MTHFS gene. What labs/testing should I consider to continually monitor my health?

- ✓ *Homocysteine (blood test)*— I prefer to see homocysteine below 8 on blood work. Homocysteine is an excellent test to easily measure how much damage is occurring in the body due to having one or more risk allele(s) in the methylation genes.

- ✓ *Blood work to test kidney function*—This includes testing for creatinine, BUN and GFR.

- ✓ *Measure glutathione levels (blood test)*

References:

1.) Kottgen A1, Kao WH, Hwang SJ, et al. Genome-wide association study for renal traits in the Framingham Heart and Atherosclerosis Risk in Communities Studies. BMC Med Genet. 2008 Jun 3;9:49.

2.) Chowdhury S, Hobbs CA, et al. Associations between maternal genotypes and metabolites implicated in congenital heart defects. Mol Genet Metab. 2012;107:596–604.

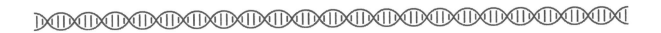

Christy L. Sutton D.C.

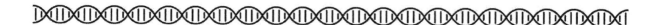

Vitamin B-12 Methylation Genes

The following genes are important for your body to correctly methylat (activate) and metabolize vitamin B-12. If you've inherited these "bad" genes, or risk alleles, from your parents, you might benefit from supplementing with vitamin B-12 in one of the activated forms called methylcobalamin or adenosylcobalamin. Smartly supplementing with vitamin B-12 may help protect you from health problems that might otherwise occur if you inherited the "bad" risk allele for these genes.

MTR gene

5-methyltetrahydrofolate-homocysteine methyltransferase gene

Names of MTR genetic variants (SNP identification)	rsnumber	Risk allele
MTR A2756G	rs1805087	G

What does the MTR gene do?

The methionine synthase (MTR) gene is essential for the body to be able to produce the methionine synthase enzyme. MTR gene issues can lead to problems with the methylation cycle and subsequent health struggles. MTR makes the important chemical methionine by combining methylated folate and homocysteine. However, the MTR enzyme won't work without adequate levels of vitamin B-12 in the activated form (methylcobalamin). The proper recycling of the highly inflammatory chemical homocysteine is highly dependent on the MTR enzyme and having adequate levels of activated vitamin B-12 (methylcobalamin).

What does a risk allele in the MTR gene mean for my health?

The MTR risk allele causes the MTR enzyme to work at a *faster* rate than normal. Having this risk allele hastens the speed at which MTR enzymes lower homocysteine. If you're deficient in the activated form of vitamin B-9 or vitamin B-12, the MTR enzyme won't be able to remove homocysteine from your body, and you'll be more likely to develop health problems such as cardiovascular disease.

Under the correct circumstances, having this MTR risk allele can be good for your health.

Low in B12? It could be your digestive system

B12 absorption requires a healthy stomach because the stomach produces intrinsic factor, a protein necessary for vitamin B-12 absorption. As we age, our stomach produces less intrinsic factor, which can lead to vitamin B-12 deficiencies—even if adequate levels of vitamin B-12 are being consumed. Anyone at high risk for vitamin B-12 deficiencies should consider vitamin B-12 shots and oral intrinsic factor.

Conditions that increase your risk of being vitamin B-12 deficient:

- Crohn's disease
- Celiac disease
- Intestinal malabsorption
- Taking acid-blocking medications
- Aging
- Being a vegetarian (B12 is only found naturally in animal products)

If adequate levels of the activated form of vitamins B-9 and B-12 are present, this MTR risk allele can be *good* for your health. One of the benefits of having this MTR risk allele is that it will help you metabolize homocysteine faster, thus lowering your homocysteine level. A high homocysteine level is associated with an increased risk for developing cardiovascular disease, stroke, Alzheimer's, clotting disorders, pregnancy-related problems and other dangerous conditions.

I have one or more risk alleles for the MTR gene. What should I talk to my doctor about doing so that I can reduce my health risks?

Consider supplementing with the methyl-activated forms of both vitamin B-9 (Quatrefolic acid or L-5-MTHF) and vitamin B-12 (methylcobalamin). It's important to take vitamins B-9 and B-12 together because taking only one can mask a deficiency in the other.

I have one or more MTR risk allele(s). What labs/testing should I consider to continually monitor my health?

- ✓ *Complete blood count (CBC) (blood test)*—A CBC shows the size of your red blood cells. Large red blood cells are a symptom of being deficient in B9 or B12.

- ✓ *Methylmalonic acid (blood test)*—This is the most accurate functional blood test for diagnosing B-12 deficiencies.

- ✓ *Homocysteine (blood test)* —This is a good, simple test to easily measure how much damage an MTR risk allele is causing your body. I prefer to see homocysteine below 8 on blood work.

- ✓ *Serum B12 level (blood test)*—This is my least-favorite blood test because you must be dangerously low in B-12 before this test flags you as having a problem.

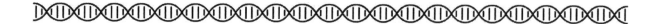

MTRR gene

5-methyltetrahydrofolate-homocysteine methyltransferase reductase gene

Names of MTRR genetic variants (SNP identification)	rsnumber	Risk allele
MTRR A66G	rs1801394	Risk allele is G
MTRR K350A	rs162036	Risk allele is G
MTRR R415T	rs2287780	Risk allele is T

What does the MTRR gene do?

The MTRR gene plays an important role in the body's ability to convert inactive vitamin B-12 (cobalamin) into the activated form of B12, called methylcobalamin. Having risk alleles in the MTRR gene causes your body to produce a defective MTRR enzyme. This defective MTRR enzyme is incapable of producing adequate levels of activated vitamin B-12 (methylcobalamin) *and* assisting in the conversion of homocysteine into methionine.

What type of health problems are associated with having a risk allele (s) for the MTRR gene?

- *Low levels of activated vitamin B-12 (methylcobalamin) can lead to:*

  - Cardiovascular disease
  - Neuropathy
  - Anemia
  - Cancer
  - Neurological problems
  - Alzheimer's
  - Fatigue
  - Depression
  - MTR enzyme no longer functioning
  - A high homocysteine level

- *Disruption in the body's ability to methylate (turn genes on and off)*—
  Methylation is a key step in the body's ability to turn both genes and bodily functions on and off. If you're low in the activated form of vitamin B-12 (methylcobalamin), it greatly hinders the body's ability to produce SAMe. SAMe is what ultimately does the turning on and off of many genes—and what the body ultimately is trying to make using the activated forms of vitamins B-9 and B-12.

Christy L. Sutton D.C.

- **Decreased ability to detoxify**—Being able to create the activated form of vitamin B-12 is essential for your body's Phase II methylation detox pathways. You can think of MTRR as a rotating door that removes toxins from your body. If you have MTRR risk alleles, your rotating door is not working as efficiently as it should, making you more likely to build up toxins and develop health problems as a result.

I have one or more risk allele(s) for the MTRR gene. What should I talk to my doctor about doing so that I can reduce my health risks?

- **Consider supplementing with activated B-12 (methylcobalamin) when appropriate**—If you have the risk allele for the MTRR gene, you may consider supplementing with vitamin B-12 in the activated form (methylcobalamin) to help your body compensate for its inability to make adequate levels of activated B-12 naturally.

- **Prevent zinc deficiencies**—Zinc is required for the MTRR enzyme to function properly; therefore, preventing zinc deficiencies will also help prevent a sluggish MTRR pathway. Foods high in zinc include oysters, beef, wheat germ, spinach, cashews, chocolate, beans and white meats.

- **Support healthy detoxification pathways by eating a clean diet, exercising and getting proper hydration.**

It's important to take vitamins B-9 and B-12 together because taking only one can mask a deficiency in the other

---

A recipe for a serious vitamin B-12 deficiency

Having the risk alleles for *both* **MTR A2756G (rs1805087)** *and* **MTRR A66G (rs1801394)** significantly increases your risk of becoming deficient in the activated form of vitamin B-12 (methylcobalamin). If you have both risk alleles, keep a watchful eye on your methylcobalamin (B12) levels, and consider doing more thorough testing to ensure that you're not vitamin B-12 deficient.

I have one or more MTRR risk allele(s). What labs/testing should I consider to continually monitor my health?

✓ *CBC (blood test)*—A CBC shows the size of your red blood cells. Large red blood cells are a symptom of being deficient in vitamins B-9 or B-12.

✓ *Methylmalonic acid (blood test)*—This is the most accurate functional blood test for measuring vitamin B-12 levels.

✓ *Homocysteine (blood test)*—This can measure how much damage an MTRR risk allele is causing your body. I prefer homocysteine to be below 8.

✓ *Serum B12 level (blood test)*—This is my least-favorite test because you must be dangerously low in B-12 before this test flags you as having a problem.

✓ *Measure zinc levels*

> *Zinc blood test or taste test*—The zinc taste test is an easy and accurate test that involves putting some liquid zinc in your mouth. If the zinc tastes like water, that indicates a deficiency

---

Laughing gas is no laughing matter

Having a risk allele in the MTRR gene can lead to low levels of methylcobalmin (B12 in the activated form). If you have the risk allele for the MTRR gene and are exposed to laughing gas (nitric oxide), you're creating a perfect storm for serious problems.

For people with risk alleles in either the MTRR or the MTHFR gene, being exposed to laughing gas can be very dangerous — **especially for infants and young children.**

Laughing gas slowly and irreversibly inactivates methylcobalamin (vitamin B-12) in the MTR enzyme. The MTR enzyme requires the activated form of vitamin B-12 (methylcobalamin) and vitamin B-9 (methyl-activated Quatrefolic acid or L-5-MTHF) to function, and will no longer function once laughing gas inactivates the vitamin B-12.

This increased risk for side effects from anesthesia is a good reason to perform specific genetic tests on infants and young children before they undergo anesthesia. There are documented cases of children dying from anesthesia, and their deaths being attributed to having risk alleles that could have been easily bypassed with proper nutritional support[1].

Christy L. Sutton D.C.

Reference:

1.) Kohlmeier, Martin Nutrigenetics, Applying the Science of Personal Nutrition. 2013. Academic Press. Pg.183-184.

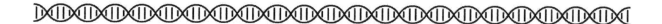

MMAB gene
Methylmalonic aciduria (cobalamin deficiency) cblB type gene

Names of MMAB genetic variants (SNP identification)	rsnumber	Risk allele
MMAB G16110A	rs7134594	Risk allele is C

What does the MMAB gene do?

The MMAB gene assists in the body's ability to make vitamin B-12 in the form called adenosylcobalamin (AdoCbl). The MMAB gene provides the body's instructions to make an enzyme involved in making adenosylcobalamin (AdoCbl).

What type of health problems are associated with having the risk allele for the MMAB gene?

Methylmalonic aciduria—Having the MMAB risk allele can lead to deficiencies in the form of vitamin B-12 known as adenosylcobalamin (AdoCbl). Deficiencies in AdoCbl can create problems breaking down cholesterol, proteins and fats. This is largely due to the fact that the enzyme called methylmalonyl CoA, which is made from the MUT gene, requires vitamin B-12 in the form called adenosylcobalamin (AdoCbl).

I have the risk allele for the MMAB gene. What should I talk to my doctor about doing so that I can reduce my health risks?

The best way to reduce your health risk is to talk to your doctor about supplementing with vitamin B-12 in the form called adensylcobalamin (AdoCbl).

I have the risk allele for the MMAB gene. What labs/testing should I consider to continually monitor my health?

✓ *Monitor cholesterol and triglyceride levels (blood test)*—This includes LDL cholesterol, HDL cholesterol, VLDL cholesterol and triglycerides.

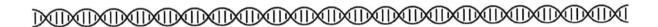

The type of B-12 you feel best with could depend on your genes

Certain genotypes may benefit from taking vitamin B-12 in the form called adenosylcobalamin (AdoCbl), rather than methylcobalamin. Those genes that are most likely to benefit from taking vitamin B-12 in the form called AdoCbl rather than methylcobalamin include:

MMAB gene—If you have an MMAB risk allele, you have a hindered ability to make vitamin B-12 in the form of *adenosylcobalamin* (Ado Cbl). If you have the MMAB risk allele, you should consider taking a combination of both adenosylcobalamin and methylcobalamin, rather than just methylcobalamin.

COMT genes—If you have the risk allele in the COMT gene, you may feel more mentally balanced taking vitamin B-12 in the form called *adenosylcobalamin* instead of methylcobalamin, or taking a combination of both adenosylcobalamin and methylcobalamin, rather than just the methylcobalamin. More information about the COMT gene is available on page 181.

Christy L. Sutton D.C.

MUT gene
Methylmalonyl-CoA mutase gene

Names of MUT genetic variants (SNP identification)	rsnumber	Risk allele
MUT (also known as MCM)	rs6458690	Risk allele is G

What does the MUT gene do?

The MUT gene provides the body's instructions to make enzymes called methylmalonyl CoA mutase, which are responsible for a particular step in the breakdown of several amino acids; specifically isoleucine, methionine, threonine and valine[1]. The methylmalonyl CoA enzyme that the MUT gene makes also helps break down certain types of fats and cholesterol[1].

What type of health problems are associated with having the risk allele for the MUT gene?

Having this risk allele is associated with high cholesterol and triglyceride levels.

I have the MUT gene risk allele. What should I talk to my doctor about doing so that I can reduce my health risks?

- *Consider supplementing with B12 in the form called adenosylcobalamin (AdoCbl) when necessary*—The MUT enzyme requires the AdoCbl to function. Therefore, supplementing with adenosylcobalamin may enable the MUT enzyme to break down cholesterol and protein faster.

- *Support healthy cholesterol levels*—Natural ways to help lower cholesterol include supplementing with niacin (vitamin B-3), eating or supplementing with garlic, getting regular exercise, and eating a diet high in raw vegetables and low in saturated fat.

- *Support healthy triglyceride levels*—Natural ways to help lower triglycerides include eating a diet low in sugar and exercising regularly.

I have a risk allele for the MUT gene. What labs/testing should I consider to continually monitor my health?

✓ ***Monitor cholesterol and triglyceride levels (blood test)***—This includes LDL cholesterol, HDL cholesterol, VLDL cholesterol and triglycerides.

References:

1.) Genetic home reference- your guide to understanding genetic conditions. MUT gene. Retrieved from https://ghr.nlm.nih.gov/gene/MUT.

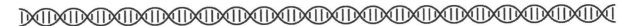

Christy L. Sutton D.C.

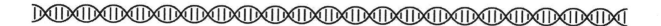

Methylation Regulation and SAMe Synthesis Genes

MAT1A gene
MAT1A-methionine adenosyltransferase gene

Names of MAT1A genetic variants (SNP identification)	rsnumber	Risk allele
MAT1A C1131T	rs2993763	A
MAT1A C15656T	rs4934028	A
MAT1A T*1297C	rs1985908	G

What does the MAT1A gene do?

The MAT1A gene provides instructions for the body to make the MAT enzyme, which converts methionine into SAMe. SAMe plays a vital role in turning genes on and off, brain and joint health, sleep, and many more critical bodily functions. SAMe is the most important methylator in the body[1].

What health problems are associated with having a risk allele in the MAT1A gene?

Low levels of SAMe—If you have a MAT1A risk allele, you can be low in SAMe even when you're high in all the raw ingredients the body needs to make SAMe, such as methionine, vitamins B-12 and B-9.

Conditions associated with low SAMe levels include:

- Depression
- Osteoarthritis
- Fibromyalgia
- Liver disease
- Sleeping problems
- Disruption of neurotransmitter metabolism
- Disruption of carnitine synthesis
- Disruption of the synthesis of CoQ10
- Disruption of the synthesis of DNA
- Disruption in the turning on and off of genes as needed

Christy L. Sutton D.C.

I have one or more MAT1A risk alleles. What should I talk to my doctor about doing so that I can reduce my health risks?

- ***Consider supplementing with SAMe when levels are low***—If you have MAT1A risk alleles, your body doesn't make SAMe efficiently and supplementing with SAMe may be necessary.

- ***Ensure you have adequate levels of the raw ingredients your body needs to make SAMe naturally***—The body needs methionine, vitamin B-9 and vitamin B-12 to naturally make SAMe.

- ***Increase your glutathione levels to help naturally increase SAMe levels***— Low glutathione levels decrease the levels of SAMe by suppressing the body's ability makes SAMe[3]. Topical glutathione creams, NAC, and milk thistle have been shown to help the body naturally increase glutathione levels. Read more about increasing glutathione levels in the section on glutathione (pg. 57).

I have one or more MAT1A risk allele(s). What labs/testing should I consider to continually monitor my health?

- ✓ ***Measure SAMe levels (blood test)***—The most accurate lab to consider for anyone with an MAT1A risk allele is to do lab tests that measure SAMe levels.

- ✓ ***Homocysteine (blood test)***—I prefer homocysteine to be below 8 on blood work.

References:

1.) Markham GD, Pajares MA (2009). "Structure-function relationships in methionine adenosyltransferases.". Cell Mol Life Sci 66 (4): 636–48.

2.). Gil B1, Pajares MA, Mato JM, Alvarez L. Glucocorticoid regulation of hepatic S-adenosylmethionine synthetase gene expression. Endocrinology. 1997 Mar;138(3):1251-8

3.) Pajares MA, Duran C, et al. Modulation of rat liver S-adenosylmethionine synthetase activity by glutathione. J. Biol. Chem. 1992; 267:17598–17605.

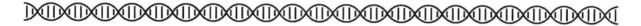

ADK gene
ADK-adenosine kinase

Names of ADK genetic variants (SNP identification)	rsnumber	Risk allele
ADK G509567T	rs1538311	Risk allele is T

What does the ADK gene do?

The ADK gene provides the body's instructions to make the ADK enzyme, which is important in regulating methylation, and thus the turning on and off of genes and bodily functions.

What health problems are associated with having a risk allele in the ADK gene?

High levels of S-adenosylhomocysteine (SAH), leading to low levels of SAMe— The health problems associated with having a risk allele in ADK largely revolve around a buildup of a chemical called S-adenosylhomocysteine (SAH). Think of SAH as the anti-methylation cycle chemical because it inhibits the body's ability to make SAMe, which can cause a lot of health problems. SAMe is the body's most important methylator, and is key for turning bodily functions on and off.

Conditions associated with low SAMe levels include:

- Depression
- Osteoarthritis
- Fibromyalgia
- Liver disease
- Sleeping problems
- Disruption of neurotransmitter metabolism
- Disruption of carnitine synthesis
- Disruption of the synthesis of CoQ10
- Disruption of the synthesis of DNA
- Disruption of turning genes on and off as needed

Christy L. Sutton D.C.

I have one or more ADK gene risk alleles. What should I talk to my doctor about doing so that I can reduce my health risks?

- ***Ensure adequate magnesium levels***—The ADK enzyme, which is made from the ADK gene, requires magnesium. Therefore, having adequate levels of magnesium could prevent methylation cycle disruption that might result from having an ADK risk allele.

- ***Lower your homocysteine level as much as possible***—A high homocysteine level further exacerbates ADK risk allele health problems because a high homocysteine level causes higher levels of SAH to build up, ultimately disrupting the methylation cycle. This ultimately causes the body to produce less SAMe. Vitamin B-9 (methyl-activated Quatrefolic acid or L-5-MTHF), vitamin B-12 (methylcobalamin), vitamin B-6 (p-5-p), vitamin B-2, TMG, phosphatidylserine, phosphatidylcholine and zinc supplementation can significantly reduce homocysteine levels.

- ***Consider supplementing with SAMe if necessary***—Having this ADK risk allele can lead to low levels of SAMe. If you have symptoms of low SAMe levels, or labs that indicate low levels of SAMe, consider supplementing with SAMe.

I have one or more ADK risk allele(s). What labs/testing should I consider to continually monitor my health?

- ✓ ***Methylation profile (blood test)***—This can be done through a lab called Doctor's Data. This test will give you a clear idea as to how well your body's methylation cycle is functioning. Some things that are included in the methylation profile include:

  - ➢ ***Homocysteine***—Having this ADK risk allele can cause a high homocysteine level, which is a sign of inflammation. I prefer homocysteine to be at or below 8 on blood work. High homocysteine can lead to lower levels of SAMe and higher levels of SAH, which ultimately suppress methylation in the body.

  - ➢ ***SAH***—Having the risk allele for ADK can cause high SAH. High SAH can be bad for your health because it decreases the body's ability to make SAMe.

> ➤ **SAMe**—Having an ADK risk allele can lead to lower levels of SAMe, causing many health problems. SAMe is the most important methylator in the body because it turns on and off vital biochemical pathways in the body.

AHCY gene

AHCY- adenosylhomocysteinase gene

Names of AHCY genetic variants (SNP identification)	rsnumber	Risk allele
AHCY 01	rs819147	Risk allele is C

What does the AHCY gene do?

The AHCY gene provides the body's instructions to make the enzyme S-adenosylhomocysteine hydrolase (SAHH), which controls the step that converts the compound S-adenosylhomocysteine (SAH) to the compounds adenosine and homocysteine. This gene plays an important role in regulating methylation.

What health problems are associated with having an AHCY risk allele?

High levels of S-adenosylhomocysteine (SAH), leading to low levels of SAMe—
The health problems associated with having a risk allele in AHCY largely revolve around a buildup of a chemical in the body called S-adenosylhomocysteine (SAH). Think of SAH as the anti-methylation cycle chemical because it inhibits the body's ability to make SAMe, which can cause a lot of health problems. SAMe is the body's most important methylator, and is key for turning bodily functions on and off.

Christy L. Sutton D.C.

Conditions associated with low SAMe levels include:

- Depression
- Osteoarthritis
- Fibromyalgia
- Liver disease
- Sleeping problems
- Disruption of neurotransmitter metabolism
- Disruption of carnitine synthesis
- Disruption of the synthesis of CoQ10
- Disruption of the synthesis of DNA
- Disruption of turning genes on and off as needed

I have one or more AHCY risk alleles. What should I talk to my doctor about doing so that I can reduce my health risks?

- ***Ensure adequate levels of vitamin B-3 and selenium***—The AHCY gene produces the SAHH enzyme, which requires vitamin B-3 and selenium to work properly. Therefore, having adequate levels of vitamin B-3 and selenium will ensure that nutritional deficiencies don't further exacerbate this genetic problem. I recommend taking a high-quality B-complex that contains the activated forms of both B-vitamins and TMG.

    - ➢ ***Natural sources of vitamin B-3 and selenium include:***

        - ○ Vitamin B3 is naturally high in fish, chicken, pork, beef, mushrooms and peas.

        - ○ Selenium is naturally high in Brazil nuts, seafood, fish, sunflower seeds and pork.

- ***Ensure adequate levels of SAMe***—Having an AHCY risk allele can lead to low levels of SAMe. If you have symptoms of low SAMe or labs that indicate low SAMe levels, consider supplementing with SAMe.

- ***Ensure adequate levels of carnitine***—Having the risk allele for the AHCY gene can lead to low levels of carnitine.

I have one or more AHCY risk alleles. What labs/testing should I consider to continually monitor my health?

- ✓ *Methylation profile (blood test)*—This can be done through a lab called Doctor's Data. This test will give you a clear idea as to how your body's methylation cycle is functioning. Some things that are included in the methylation profile are:

  - ➢ *Homocysteine*—Having this AHCY risk allele can cause a high homocysteine level, which is bad for your health. I prefer homocysteine to be below 8 eight on blood work. High homocysteine can lead to lower levels of SAMe and higher levels of SAH, which can suppress methylation.

  - ➢ *SAH*—Having the risk allele for AHCY can cause high SAH, which is bad for your health because it decreases the body's ability to make SAMe. SAMe is the most important methylator in the body, and it is what ultimately turns on and off vital biochemical pathways.

  - ➢ *SAMe*—SAMe can become low if you have an AHCY risk allele. Low SAMe can lead to many health problems.

- ✓ *Nutreval by Genova Diagnostic's (blood and urine)*—This measures your levels of vitamins, minerals, heavy metals, toxins and amino acids. It provides a valuable and overarching look at how your overall environment is affecting your health.

- ✓ *Carnitine panel (blood test)*—Having an AHCY risk allele can lead to low carnitine levels. Carnitine is important for proper fatty acid metabolism.

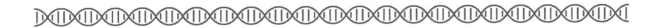

BHMT gene
Betaine—Homocysteine S-Methyltransferase gene

Names of BHMT genetic variants (SNP identification)	rsnumber	Risk allele
BHMT R239Q	rs3733890	Risk allele is A
BHMT-02 C13813T	rs567754	Risk allele is T

What does the BHMT gene do?

The BHMT gene provides the body's instructions to make the enzyme betaine-Homocysteine S-methyltransferase (BHMT), which is essential for a lower homocysteine level. Generally, the BHMT enzyme lowers homocysteine by providing a "short cut" or "back door" through the methylation cycle. Specifically, the BHMT enzyme converts betaine and homocysteine to dimethylglycine and methionine.

What type of health problems are associated with having the risk alleles for the BHMT gene?

High homocysteine level—Having a BHMT risk allele can lead to high homocysteine levels. Health problems associated with high homocysteine levels include:

- Increased inflammation
- Increases coronary artery disease risk
- Increases Alzheimer's disease risk
- Increased stroke risk
- Increased deep vein thrombosis (DVT) and pulmonary embolism risk
- Increased atherosclerosis (narrowing of blood vessels) risk
- Pregnancy problems: high homocysteine levels during pregnancy may be associated with fetal abnormalities, placenta abruption and pre-eclampsia

I have a risk allele in the BHMT gene. What should I talk to my doctor about doing so that I can reduce my health risks?

- *Reduce stress*—Stress and high cortisol levels suppress the BHMT enzyme, leading to high inflammation and homocysteine levels. Decreasing stress and stress hormone levels, such as cortisol, can help the BHMT enzyme work more efficiently—thus preventing health problems that might result from having this risk allele.

> **Methods to help promote lower levels of stress and cortisol:**

   o *Stress management techniques*—These include regular relaxing exercise, talking about things that cause stress rather than bottling up your feelings, meditation, prayer, living below your means and having nurturing relationships.

   o *Keep your blood sugar stable*—A stable blood sugar helps prevent cortisol from getting too high or too low while giving your adrenal glands a chance to rest. The best way to keep your blood sugar stable is by eating a diet high in protein, fat, and fiber and low in refined sugar. Eating small meals throughout the day also helps keep your blood sugar stable.

   o *Consider supplementing with phosphatidylserine and phosphatidylcholine to lower cortisol levels*—These nutrients will help lower the stress hormone cortisol, thus helping the BHMT enzyme work more efficiently.

• *Consider supplementing with the nutrients zinc and TMG*—The BHMT enzyme requires zinc and TMG (betaine) to function; therefore, having adequate levels of zinc and TMG will help prevent further problems in the BHMT pathway.

   > *Foods high in zinc*—Oysters, beef, spinach and cashews

   > *Foods high in TMG*—Quinoa, spinach, lamb and beets

I have one or more BHMT gene risk allele(s). What labs/testing should I consider to continually monitor my health?

✓ *Homocysteine (blood test)*—Homocysteine can become high in people with a risk allele for the BHMT gene. High homocysteine can be a sign of inflammation and is associated with many health problems. I prefer homocysteine to be at or below 8 on blood work.

✓ *Adrenal hormone testing (saliva)*—This test measures the adrenal stress hormone cortisol throughout the entire day, which helps you understand how stress affects you, particularly your sleep. High cortisol can further hinder the ability for the BHMT enzyme to work properly; therefore, it's important for anyone with a BHMT risk allele to monitor and promote healthy cortisol levels.

✓ **Measure zinc levels (blood or taste test)**—Low zinc levels can prevent the BHMT enzyme from functioning efficiently.

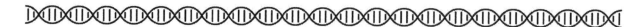

CBS gene
Cystathione Beta Synthase gene

Names of CBS genetic variants (SNP identification)	rsnumber	Risk allele
CBSC699T	rs234706	Risk allele is A
CBS A13637G	rs2851391	Risk allele is T

What does the CBS gene do?

The CBS gene provides the body's instructions to make the CBS enzyme (cystathionine-beta-synthase), which helps lower your homocysteine level by converting homocysteine into cystathione.

What type of health problems are associated with having a risk allele for the CBS gene?

Having the risk allele for the CBS gene can cause an *increased* speed of the CBS enzyme, which means that the enzyme will *remove homocysteine at a faster rate in people with the risk allele*. This faster rate is both good and bad.

- **The GOOD**—Having the risk allele for CBS can be good because it's associated with a decreased risk of coronary artery disease, as people with the risk allele for CBS remove homocysteine at a faster rate. A high homocysteine level can increase your risk of developing coronary artery disease.

- **The BAD**—Having the risk allele for CBS can have some bad health effects, including:

> - ***A potential for higher glutamate levels***—Some side effects of high glutamate levels include an increased risk of anxiety and an increased risk of headaches or stomach aches when exposed to MSG or high levels of glutamate.

> - ***Potential for increased level of ammonia***—Ammonia build-up is a sign of liver problems and is very bad for your health.

> - ***Potential for increased levels of sulfites and possible sulfite sensitivities***

The possible negative effects of having the risk alleles for CBS are thought to lie in the biochemical pathway that occurs further downstream within the cystathionine pathway. I don't believe there is enough high-quality data available to make any general statements regarding these side effects. However, I do believe there are some intelligent ways to monitor and prevent health problems that could potentially result from having the CBS risk allele(s).

I have one or more risk allele(s) for the CBS gene. What should I talk to my doctor about doing so that I can reduce my health risks?

- ***Divert homocysteine away from the CBS pathway and toward other methylation cycle pathways by:***

  > - ***Diverting homocysteine toward BHMT and away from CBS***—It is possible to divert homocysteine away from CBS and towards the BHMT pathway by supplementing with TMG, zinc, phosphatidylserine and phosphatidylcholine. Stress reduction is also helpful.

  > - ***Diverting homocysteine toward the MTR / MTRR / MTHFR enzymes and away from the CBS enzyme***—Vitamin B-9 (methyl-activated Quatrefolic acid or L-5-MTHF) and vitamin B-12 in the forms of both adenosylcobalamin and methylcobalamin are necessary to divert homocysteine away from the CBS enzyme and toward the MTR / MTRR / MTHFR part of the methylation cycle.

- ***Monitor the CBS pathway for problems resulting from over activity by:***

> ***Checking sulfite (not sulfate) levels***—If sulfite is high, consider supplementing with molybdenum. High sulfite levels can be a negative side effect of having a risk allele in the CBS gene. Many people confuse sulfite and sulfate. High *sulfite* can be bad for one's health, while high *sulfate* can be good. Sulfate is needed for Phase II sulfation detox pathways (pg. 76). If your sulfite levels are high, consider checking to see if you have the risk allele for the SUOX gene, which converts sulfite (bad) into sulfate (good). More about the SUOX gene is covered in (pg. 124).

> ***Monitor ammonia levels***—High ammonia can be a negative side effect of having a risk allele for the CBS gene. High ammonia levels can also signify liver problems. Consider supporting the liver if ammonia levels are high.

> ***If you're anxious, consider supplementing with GABA and vitamin B-6 (P-5-P)***—Vitamin B-6 in the activated form called P-5-P (pyridoxal-5'-phosphate) is necessary to convert glutamate (the excitatory and anxiety-producing neurotransmitter) into GABA (the inhibitory and calming neurotransmitter). Glutamate levels may be high and GABA levels may be low in people with CBS, which can result in high anxiety levels.

> ***Avoid MSG (monosodium glutamate)***—MSG is high in free glutamic acid, which is excitatory and can be a neurotoxin in high doses. Having a CBS risk allele can cause an increased sensitivity to MSG and an increased risk for side effects, such as anxiety, headaches and stomachaches.

MSG is the most common form of free glutamic acid but there are many other sources of free glutamic acid in our diets. Food labeling laws make it difficult to know when you're eating MSG because it has many misleading names.

Many people think MSG is only in Chinese food, but unfortunately it's in most packaged foods, and even in some organic and non-genetically modified organism (GMO) packaged foods. Go to the health food store and look at the ingredients in chips. They almost all contain "yeast extract," which is the same thing as MSG but with a friendlier name. If a package says "No MSG added," it can still have MSG in it. Labeling laws don't require all product ingredients to be on the label, but only require the ingredients that the manufacturer put into the product to be put on the label. This means that if a product contains a spice extract that already contained MSG, the label can still say "No MSG added".

Some common names for MSG used on ingredient labels to hide MSG or MSG-like ingredients include:

> - Yeast extract
> - Glutamate
> - Glutamic acid
> - Hydrolyzed anything
> - Soy protein isolates
> - Bouillon
> - Natural flavoring(s)
> - Carrageenan
> - Autolyzed anything
> - Spices
> - Broth/stock—Broths almost always have MSG or yeast extract as an ingredient

I have one or more CBS risk allele(s). What labs/testing should I consider to continually monitor my health?

✓ ***Urinary sulfite levels (urinary strip test)***—If sulfite levels are high, also look at the SUOX gene.

✓ ***Ammonia levels (blood test)***—Ammonia levels may become high with the CBS risk allele.

✓ ***Homocysteine (blood test)***—I prefer homocysteine to be below 8 on blood work.

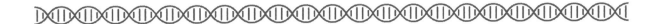

MTHFD1 gene
Methylenetetrahydrofolate dehydrogenase

Names of MTHFD1 genetic variants (SNP identification)	rsnumber	Risk allele
MTHFD1 G1958A	rs2236225	Risk allele is A

What does the MTHFD1 gene do?

The MTHFD1 gene is essential for the body to make choline. Choline is important for a healthy brain, liver, nervous system, healthy folate levels and a healthy methylation cycle. The MTHFD1 gene provides the body's instructions to make the MTHFD1 enzyme, which is called methylenetetrahydrofolate dehydrogenase 1 (MTHFD1). Specifically, the MTHFD1 enzyme links formic acid and THF together.

What health problems are associated with having the risk allele in the MTHFD1 gene?

The health problems associated with having this risk allele in the MTHFD1 gene are largely a result of the body not being able to produce enough choline, leading to choline deficiencies.

Health issues related to low choline include:

- *Mental illness, anxiety and neurological disorders*—Choline is important for brain health. Mental health issues are also known side effects of low choline, and can result from having this risk allele in the MTHFD1 gene[1,2,3].

- *Fatty liver*—Having an MTHFD1 risk allele can lead to low choline levels, possibly causing fatty liver.

- *Birth defects and possible memory problems in children*—It's very important for anyone with risk alleles in the MTHFD1 or PEMT genes to make sure they're getting adequate choline and phosphatidylcholine, especially while pregnant and/or breastfeeding. Read more about the PEMT gene on page 150.

I have the risk allele for the MTHFD1 gene. What should I talk to my doctor about doing so that I can reduce my health risks?

- *Increasing choline through diet*—Choline is naturally high in eggs, meat, chicken, cauliflower and almonds. High dietary intake of choline has been linked to an increased risk of colon cancer in men[4]. The increased risk for colon cancer may be more a result of eating foods that are high in choline rather than choline itself. For this reason, it may be better for men with an increased risk of colon cancer to consider supplementing with choline, or phosphatidylcholine, rather than solely increasing their diet in choline-high foods.

- *Consider supplementing with choline*—Supplementing with choline is a safe alternative to increasing choline through diet alone.

I have a risk allele in the MTHFD1 gene. What labs/testing should I consider to continually monitor my health?

✓ *Monitor liver health with ALT, AST, and GGT (blood test)*—ALT and AST measures liver enzymes. Low choline has been associated with high ALT levels, which indicates a liver problem[5].

✓ *Monitor triglycerides (blood test)*—High triglycerides are seen with fatty liver, a side effect associated with having this risk allele for the MTHFD1 gene.

References:

1.) Bjelland I, Tell GS, Vollset SE, et al. (October 2009). "Choline in anxiety and depression: the Hordaland Health Study". The American Journal of Clinical Nutrition 90 (4): 1056–60.

2.)Zeisel SH; da Costa KA (November 2009). "Choline: an essential nutrient for public health". Nutrition Reviews 67 (11): 615–23.

3.) Shaw GM, Carmichael SL, Yang W, et al (July 2004). "Periconceptional dietary intake of choline and betaine and neural tube defects in offspring". American Journal of Epidemiology 160 (2): 102–9.

4.) Lee JE, Giovannucci E, Fuchs CS, et al (March 2010). "Choline and betaine intake and the risk of colorectal cancer in men". Cancer Epidemiology, Biomarkers & Prevention 19 (3): 884–7.

5.) Micronutrient Information Center: Choline". Linus Pauling Institute. Retrieved from: http://lpi.oregonstate.edu/mic/other-nutrients/choline

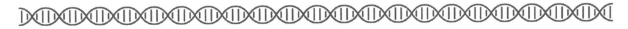

Christy L. Sutton D.C.

SUOX gene
Sulfite oxidase gene

Names of SUOX genetic variants (SNP identification)	rsnumber	Risk allele
SUOX C5444T	rs705703	Risk allele is T

What does the SUOX gene do?

The SUOX gene plays a large role in the body's ability to maintain normal sulfite levels, enabling it to properly detoxify. The SUOX gene provides the body's instructions to make the SUOX enzyme, which converts sulfite (which is harmful to the body) to sulfate (which is much less toxic and necessary for detoxification).

What health problems are associated with having the risk allele for the SUOX gene?

- *High levels of sulfite and low levels of sulfate*—High sulfite can be bad for the body. Ideally the body has higher sulfate levels, which are needed for the body to detoxify properly.

- *Sulfite sensitivities*—This can manifest in allergy-like reactions from eating/drinking foods high in sulfites, including red wine, dried fruits and molasses.

I have the risk allele for the SUOX gene. What should I talk to my doctor about doing so that I can reduce my health risks?

- *Ensure adequate levels of trace minerals such as molybdenum*—Molybdenum is required for the SUOX enzyme to function properly. Foods naturally high in molybdenum include legumes and leafy green vegetables.

- *Continually monitor vitamin B-12 levels*—Vitamin B-12 may reduce sulfite sensitivity. Therefore, anyone with high sulfite levels should monitor vitamin B-12 levels and consider B-12 supplementation if necessary.

- ***Eat a diet high in onions, garlic, broccoli, cauliflower and cabbage***—These foods are naturally high in sulfate, which is important for Phase II sulfation and the glutathione detox pathway. Having the risk allele in the SUOX gene can lead to low sulfate levels and a hindered Phase II sulfation detox pathway.

I have the risk allele for the SUOX gene. What labs/testing should I consider to continually monitor my health?

Sulfite and sulfate urine tests—These simple urine tests measure sulfate and sulfite levels. If sulfite levels are high, a SUOX genetic variation may be the underlying reason.

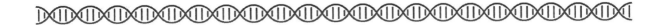

Christy L. Sutton D.C.

Phase 1 and Phase 2 Detoxification Pathways

Toxins from the environment enter the body. The toxins then go through a series of steps so that they can be detoxified and removed from the body. Some of the most important steps for detoxifying and removing toxins from the environment are called Phase 1 and Phase 2 detoxification pathways. There are genetic defects effecting the Phase 1 and Phase 2 detoxification pathways that can cause the body to not be able to detoxify properly. Some of the health problems that are associated with having these genetic defects include cancer, neurological problems, heart attack, stroke, pregnancy related problems, birth defects, autism, autoimmune diseases, and many more.

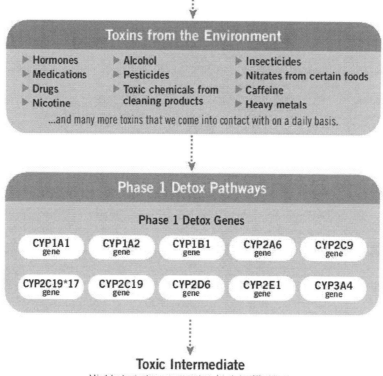

Toxins from the Environment

- Hormones
- Medications
- Drugs
- Nicotine
- Alcohol
- Pesticides
- Toxic chemicals from cleaning products
- Insecticides
- Nitrates from certain foods
- Caffeine
- Heavy metals

...and many more toxins that we come into contact with on a daily basis.

Phase 1 Detox Pathways

Phase 1 Detox Genes

CYP1A1 gene	CYP1A2 gene	CYP1B1 gene	CYP2A6 gene	CYP2C9 gene
CYP2C19*17 gene	CYP2C19 gene	CYP2D6 gene	CYP2E1 gene	CYP3A4 gene

Toxic Intermediate
Highly toxic temporary step in detoxification.
If Phase 2 detox does not work, this step can create health problems.

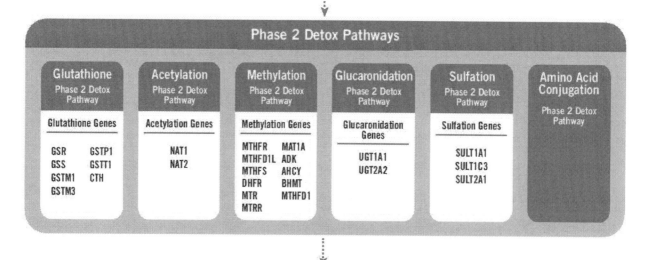

Phase 2 Detox Pathways

Glutathione Phase 2 Detox Pathway	Acetylation Phase 2 Detox Pathway	Methylation Phase 2 Detox Pathway	Glucaronidation Phase 2 Detox Pathway	Sulfation Phase 2 Detox Pathway	Amino Acid Conjugation Phase 2 Detox Pathway
Glutathione Genes GSR GSTP1 GSS GSTT1 GSTM1 CTH GSTM3	**Acetylation Genes** NAT1 NAT2	**Methylation Genes** MTHFR MAT1A MTHFD1L ADK MTHFS AHCY DHFR BHMT MTR MTHFD1 MTRR	**Glucaronidation Genes** UGT1A1 UGT2A2	**Sulfation Genes** SULT1A1 SULT1C3 SULT2A1	

Detoxified Substance Ready for Removal from the Body

Personalized genetic report found at http://geneticdetoxification.com

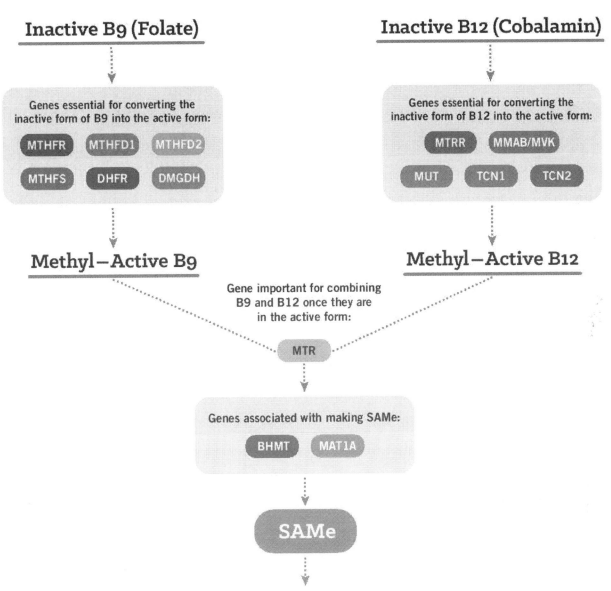

SAMe is the most important methylator in the body, and is what ultimately turn genes on and off, initiates our metabolic pathways, including some detoxification pathways.

Christy L. Sutton D.C.

Chapter 3
Genes Necessary to Initiate Detox Pathways

NR1I2 gene
Nuclear receptor subfamily 1, group I

Names of NR1I2 gene genetic variants (SNP identification)	rsnumber	Risk allele
Nuclear receptor subfamily 1, group I	rs1523127	Risk allele is A

What does the NR1I2 gene do?

Initiates Phase I and Phase II detox pathways—The NR1L2 gene provides the body's instructions to make a protein called pregnane X receptor (PXR). Its primary function is to sense the presence of foreign toxic substances and initiate the body's detox pathways. The PXR protein created from the NR1L2 gene regulates the phase I cytochrome P450 gene CYP3A4, which is important for the metabolism of many drugs[1]. The NR1L2 gene also increases phase II glutathione detox pathways[2].

What health problems are associated with having a risk allele in the NR1I2 gene?

- *Crohn's Disease*

- *Inflammatory bowel disease (IBS)*

- *Colon cancer*

I have more or more risk allele(s) in the NR1I2 gene. What should I talk to my doctor about doing so that I can reduce my health risks?

- *Avoid ingesting toxins and exposure to toxins in general*

- *Increase antioxidant intake*

- *Support Phase I and glutathione detox pathways*—Because the N21I2 gene is important in Phase I and Phase II glutathione detox pathways, supporting those detox pathways is highly recommended. You can read more about this in the section about Phase I detox and the section about glutathione (pg. 57).

Christy L. Sutton D.C.

I have one or more risk allele(s) in the NR1I2 gene. What labs/testing should I consider to continually monitor my health?

✓ **Colonoscopy**—There is an increased risk of serious digestive issues; therefore, a colonoscopy can help monitor those issues to ensure that colon cancer is not present.

✓ **Calprotectin (stool analysis)**—This test reflects the level of inflammation that is present in the digestive system.

References:

1.) Lehmann JM, McKee DD, et al. (September 1998). "The human orphan nuclear receptor PXR is activated by compounds that regulate CYP3A4 gene expression and cause drug interactions". J. Clin. Invest. 102 (5): 1016–23.

2.) Falkner KC, Pinaire JA, et al. (September 2001). "Regulation of the rat glutathione S-transferase A2 gene by glucocorticoids: involvement of both the glucocorticoid and pregnane X receptors".Mol. Pharmacol. 60 (3): 611–9. PMID.

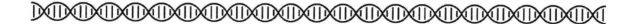

Personalized genetic report found at http://geneticdetoxification.com

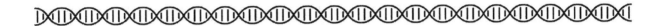

Pesticide and Herbicide Detoxification

The Phase I and Phase II detox pathways are necessary for pesticide and herbicide detoxification. However, another gene called PON1 is also crucial for the body's ability to properly detoxify pesticides and herbicides. While pesticides and herbicides are hazardous to everyone's health, certain people are genetically predisposed with sensitivities to one or both, and should put a greater emphasis on avoiding these chemicals.

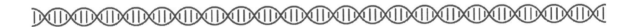

Christy L. Sutton D.C.

PON1 gene
Serum paraoxonase/arylesterase 1 gene

Names of PON1 gene genetic variants (SNP identification)	rsnumber	Risk allele
PON1 Q192R	rs662	Risk allele is C

What does the PON1 gene do?

The PON1 gene detoxifies organophosphate toxins such as pesticides, nerve gases and herbicides like Roundup, which are found on genetically modified produce. The PON1 gene provides the body's instructions to make an enzyme that helps detoxify pesticides, herbicides and other neurotoxins that damage the nervous system.

What health problems are associated with having a risk allele in the PON1 gene?

- *Increased sensitivity and toxicity when exposed to pesticides, GMO foods sprayed with roundup and other neurotoxins*—There is an increased risk of developing neurological problems in people with both the PON1 risk allele and exposure to pesticides or other neurotoxins. Because GMO foods are exposed to high levels of the herbicide Roundup, people with this PON1 risk allele should avoid GMO foods.

- *Increased risk of cardiovascular disease*—Having the risk allele for the PON1 gene is associated with an increased risk of developing coronary artery disease[1].

- *Neurological damage*—Having the risk allele may be associated with the presence of other neurological disorders such as Parkinson's disease and Gulf War Syndrome[2].

I have one or more risk allele(s) in the PON1gene. What should I talk to my doctor about doing so that I can reduce my health risks?

- *Avoid pesticides, GMO foods and neurotoxins*—Having a risk allele in the PON1 gene makes exposure to these toxins particularly dangerous. Try to eat organic and avoid GMO foods.

- *Increase antioxidant levels*—High levels of antioxidants can help protect the body from toxins and help prevent neurological damage that could result from having this risk allele.

- *Detoxify*—Consider doing a 21- or 30-day detox diet, including eating ample amounts of vegetables, adequate clean protein, fruits and healthy fats. I don't recommend doing a one-size-fits-all detox protocol. Any detoxification program needs to be tailored to the individual and monitored by a trained and licensed health care professional.

- *Exercise and sweat daily*—Sweating allows your body to bypass many detox pathways and remove toxins without causing damage. Exercise is an essential and irreparable part of keeping your body healthy and preventing cancer.

- *Drink plenty of water*—Water is necessary to help the body properly detoxify. Roundup is water-soluble; therefore, you need plenty of water to remove it from the body.

Monsanto's Roundup and how it can affect your health

Roundup is an herbicide also known as Glyphosate that is sprayed on most soy, corn and wheat. It can enter the body through the skin, drinking water contaminated with Roundup or through food that has been sprayed with Roundup.

In March 2015 the World Health Organization classified Roundup as a possible carcinogen, which means that it likely causes cancer. Cancers that are associated with exposure to Roundup include Non-Hodgkin's lymphoma, renal cancer, pancreatic cancer and skin tumors.

Roundup can lead to less good bacteria and more bad bacteria in your digestive system.

A 54-year-old man accidently sprayed himself with Roundup and developed skin lesions six hours later. One month later he developed bilateral Parkinsonian syndrome[3].

Christy L. Sutton D.C.

I have one or more risk allele(s) in the PON1 gene. What labs/testing should I consider to continually monitor my health?

- ✓ **Toxicity testing**—This provides information about your toxicity levels, as well as how quickly you're accumulating toxins in your body.

- ✓ **Cholesterol panel**—Having a risk allele in the PON1 gene has been associated with high cholesterol and an increased risk for cardiovascular events.

References:

1.) T Liu, X Zhang, J Zhang, Z Liang, et al. Association between PON1 rs662 polymorphism and coronary artery disease. European Journal of Clinical Nutrition 68, 1029-1035 (September 2014).

2.) Bharti Mackness, Paul N. Durrington, Michael I. Mackness. PON1 in Other Diseases. Paraoxonase (PON1) in Health and Disease. pp 185-195.

3.) Barbosa ER, Leiros da Costa MD, et al. Parkinsonism after glycine-derivate exposure. Mov Disord. 2001;16:565–8

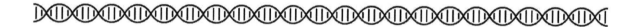

Personalized genetic report found at http://geneticdetoxification.com

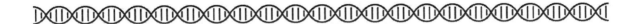

Chapter 4
Alcohol Detoxification Genes

Alcohol Detoxification

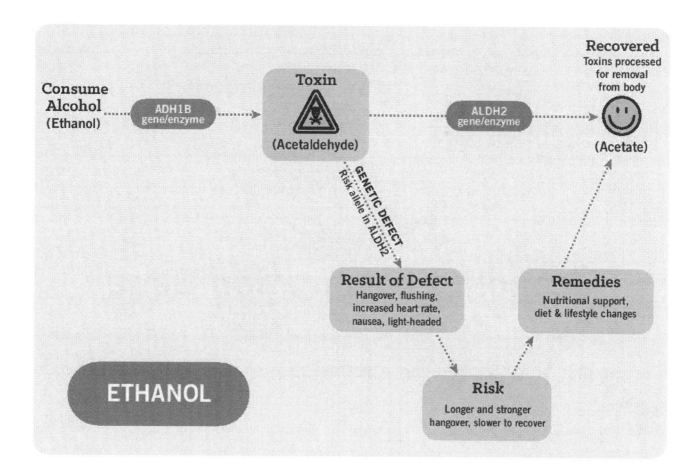

Some people are predisposed to having severe hangovers and other undesirable side effects from drinking, including facial flushing, heart palpation, and even an increased risk for developing cancer. The negative side effects from drinking alcohol result from the buildup of toxic chemicals, and in some cases a genetically hindered ability to remove the toxins created from drinking alcohol.

It's helpful to know if you have these genetic predispositions, especially if you want to live longer and healthier. In this section, you'll learn more about how you metabolize alcohol, what type of health problems you're more likely to develop and how to reduce your risk for developing these health problems.

ADH1B & ADH1C genes (ADH genes)
Alcohol dehydrogenase gene

Names of ADH genetic variants (SNP identification)	rsnumber	Risk allele
ADH1B (Alcohol dehydrogenase 1B)—*Extremely fast* at converting alcohol to the toxic chemical acetaldehyde. If you have this risk allele, you'll transform from being inebriated into having a hangover *extremely fast*.	rs1229984	Risk allele is C
ADH1B*3 (Alcohol dehydrogenase 1B)—*Fast* at converting alcohol to the toxic chemical acetaldehyde. If you have this risk allele, your transformation from being inebriated into having a hangover will be *fast*.	rs2066702	Risk allele is A
ADH1C*2 (Alcohol dehydrogenase 1C)—*Slow* to convert alcohol into the toxic chemical acetaldehyde. If you have this risk allele, you will be *slower* to move from being inebriated into having a hangover. This means you will have a longer "buzz" before developing a hangover.	rs1693482	Risk allele is T

What does the ADH (alcohol dehydrogenase) gene do?

The ADH gene provides the body's instructions to make enzymes that are essential to detoxify ethanol (alcohol). The ADH gene also plays a minor role in detoxifying and neutralizing free radicals and steroid hormones (pregnenolone, 17-OH progesterone, DHEA, cortisol, androstenedione and progesterone).

What health problems are associated with having a risk allele in the ADH1B gene?

- *Increased risk of cancer, especially when alcohol is consumed*

- *Increased sensitivity to alcohol. Some side effects from drinking include:*

  - *Facial flushing shortly after drinking*—Sometimes called the "Asian Flush" or "Oriental Flushing Syndrome"

Christy L. Sutton D.C.

> *Light-headedness*

> *Heart palpitations*

> *Nausea*

> *General "hangover" symptoms*—These symptoms are indicative of a disease known as the alcohol flush reaction.

> *Can quickly transition from the "jolly/happy" phase of drinking to the "hangover" phase*—This is especially true if you have one or more risk allele(s) for rs2066702. If you have the risk allele for rs1693482, you'll probably have a longer "jolly/happy phase" before transitioning into the "hangover" phase of drinking.

I have one or more risk allele(s) for the ADH genes. What should I talk to my doctor about doing so that I can reduce my health risks?

- *Decrease alcohol intake*—Avoiding alcohol or drinking in moderation is the most effective way to eliminate problems related to having the ADH gene risk allele.

- *Consider increasing Vitamin B-9 intake (methyl-activated Quatrefolic acid or L-5-MTHF)*—Alcohol is known to interfere with vitamin B-9 absorption and metabolism. Therefore, if you're consuming alcohol, extra vitamin B-9 could help prevent the resulting side effects. Ideally the B vitamins should be taken in a high-quality B-complex.

- *Increase antioxidant levels*—Antioxidants like vitamins C, E, A and glutathione are important for anyone with one or more ADH gene risk allele(s). High antioxidant levels help protect the body from cancer-causing free radicals that can increase as a result of having these risk allele(s), especially when alcohol is consumed.

- *Consider supporting detox pathways with liver-promoting nutrients such as milk thistle and glutathione, especially if drinking alcohol.*

- *Exercise cautiously when taking hormones (corticosteroids, estrogen, progesterone, testosterone, DHEA, etc.)*—The ADH gene plays a role in detoxifying hormones.

I have one or more ADH gene risk allele(s). What labs/testing should I consider to continually monitor my health?

The following tests are important for anyone who has both a risk allele in the ADH gene and drinks alcohol. If alcohol is not being consumed, these labs are not as important.

- ✓ *Liver enzymes (blood test)*—Liver enzymes can be high in anyone who is overtaxing their liver by drinking alcohol.

- ✓ *Hormone testing (blood or saliva test)*—Hormone levels can be high in people who have one or more risk allele(s) in an ADH gene, especially if they drink alcohol.

- ✓ *Folate and Homocysteine levels (blood test)*—Drinking alcohol can interfere with folate levels (vitamin B-9) and lead to a high homocysteine level. I prefer homocysteine to be below 8 on blood work.

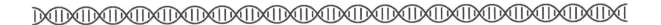

ALDH2 gene
Aldehyde dehydrogenase

Names of ALDH gene genetic variants (SNP identification)	rsnumber	Risk allele
ALDH2*2—*Slow* to convert the toxin acetaldehyde into the nontoxic chemical acetate. If you have this risk allele, then you will tend to *have longer and stronger hangovers from drinking.*	rs671	Risk allele is A
ALDH2—*Slow* to convert the toxin acetaldehyde into the nontoxic chemical acetate. If you have this risk allele, then you will tend to *have longer and stronger hangovers from drinking.*	rs4646778	Risk allele is A

What do the ALDH2 genes do?

If you have the risk allele(s) in the ALDH2 gene, then you probably tend to have pretty bad hangover symptoms after drinking. ALDH2 are the most important enzymes for detoxing alcohol by converting acetaldehyde (a toxic byproduct from drinking) into acetate (a less-toxic substance). Having a risk allele in the ALDH2 genes can lead to an increased level of toxicity and increased side effects from drinking. The increased level of toxicity is a result of having excess amounts of acetaldehyde—the highly toxic byproduct of drinking.

What health problems are associated with having a risk allele in the ALDH2 gene?

These health problems are only an issue if you drink alcohol. If you don't drink, then you can have the risk allele and <u>not</u> be at an increased risk of developing these health problems.

- *Increased risk of cancer, especially when alcohol is consumed.*

  - If you have the risk allele ALDH2*2 (rs671) and drink regularly, then you're at a significantly increased risk of developing cancer of the *oropharynx and esophagus.*

- ***Increased risk of Parkinson's disease[1]***

- ***Facial flushing "Asian Flush" or "Oriental Flushing Syndrome"***

- ***Light-headedness***

- ***Heart palpitations***

- ***Nausea***

- ***More intense "hangover" symptoms***—These symptoms are indicative of a disease known as the alcohol flush reaction, or the "Oriental flush."

  ➢ If you have one or more risk alleles(s) for the ALDH2 gene, then you probably have a more severe "hangover phase" because your body is slow to remove the toxic chemical acetaldehyde, which is responsible for the "hangover" phase.

If you have this genetic combination, you probably get horrible hangovers

If you have the risk alleles for both ADH1B (rs1229984) and ALDH2*2 (rs671), you're genetically more likely to have more significant hangovers from drinking.

This genetic combination is very fast to transition from the "happy/jolly" phase of drinking to the "hangover" phase.

However, these people are slow to transition out of the "hangover" phase. Besides the bad hangovers, there is also a significant risk of developing cancer if alcohol is regularly consumed by anyone with this genetic combination.

Christy L. Sutton D.C.

I have more or more risk allele(s) in the ALDH2 gene. What should I talk to my doctor about doing so that I can reduce my health risks?

- *Limit or avoid alcohol consumption*—Avoiding alcohol is the most effective way to eliminate problems associated with having a risk allele in the ALDH2 gene.

- *Increased intake of Vitamin B3 and magnesium*—The ALDH2 enzyme, made from the ALDH2 gene, requires vitamin B3 and magnesium. If you drink, then maintaining high levels of vitamin B3 and magnesium will help minimize problems related to having these risk alleles. Ideally the B vitamins should be taken in a high-quality B-complex that consists of the activated forms of all B vitamins.

- *Support detox pathways with liver promoting-nutrients such as milk thistle and glutathione, especially if drinking alcohol.*

I have one or more risk allele(s) in the ALDH2 gene. What labs/testing should I consider to continually monitor my health?

If you aren't consuming alcohol, then these labs aren't as important.

- ✓ *Liver enzymes (blood test)*—Liver enzymes can be high in anyone who is overtaxing their liver by drinking more alcohol than they're able to metabolize.

- ✓ *Nutreval by Genova diagnostics (blood and urine)*—The Nutreval test measures levels of Vitamin B-3 and magnesium. Having the risk allele for the ALDH2 gene while also having a vitamin B-3 or magnesium deficiency can lead to even worse problems from drinking alcohol.

- ✓ *Folate and Homocysteine levels (blood test)*—Drinking alcohol can interfere with folate levels (vitamin B-9) absorption and metabolism and lead to a high homocysteine level. I prefer homocysteine to be at or below 8 on blood work.

References:

1.) Fitzmaurice AG1, Rhodes SL, Cockburn M, Ritz B, JM. Aldehyde dehydrogenase variation enhances effect of pesticides associated with Parkinson disease.. Neurology. 2014 Feb 4;82(5):419-26.

Personalized genetic report found at http://geneticdetoxification.com

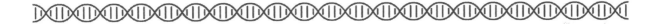

For more information on detoxification genes, consult the following pages:

- **NQO1 gene:** pg 255

- **CYP2C19 gene**: pg 331

- **VDR gene**: pg 368

- **GC gene:** pg 370

Christy L. Sutton D.C.

Part 2
Mental Health Genes

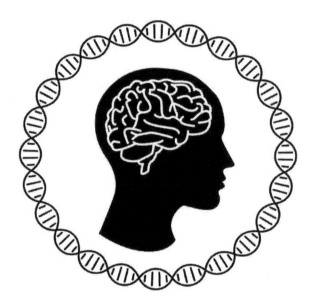

Mental health, like many other aspects of our health, is a function of much more than just genes. The genes that we inherit can increase our risk for cognitive decline, Alzheimer's disease, mental illness, depression, schizophrenia, bipolar disorder, ADHD, autism and many other brain-based conditions.

However, the environment that we're exposed to throughout our life can tip the scale toward a brain that is healthy enough to allow us to function — or a brain that is not. This section of the book is focused on how to tip the scale toward a healthy brain by tailoring your environment to protect your brain from your specific genetic vulnerabilities.

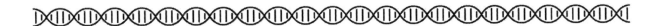

Chapter 5
Cognitive Acuity

BDNF gene

Brain-derived neurotrophic factor gene

Names of BDNF gene genetic variants (SNP identification)	rsnumber	Risk allele
BDNF T64089C	rs11030104	Risk allele is A
BDNF V81M	rs6265	Risk allele is T

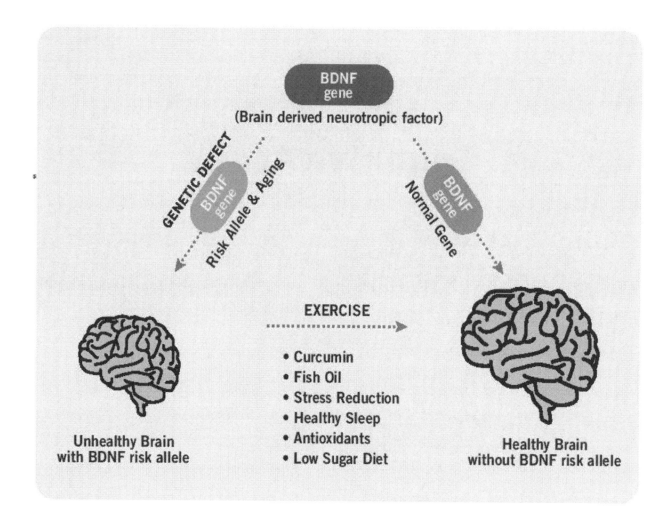

What does the BDNF gene do?

BDNF is essential for brain health because it helps the brain grow and stay healthy. The gene creates a protein called brain-derived neurotrophic factor (BDNF), which you can think of as "brain fertilizer." BDNF helps the brain develop new connections, repair failing brain cells and protect healthy brain cells[3].

BDNF increases the brain's level of excitement by preventing calming GABAergic-signaling activities[1].

What health problems are associated with having a risk allele for the BDNF gene?

- *Having a risk allele in the BDNF gene can cause lower levels of BDNF, which has been associated with:*

    ➢ Cognitive decline

    ➢ Depression

    ➢ Neurological disorders

    ➢ Impaired motor skills

    ➢ Impaired learning

    ➢ Being an introvert

- *BDNF doesn't just affect brain health, but can actually affect the health of our entire body*—This is because the entire body is controlled by the nervous system. Healthy brains and healthy bodies aren't mutually exclusive. You can't have a healthy brain without being healthy, eating well and exercising.

I have one or more risk allele(s) in the BDNF gene. What should I talk to my doctor about doing so that I can reduce my health risks?

- *Exercise*—This is the best way to increase BDNF and thus promote brain health. In fact, exercise has been shown to reverse the age-related cognitive decline associated with declining BDNF levels. Exercise not only prevents cognitive decline in older people, but also benefits the brains of younger people by increasing BDNF levels, which ultimately improves learning and memory.

Christy L. Sutton D.C.

- *Avoid and minimize stress*—Exposure to chronically high stress levels and the stress hormone cortisol have been shown to decrease the expression of BDNF in rats[2]. This is why avoiding high levels of stress through meditation, relaxing exercise, talking, nurturing relationships and vacations can be so good for your brain.

  ➢ *Lower your cortisol levels if it's high*—High levels of stress can lead to high levels of cortisol, which can be bad for the brain. Phosphatidylserine can help lower cortisol, protect the brain from stress and help you deal with stress.

- *Ways to boost BDNF naturally[3]:*

  ➢ Exercise

  ➢ Mental stimulation

  ➢ Intermittent fasting (12 hours)—Late dinner and early breakfast.

  ➢ A low-sugar diet

  ➢ Nurturing relationships

  ➢ Seven hours of sleep nightly

  ➢ Antioxidants (try red grapes or resveratrol)

  ➢ Favorite forms of relaxation to reduce stress

  ➢ Omega-3 fatty acids found in fish or fish oil

  ➢ Avoid high fructose corn syrup and processed foods

  ➢ Turmeric consumption (Curcumin, which is found in turmeric and to a lesser extent in curry, has shown to increase BDNF and even prevent Alzheimer's disease[3]).

  ➢ Consider supplementing with Vinpocetine—Vinpocetine has been shown to increase blood flow to the brain, and improve both memory and concentration[4].

I have one or more risk allele(s) in the BDNF gene. What labs/testing should I consider to continually monitor my health?

At this time there are no credible labs for measuring BDNF. However, there are many ways to monitor and measure brain health. Some tests that can help include:

- ✓ **Smell test**—Loss of sense of smell is one of the first signs of brain decline. Therefore, testing your smell is a great way to monitor brain health.

- ✓ **Memory recall testing**

Why is aging bad for your brain?

As you age, your body naturally makes less BDNF protein, which can lead to a decline in memory and cognitive acuity.

Having a BDNF gene risk allele can further accelerate age-related cognitive decline. About one in three Americans has a risk allele in the BDNF genes[1].

You can dramatically increase BDNF protein through exercise, diet and lifestyle. By boosting BDNF protein you can also decrease your risk of developing Parkinson's and Alzheimer's[3].

References:

1.) Henneberger C, Jüttner R, Rothe T, Grantyn R (2002). "Postsynaptic action of BDNF on GABAergic synaptic transmission in the superficial layers of the mouse superior colliculus". J. Neurophysiol. 88 (2): 595–603.

2.) Warner-Schmidt JL, Duman RS (2006). "Hippocampal neurogenesis: opposing effects of stress and antidepressant treatment". Hippocampus 16(3): 239–49.

3.) Day, John. 10 Ways to Boost Brain Function With BDNF. Retrieved from: http://drjohnday.com/10-ways-to-boost-brain-function-with-bdnf/

4.) Ogunrin, AO. (2014) Effect of Vinpocetine on Cognitive Performance of a Nigerian Population. .Ann Med Health Sci Res. 2014 Jul-Aug; 4(4): 654–661.

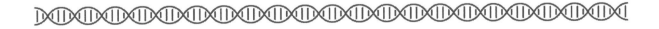

Christy L. Sutton D.C.

PEMT gene
Phosphatidyl ethanolamine methyltransferase gene

Names of PEMT genetic variants (SNP identification)	rsnumber	Risk allele
PEMT G634A	rs7946	T
PEMT T17020543A	rs4646406	A
PEMT T17023592G	rs4244593	T

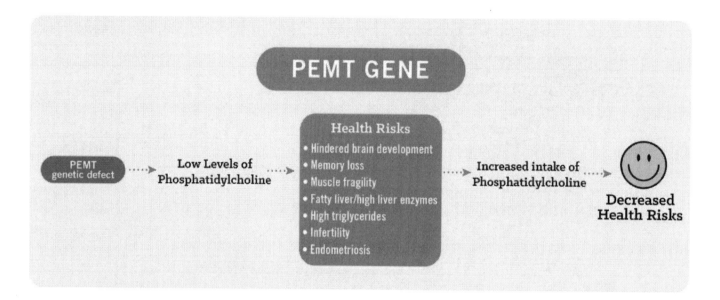

What does the PEMT gene do?

The PEMT gene is essential for synthesis of phosphatidylcholine, which is necessary for a healthy brain and liver, good memory, low triglyceride levels and adrenal health.

What health problems are associated with having the risk allele(s) for the PEMT gene?

Having the risk allele in the PEMT gene can create a phosphatidylcholine deficiency. Low choline and phosphatidylcholine levels can increase your chances of health problems. Some health problems related to having a risk allele in the PEMT gene include:

- *Hindered brain development, especially for infants and young children*

- *Muscle fragility*

Personalized genetic report found at http://geneticdetoxification.com

- *"Pregnancy brain"—Pregnancy related memory problems*

- *Alzheimer's and schizophrenia*[4,5]

- *Endometriosis*[3,6]

- *Infertility*[6]

- *High triglycerides* (which eventually develop into fatty liver[2])

  > If you have one or two risk alleles for PEMT *G634A (rs7946), you're significantly more likely to develop fatty liver* than a person with no risk alleles[1].

Having a PEMT gene risk allele can create pregnancy problems

Pregnant and lactating women with a PEMT risk allele are more likely to have memory problems while pregnant and post-pregnancy, and also more likely to have children with decreased brain development. It's important for pregnant and lactating women to increase consumption of choline-rich foods (meat, eggs, bacon, sunflower seeds), and consider supplementing with phosphatidylcholine while pregnant and/or breastfeeding.

Having adequate choline and phosphatidylcholine levels while pregnant and/or lactating is essential for fetal brain development. During pregnancy and lactation, PEMT pathway activity is greatly increased so that the mother can make more choline and phosphatidylcholine for the baby's developing brain.

I've seen women experience significant relief from memory loss while pregnant and postpartum ("pregnancy brain") from taking phosphatidylcholine.

It's also important to look at the MTHFD1 gene during pregnancy and lactation because the MTHFD1 gene is also involved in synthesis of choline and brain health, especially in the developing brain of a child (Pg. 122).

Christy L. Sutton D.C.

I have one or more risk allele(s) for the PEMT gene. What should I talk to my doctor about doing so that I can reduce my health risks?

➤ *Consider phosphatidylcholine supplementation*—Supplementing with phosphatidylcholine is the best way to bypass health problems related to having a risk allele in the PEMT gene. If have a PEMT risk allele, you will be limited in your ability to make phosphatidylcholine, which can lead to liver problems and high triglyceride levels.

➤ *Consider phosphatidylcholine consumption*—If you have a PEMT risk allele, then you're genetically hindered in your ability to naturally convert choline into phosphatidylcholine; therefore, supplementing with phosphatidylcholine may be necessary. Phosphatidylcholine accounts for about 95 percent of total choline in the body—meaning that it's important for the body to be able to convert choline into phosphatidylcholine[7].

Choline, which is required for the body to make phosphatidylcholine, is naturally highest in meat and eggs. If you have a PEMT risk allele, you can try to eat more meat and eggs. But you should also consider supplementing with phosphatidylcholine, especially if you have high cholesterol or triglyceride levels. When you eat foods high in choline, your body still has to convert the choline into phosphatidylcholine.

➤ *Consider SAMe supplementation (if labs indicate SAMe levels are low)*— SAMe is required for the PEMT enzyme to function properly. Supplementing with additional vitamin B-9 in the methy-activated form called Quatrefolic acid and vitamin B-12 in the form called methylcobalamin can also naturally boost SAMe levels.

I have one or more risk allele(s) for the PEMT gene. What labs/testing should I consider to continually monitor my health?

✓ *Triglycerides (blood test)*—Having a risk allele in the PEMT gene can cause high triglyceride levels, which can cause fatty liver.

✓ *Creatinine kinase (blood test)*—This lab test is especially important for anyone with muscle fragility, which can result from having a PEMT gene risk allele.

✓ ***A methylation profile (blood test)***—This lab test reveals the health of your methylation cycle by measuring your levels of folate, cystathione, cysteine, homocysteine, methionine, SAMe (S-Adenosyl-L-methionine), and SAH (S-adnosylmethionine). SAMe is important for the PEMT pathway to function properly.

➢ SAMe is required for the PEMT enzyme to covert choline to phosphatidylcholine. Having a PEMT gene risk allele is further exacerbated by low SAMe levels, so monitoring these levels is important.

✓ ***Estrogen levels (blood or saliva)***—Estrogen increases PEMT enzyme efficiency. Therefore, anyone with low estrogen is more likely to have low levels of phosphatidylcholine.

References:

1.) Song J., da Costa K. A., et al. 2005. Polymorphism of the PEMT gene and susceptibility to nonalcoholic fatty liver disease (NAFLD). FASEB J.19: 1266–1271

2.) Da-Costa K.A., Kozyreva O.G. et al. Common genetic polymorphisms affect the human requirement for the nutrient choline. FASEB J. 2006;20:1336–1344.

3.) Szczepańska M1, Mostowska A, et al. Polymorphic variants of folate and choline metabolism genes and the risk of endometriosis-associated infertility.Eur J Obstet Gynecol Reprod Biol. 2011 Jul;157(1):67-72. Epub 2011 Mar 22.

4.) Liu Y, Zhang H, Ju G,et al. A study of the PEMT gene in schizophrenia. Neuroscience Letters. 2007;424:203–206.

5.) Bi X-H, Zhao H-L, Zhang Z-X, Zhang J-W. PEMT G523A (V175M) is associated with sporadic Alzheimer's disease in a Chinese population. J Mol Neurosci. 2011;46:505–508

6.) Szczepańska M1, Mostowska A, et al. Polymorphic variants of folate and choline metabolism genes and the risk of endometriosis-associated infertility. Eur J Obstet Gynecol Reprod Biol. 2011 Jul;157(1):67-72.

7.) Ueland P. M. Choline and betaine in health and disease. J Inherit Metab Dis 34, 3–15 (2011).

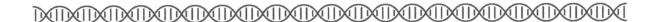

Christy L. Sutton D.C.

FADS2 gene
Fatty acid desaturase 2 gene

Names of FADS2 gene genetic variants (SNP identification)	rsnumber	Risk allele
FADS2	rs174575	Risk allele is G

What does the FADS2 gene do?

The FADS2 gene helps produce fatty acids that are important for brain function, including DHA (docosahexaenoic acid) and AA (arachidonic acid).

What health problems might be associated with having an FADS2 risk allele?

Infants with lower I.Q.—Children with the (G/G) genotype that were breastfed had higher I.Q.s than children that were formula-fed[3]. It appears as though infants with the (G/G) genotype don't make enough DHA and AA fatty acids to support their rapidly growing brains. It may be more urgent for infants with a (G/G) genotype to receive a DHA supplement, especially if they aren't being breastfed. It's important for any woman who is nursing to be supplementing with a high-quality/high-potency fish oil with extra DHA, especially if the nursing mother or her spouse has the G risk allele.
Infants with the C allele had around a seven-point increase in I.Q. when they were breastfed[1,2].

I have one or more risk allele(s) in the FADS2 gene. What should I talk to my doctor about doing so that I can reduce my health risks?

Having spent a large amount of time breastfeeding my daughter, I am intimately aware of how difficult that process can be. Because many women cannot breastfeed or choose not to for a variety of reasons, this information should be used to help parents understand how important it is to provide infants with adequate levels of DHA and healthy fats, rather than shaming women for not being able to or choosing not to breastfeed.

While it can be very beneficial for an infant to receive a high-quality DHA supplement, it may be even more urgent for infants with a FADS2 (G/G) genotype to receive a DHA supplement, especially if they are not being breastfed. It's important for all nursing women to consider supplementing with a high-quality/high-potency omega-3 fish oil with extra DHA, especially if they have this G risk allele. It's also important for nursing mothers to consider eating ample amounts of low mercury fish, meat, chicken, olive oil and butter. These foods are high in the fats that are most important for brain development. Low mercury fish tend to be the smaller fish like salmon, cod, tilapia, herring, anchovies, perch, and flounder. Fish that are high in mercury include tuna, orange roughy, mackerel, marlin, tilefish, grouper, and sea bass.

I have one or more risk allele(s) in the FADS2 gene. What labs/testing should I consider to continually monitor my health?

There are no labs that I would recommend for an infant with the FADS2 risk allele. However, children over the age of two and adults with the risk allele could do the Nutreval from Genova Diagnostics test.

- ✓ **Nutreval by Genova Diagnostics (blood and urine test)**—This test measures the fatty acids that are most affected by having an FADS2 risk allele, including DHA, AA and EPA, among others. This test also measures antioxidant levels (including glutathione and CoQ10) of vitamins, minerals, amino acids, heavy metals and some toxins. The Nutreval test provides a valuable and overarching look at how your environment impacts your overall health.

References:

1.) Duke University. (2007. Nov 5th). Gene governs IQ boost from breastfeeding. Retrieved from: http://www.eurekalert.org/pub_releases/2007-11/du-ggi110107.php

2. Caspi A, Williams B, Kim-Cohen J, et al. November 2007). "Moderation of breastfeeding effects on the IQ by genetic variation in fatty acid metabolism". Proc. Natl. Acad. Sci. U.S.A. 104 (47): 18860–5.

3.) Steer CD, Davey Smith G, Emmett PM, eta l. (2010). "FADS2 polymorphisms modify the effect of breastfeeding on child IQ"

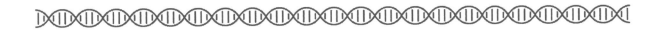

Christy L. Sutton D.C.

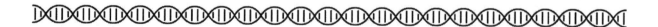

Chapter 6
Alzheimer's Genes

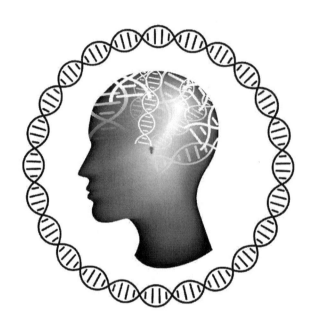

Do you know that there are specific genes related to developing Alzheimer's disease? Just because you have these genes doesn't necessarily mean that you'll develop Alzheimer's, but it does mean that you're at an increased risk. Translation: You can decrease your risk by developing a healthy lifestyle.

Proven ways to reduce the risk of developing Alzheimer's disease

- **Exercise**—Physical exercise reduces your risk of Alzheimer's by 50 percent[6]. The best exercise program for Alzheimer's prevention includes aerobic exercise (30 minutes a day at least five times a week) combined with moderate weight resistance training (two to three strength sessions of moderate resistance training a week). Try adding yoga or tai chi to improve balance and coordination and prevent falling.

- **Don't drink or smoke**—It's bad for your brain and will increase your chances of developing Alzheimer's.

- **Keep your blood sugar stable**—Having blood sugar that fluctuates from one extreme to the other is very hard on the brain. Eating four to six small, healthy meals daily helps promote a stable blood sugar, which helps with overall brain function. Don't skip meals. Make sure your meals are filled with plenty of protein, healthy fats and fiber. Don't eat large amounts of sugar.

- **Keep your brain active**—If you don't use it, you lose it. Continue learning; practice memorization; and enjoy regular puzzles, riddles, and strategy games. Maintain an active social life, regardless of your age. Try a new route to your destination, for example. It will make your brain work harder.

- **Get quality sleep and regular relaxation time**—Chronic stress and sleep deprivation increase your risk of developing Alzheimer's. Sleep is when your body clears out many of the toxins that build up in your body while you're awake. One of these is beta amyloid, which is damaging to the brain and forms the plaques that appear in the brains of Alzheimer's patients[7].

- **Control high blood pressure**

- **Ensure adequate levels of omega-3 fatty acids[1]**—Omega-3-fatty acids are important for brain health and are highest in fish. Eating fish or supplementing with fish oil can protect the brain and promote brain health.

- **Follow a Mediterranean diet**—This diet, rich in fish, nuts, olive oil and fresh produce, has been shown to promote brain health.

- **Avoid head injuries**—Head injuries, especially concussions, increase your risk of developing Alzheimer's. Avoid sports that increase risk of head injuries, wear helmets, buckle up, hold on to railings when going up or down stairs, and avoid ladders whenever possible.

> **Maintain adequate vitamin D levels**—Vitamin D-3 has shown to have neuroprotective effects that may preserve cognitive function.

> **Consider increasing curcumin intake**—Curcumin from turmeric may help prevent Alzheimer's-related plaques from forming in the brain[2,3,4].

> **Maintain high antioxidant levels**—Antioxidants protect the brain. Foods high in antioxidants include fruits, vegetables and green tea. These foods have been shown to also prevent damage to the neurons in the brain and thus prevent Alzheimer's[1]. Some antioxidants include vitamin C, vitamin E, vitamin A, glutathione and alpha-lipoic acid.

> **Consider supplementing with a high-quality B-complex**—Essential for brain health.

> **Consider supplementing with Huperzine**—Huperzine had been shown to potentially increase cognitive function[5], and reduce plaquing in brain[16].

> **Consider supplementing with Vinpocetine**—Vinpocetine has been shown to increase blood flow to the brain, and improve both memory and concentration[8,9].

> **Consider supplementing with Acetyl L-carnitine**—This has been shown to help with memory and helps with the production of acetylcholine.

> **Consider supplementing with Ginkgo Biloba**—This increases blood flow to the brain, protects overall neuronal function, scavenges free radicals, supports mitochondrial function, and inhibits chemical pathways that lead to brain decline by reducing the overstimulation of neurons that cause brain fatigue[10, 11, 12, 13, 14]. Ginkgo has been shown to support memory in animals and humans[15].

> **Intermittent fasting**—Intermittent fasting helps to break down plaquing associated with Alzheimer's. This consists of reduced calorie intake or full fasting for 16–24 hours, followed by regular eating. Fasting is not safe for everyone and should be performed under the care of an experienced health care provider.

Why having stable blood sugar is so important for brain health

Maintaining a stable blood sugar that is within a normal range is essential for a healthy brain. When your blood sugar is too low, there isn't enough fuel for your brain to work.

When blood sugar is too high, it can cause inflammation and damage to your brain and body.

References:

1.) Lara HH, Alanís-Garza EJ, et al. Nutritional approaches to modulate oxidative stress that induce Alzheimer's disease. Nutritional approaches to prevent Alzheimer's disease. 2015 Mar-Apr;151(2):245-51.

2.) Yang F., Lim G. P., et al. (2005) Curcumin inhibits formation of amyloid β oligomers and fibrils, binds plaques, and reduces amyloid in vivo. J. Biol. Chem. 280, 5892–5901.

3.) Begum A. N., Jones M. R., et al. (2008) Curcumin structure-function, bioavailability, and efficacy in models of neuroinflammation and Alzheimer's disease. J. Pharmacol. Exp. Ther. 326, 196–208.

4.) Garcia-Alloza M., et al.(2007) Curcumin labels amyloid pathology in vivo, disrupts existing plaques, and partially restores distorted neurites in an Alzheimer mouse model. J. Neurochem. 102, 1095–1104.

5.) Li J, Wu HM, Zhou RL, et al. Huperzine A for Alzheimer's disease. Cochrane Database Syst Rev. 2008;2

6.) HelpGuide.org. Alzheimer's and Dementia Prevention. Retrieved from: http://www.helpguide.org/articles/alzheimers-dementia/alzheimers-and-dementia-prevention.htm

7.) Hamilton, John. Snooze Alert: A Sleep Disorder May Be Harming Your Body and Brain. (2015. Aug 24th). Retrieved from: http://www.npr.org/sections/health-shots/2015/08/24/432764792/snooze-alert-a-sleep-disorder-may-be-harming-your-body-and-brain.

8.) Ogunrin, AO. (2014) Effect of Vinpocetine on Cognitive Performance of a Nigerian Population. .Ann Med Health Sci Res. 2014 Jul-Aug; 4(4): 654–661.

9.) Valikovics A. Investigation of the effect of vinpocetine on cerebral blood flow and cognitive functions [in Hungarian]. Ideggyogy Sz. 2007 Jul;60(7-8):301- 10.

10.) Ahlemeyer B, Krieglstein J. Neuroprotective effects of Ginkgo biloba extract. Cell Mol Life Sci. 2003 Sep;60(9):1779- 92.

11.) Ahlemeyer B, Krieglstein J. Pharmacological studies supporting the therapeutic use of Ginkgo biloba extract for Alzheimer's disease. Pharmacopsychiatry. 2003 Jun;36 Suppl 1:S8-14. Review.

12.) Ponto LL, Schultz SK. Ginkgo biloba extract: review of CNS effects. Ann Clin Psychiatry. 2003 Jun;15(2):109-19.

14.) Sierpina VS, Wollschlaeger B, Blumenthal M. Ginkgo biloba. Am Fam Physician. 2003 Sep 1;68(5):923-6.

15.) Polich J, Gloria R. Cognitive effects of a Ginkgo biloba/ vinpocetine compound in normal adults: systematic assessment of perception, attention and memory. Hum Psychopharmacol. 2001 Jul;16(5):409-4

16.) Huang XT, Qian ZM, He X, et al. Reducing iron in the brain: a novel pharmacologic mechanism of huperzine A in the treatment of Alzheimer's disease. Neurobiol Aging. 2014;35(5):1045–54.

Christy L. Sutton D.C.

<u>ApoE 4 gene</u>
Apolipoprotein epsilon 4 gene

Names of ApoE 4 gene genetic variants (SNP identification)	rsnumber	Risk allele
ApoE 4	rs429358	Risk allele is C

GENETIC VARIANT IN ApoE 4 GENE **NORMAL ApoE 4 GENE**

EXERCISE

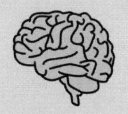

- Curcumin
- Fish Oil
- Stress Reduction
- Healthy Sleep
- Antioxidants

- Stable Blood Sugar
- Don't Drink or Smoke
- Healthy Diet and Lifestyle
- B Vitamins, Huperzine, Vinpocetine

Increased Alzheimer's Risk

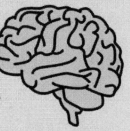

Decreased Alzheimer's Risk

+ +

High Cholesterol Levels

EXERCISE

- Niacin (Vitamin B3)
- Fiber
- Berberine

- Fish Oil
- Plant Based Diet
- No Trans Fats

Lower Cholesterol Levels

+ +

Weaker Bones

VITAMIN D3/K2

Stronger Bones

What does the ApoE 4 gene do?

The ApoE 4 gene is essential in carrying cholesterol in the brain. It can play a role in plaque building up in the brain, a key factor in developing Alzheimer's disease.

What health problems might be associated with having an ApoE 4 risk allele?

- *Significantly increased Alzheimer's risk*—Having an ApoE 4 risk allele is associated with developing late-onset Alzheimer's disease. People with the (C/C) genotype are about **10-30 times more likely to develop Alzheimer's disease**[5]. Some reports suggest that the influence of ApoE 4 on Alzheimer's disease *might be largely mitigated by routine exercise*[6]. Having this risk allele doesn't mean that you will definitely develop Alzheimer's, but it does warrant taking extra precautions to prevent the disease. Developing Alzheimer's is multifactorial and greatly depends on your environment and lifestyle. There are people that develop Alzheimer's disease without having the ApoE 4 gene, and there are people that have the gene and do not develop Alzheimer's disease.

- *Increase in blood cholesterol levels*—Having risk alleles for both ApoE 4 (rs429358) and ApoE 2 (rs7412, risk allele T) elicit a stronger rise in blood cholesterol[1,2].

- *Lower bone density due to lower vitamin K2 levels*—People with the ApoE 4 risk allele are more likely to have low levels of vitamin K2, and thus an increased risk of bone fractures[3]. Vitamin K2 is essential for minerals to be deposited into the bones. Vitamin K2, the type of vitamin K that is most important for strong bones, is made by good bacteria in the digestive system. This should not be confused with vitamin K1, which is from green leafy vegetables and is associated with increasing blood clotting.

- *Increased levels of inflammation*- Having the C risk allele is associated with high levels of the inflammatory marker CRP.

I have one or more risk allele(s) in the ApoE 4 gene. What should I talk to my doctor about doing so that I can reduce my health risks?

- *Exercise*—Some reports suggest that the influence of an ApoE 4 risk allele on Alzheimer's disease might be largely mitigated by routine exercise[6].

Christy L. Sutton D.C.

- **Support bone health**—The best way for people with the ApoE 4 risk allele to support bone health is with weight-bearing exercise, Vitamin D3 and Vitamin K2 supplementation, probiotics, and adequate mineral intake.

- **Support health cholesterol levels naturally**—The ApoE 4 risk allele can cause high cholesterol levels. People with this risk allele appear to respond well to dietary intervention for lowering cholesterol. The best diet for anyone with both high cholesterol and the ApoE 4 risk allele is a low-fat, low-cholesterol diet. Ways to support healthy cholesterol levels naturally include:

  > *Limiting alcohol because it has LDL cholesterol-raising effects[2].*

  > *Eat a diet that high in good fats and low in bad fats, including plenty of fish, olive oil, avocados and nuts. Minimize margarine, trans-fats, and processed and fried foods.*

  > *Consider supplementing with fish oil and vitamin B-3 (niacin).*

  > *Follow a high-fiber diet, including plenty of fruits, vegetables and nuts.*

  > *Exercise regularly.*

  > *Exercise caution with taking statin drugs to reduce cholesterol*—This is because statins can lead to memory problems, muscle pain, and CoQ10 and vitamin D deficiencies. Talk to your doctor before changing any medications.

- **Adequate vitamin B intake**—B vitamins are necessary for brain health and keeping your homocysteine level low. Having high homocysteine on lab work is associated with an increased risk of developing Alzheimer's disease.

* Read the section titled, "Proven ways to reduce the risk of developing Alzheimer's disease" on page 157 for more information.

I have one or more risk allele(s) in the ApoE 4 gene. What labs/testing should I consider to continually monitor my health?

  ✓ *Lipid / Cholesterol panel (blood test)*

✓ **Bone density testing**—Having the ApoE 4 risk allele can increase your risk of a bone fracture.

✓ **Smell test**—Loss of sense of smell is one of the first signs of Alzheimer's. Therefore, testing your sense of smell is a great way to monitor your brain health.

✓ **Memory recall testing**

✓ **Vitamin D levels (blood test)**—Vitamin D is important for brain health. I prefer to see vitamin D level around 70 to 100 on lab work.

✓ **Homocysteine (blood work)**—High homocysteine is associated with an increased risk of developing Alzheimer's. I prefer homocysteine to be below 8 on blood work.

✓ **CRP (blood work)**—*This is an inflammatory marker that is associated with being elevated in people with the risk allele.*

✓ **Calcium score test**—This test is used to check for heart disease in an early stage and to determine how severe it is. It monitors for buildup of calcium in plaque on the walls of the arteries in the heart. This test does emit a low level of radiation, so antioxidants should be greatly increased before and after this test is performed. ApoE 4 risk alleles are associated with higher levels of cholesterol.

Preventing Alzheimer's is key, but there is hope for a cure

There have been some studies done on mice that have shown to improve brain function in Alzheimer's disease.
The studies used ultrasound on their brains[1]. The ultrasound is thought to help remove the plaque that occurs in the brains of people affected with Alzheimer's disease[1].

References:

1.) Jeffrey, Colin. (2015, March 11). Non-invasive Alzheimer' treatment restores memory using ultrasound. Retrieved from: http://www.gizmag.com/alzheimers-dementia-treatment-ultrasound/36510/

References:

1.) Masson LF, McNeill G, Avenell A. Genetic variations and the lipid response to dietary intervention: a systemic review. Am J Clin Nutr 2003;77 (5):1098-111.

Christy L. Sutton D.C.

2.) Sarkkinen E, Korhonen M, Erkkila A, et al. Effect of apolipoprotein E polymorphism on serum lipid response to the separate modification of dietary fat and dietary cholesterol. Am J. Clinical Nutr 1998;68(6):1215-22.

3.) Kohlmeier M, Saupe J, Schaefer K, Asmus G (1998) Bone fracture history and prospective bone fracture risk of hemodialysis patients are related to apolipoprotein E genotype. Calcif Tissue Int 62: 278-281.

4.) Ordovas JM. Gene-diet interaction and plasma lipid responses to dietary intervention. Biochem Soc Trans2002; 30:68–73.

5.) Estep, Preston. (2012. Aug 1). The predominant variant of the APP gene greatly increases risk for Alzheimer's Disease and cognitive decline. Retrieved from: http://blog.personalgenomes.org/2012/08/01/the-predominant-variant-of-the-app-gene-greatly-increases-risk-for-alzheimers-disease-and-cognitive-decline/.

6.) Head, D., Bugg, J.M., Goate, A.M., et al. (2012) Exercise Engagement as a Moderator of the Effects of APOE Genotype on Amyloid Deposition. Archives of neurology, Epub ahead of print.

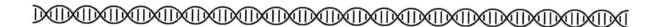

ApoE 2 gene
Apolipoprotein epsilon 2

Names of ApoE 2 gene genetic variants (SNP identification)	rsnumber	Risk allele
ApoE 2	rs7412	Risk allele is T

The health effects of having an ApoE 2 genetic variant is unclear regarding Alzheimer's risks. However, it known that having a risk allele in the ApoE 2 gene is associated with more normal cholesterol levels unless it's in combination with having the risk allele for ApoE 4[1,2]. If you have the risk allele for the ApoE 2 gene and you have high cholesterol levels, then eating a diet high in fat and low in carbohydrates may be very beneficial— including oat bran, tea, vegetables and fruits.

Read the section titled, "Proven ways to reduce the risk of developing Alzheimer's disease" on page 157 for more information.

References:

1.) Masson LF, McNeill G, Avenell A. Genetic variations and the lipid response to dietary intervention: a systemic review. Am J Clin Nutr 2003;77 (5):1098-111.

2.) Sarkkinen E, Korhonen M, Erkkila A, et al. Effect of apolipoprotein E polymorphism on serum lipid response to the separate modification of dietary fat and dietary cholesterol. Am J. Clinical Nutr 1998;68(6):1215-22.

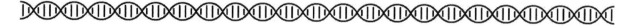

TOMM40 gene
Translocase of outer mitochondrial membrane 40

Names of TOMM40 gene genetic variants (SNP identification)	rsnumber	Risk allele
TOMM40 A45395619G	rs2075650	Risk allele is G
TOMM40 G45395266A	rs157580	Risk allele is G

What does the TOMM40 gene do?

The TOMM40 gene is associated with developing Alzheimer's disease. Having the risk allele does not mean that you will develop Alzheimer's, but it does warrant taking extra precautions to prevent the disease. Developing Alzheimer's is multifactorial and greatly depends on your environment and lifestyle.

The TOMM40 gene creates a protein that helps nutrients move in and out of the mitochondria. Mitochondria are important for energy production and are known to play an important role in developing Alzheimer's disease; however, the exact role that mitochondria play in Alzheimer's is still not fully understood[1].

What health problems are associated with having the TOMM40 risk allele?

- *Alzheimer's disease*[2]
  - ➢ The TOMM40 gene appears to significantly increase susceptibility to developing Alzheimer's when combined with having the risk allele for the ApoE 4 gene[4]. However, having a TOMM40 risk allele does appear to play a role in memory decline independent of having the ApoE 4 risk allele. The memory decline related to TOMM40 appears to be most noticeably related to verbal learning after age 60.

- *High triglycerides*—Having the risk allele for TOMM40 G45395266A (rs157580) is associated with high triglyceride levels in genome-wide association studies[3].

I have one or more TOMM40 gene risk allele(s). What should I talk to my doctor about doing so that I can reduce my health risks?

- *Exercise*—Exercise is one of the best ways to prevent Alzheimer's disease.

- **Support healthy triglyceride levels**—A low- sugar diet is essential for low triglyceride levels.

  Read the section titled, "Proven ways to reduce the risk of developing Alzheimer's disease" on page 157 for more information.

I have one or more risk allele(s) in the TOMM40 gene. What labs/testing should I consider to continually monitor my health?

- ✓ **Triglycerides and hemoglobin A1C (blood test)**—TOMM40 risk alleles are associated with high triglyceride levels. Hemoglobin A1C is the best way to monitor blood sugar. High blood sugar will lead to high triglyceride levels.

- ✓ **Smell test**—Loss of sense of smell is one of the first signs of Alzheimer's. Therefore, testing one's smell is a great way to monitor one's brain health.

- ✓ **Memory recall testing**

- ✓ **Vitamin D levels (blood test)**—Vitamin D is important for brain health. I prefer to see vitamin D level around 70 to 100 on lab work.

- ✓ **Homocysteine (blood work)**—High homocysteine is associated with an increased risk of developing Alzheimer's disease. I prefer homocysteine to be below 8 on blood work.

References:

1.) Devi L, Prabhu BM, Galati DF, et al. (August 2006). "Accumulation of amyloid precursor protein in the mitochondrial import channels of human Alzheimer's disease brain is associated with mitochondrial dysfunction". J. Neurosci. 26 (35): 9057–68.

2.) Potkin SG, Guffanti G, Lakatos A et al. (2009). et al. "Hippocampal Atrophy as a Quantitative Trait in a Genome-Wide Association Study Identifying Novel Susceptibility Genes for Alzheimer's Disease".PLoS ONE 4 (8): e6501.

3.)Jiang R1, Brummett BH, et al. Chronic family stress moderates the association between a TOMM40 variant and triglyceride levels in two independent Caucasian samples.Biol Psychol. 2013 Apr;93(1):184-9.

4.) Bright Focus Foundation. Risk factors and prevention of Alzheimer's. Retrieved from: http://www.brightfocus.org/alzheimers/about/risk/?referrer=https://www.google.com/

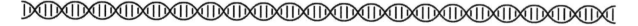

ABCA2 gene
ATP-binding cassette sub-family A member 2 gene

Names of ABCA2 gene genetic variants (SNP identification)	rsnumber	Risk allele
ABCA2	rs908832	Risk allele is A

What health problems might be associated with having an ABCA2 risk allele?

Increased risk for developing early onset Alzheimer's disease[1]. If you have the (A, A) genotype for the ABCA2 gene, you're *3.8 times* more likely to develop early onset Alzheimer's disease. Having the (A, A) genotype for the ABCA2 gene doesn't mean that you will definitely develop Alzheimer's, but it does warrant taking extra precautions to prevent it. Developing Alzheimer's is multifactorial and greatly depends on one's environment and lifestyle.

I have one or more risk allele(s) in the ABCA2 gene. What should I talk to my doctor about doing so that I can reduce my health risks?

- *Control cholesterol levels*—The ABCA2 gene plays a role in cholesterol transport. Ways to naturally lower cholesterol include:

  - *Limit alcohol*—It has LDL-cholesterol-raising effects[2].

  - *Eat a diet high in good fats and low in bad fats*—This includes eating plenty of fish, olive oil, avocadoes, and nuts. Minimize margarine, trans fats, and processed and fried foods.

  - *Consider supplementing with fish oil and vitamin B-3 (niacin)*

  - *Eat a high-fiber diet*—This includes plenty of fruits, vegetables and nuts.

  - *Exercise*

  - *Exercise caution with taking statins to reduce cholesterol*—Statins can lead to memory problems, muscle pain, and CoQ10 and vitamin D deficiencies.

Christy L. Sutton D.C.

Read the section titled, "Proven ways to reduce the risk of developing Alzheimer's disease" on page 157 for more information.

I have one or more risk allele(s) in the ABCA2 gene. What labs/testing should I consider to continually monitor my health?

✓ ***Monitor cholesterol levels (blood test)***

✓ ***Smell test***—Loss of sense of smell is one of the first signs of Alzheimer's. Therefore, testing your sense of smell is a great way to monitor your brain health.

✓ ***Memory recall testing***

✓ ***Vitamin D levels (blood test)***—Vitamin D is important for brain health. I prefer to see vitamin D level around 70 to 100 on lab work.

✓ ***Homocysteine (blood work)***—High homocysteine is associated with an increased risk of developing Alzheimer's disease. I prefer homocysteine to be below 8 on blood work.

References:

1.) Mace S, Cousin E, Ricard S, Genin E, et al. ABCA2 is a strong genetic risk factor for early-onset Alzheimer's disease. Neurobiol Dis. 2005;18:119–125.

2.) Ordovas JM. Gene-diet interaction and plasma lipid responses to dietary intervention. Biochem Soc Trans2002;30:68–73.

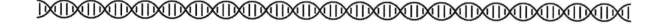

Personalized genetic report found at http://geneticdetoxification.com

A2M gene
Alpha-2-macroglobulin

Names of A2M gene genetic variants (SNP identification)	rsnumber	Risk allele
A2M	rs11609582	Risk allele is T

What health problems might be associated with having an A2M risk allele?

Alzheimer's disease[1]— Having the risk allele does not mean that you'll definitely develop Alzheimer's, but it does warrant taking extra precautions to prevent the disease. Developing Alzheimer's is multifactorial and greatly depends on your environment and lifestyle.

- Having the A2M (A/T) genotype makes you 1.78 times more likely to develop Alzheimer's disease.

- Having the A2M (T/T) genotype makes you 1.86 times more likely to develop Alzheimer's disease.

I have one or more risk allele(s) in the A2M gene. What should I talk to my doctor about doing so that I can reduce my health risks?

Read the section titled, "Proven ways to reduce the risk of developing Alzheimer's disease" on page 157 for more information.

I have the A2M risk allele. What labs/testing should I consider to continually monitor my health?

✓ *Smell test*—Loss of sense of smell is one of the first signs of Alzheimer's. Therefore, testing your sense of smell is a great way to monitor your brain health.

✓ *Memory recall testing*

✓ *Vitamin D levels (blood test)*—Vitamin D is important for brain health. I prefer to see vitamin D level around 70 to 100 on lab work.

Christy L. Sutton D.C.

✓ **Homocysteine (blood work)**—High homocysteine is associated with an increased risk of developing Alzheimer's disease. I prefer homocysteine to be at or below 8 on blood work.

References:

1.) Saunders AJ, Bertram L, Mullin K, et al. Genetic association of Alzheimer's disease with multiple polymorphisms in alpha-2-macroglobulin. Human molecular genetics. 2003;12(21):2765–76.

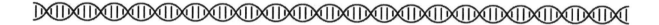

APBB2 gene
Amyloid beta A4 precursor protein-binding family B member 2 gene

Names of APBB2 gene genetic variants (SNP identification)	rsnumber	Risk allele
APBB2	rs13133980	Risk allele is G

What health problems might be associated with having an APBB2 risk allele?

An increased risk for developing Alzheimer's disease[1]—Having the risk allele doesn't mean that you will develop Alzheimer's, but it does warrant taking extra precautions to prevent the disease. Developing Alzheimer's is multifactorial and greatly depends on your environment and lifestyle.

I have one or more risk allele(s) in the APBB2 gene. How can I reduce my health risks?

Read the section titled, "Proven ways to reduce the risk of developing Alzheimer's disease" on page 157 for more information.

I have one or more risk allele(s) in the APBB2 gene. What labs/testing should I consider to continually monitor my health?

- ✓ **Smell test**—Loss of sense of smell is one of the first signs of Alzheimer's. Therefore, testing your sense of smell is a great way to monitor your brain health.

- ✓ **Memory recall testing**

- ✓ **Vitamin D levels (blood test)**—Vitamin D is important for brain health. I prefer to see vitamin D level around 70 to 100 on lab work.

- ✓ **Homocysteine (blood work)**—High homocysteine is associated with an increased risk of developing Alzheimer's disease. I prefer homocysteine to be at or below 8 on blood work.

References:

1.) Golanska E1, Sieruta M, Gresner SM, et al.APBB2 genetic polymorphisms are associated with severe cognitive impairment in centenarians. Exp Gerontol. 2013 Apr;48(4):391-4.

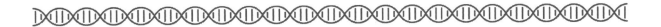

BCHE gene
Butyrylcholinesterase gene

Names of BCHE gene genetic variants (SNP identification)	rsnumber	Risk allele
BCHE	rs1803274	Risk allele is T

What does the BCHE gene do?

The BCHE gene provides the body's instructions for making an enzyme that breaks the memory- enhancing neurotransmitter acetylcholine down into choline and acetic acid.

 Christy L. Sutton D.C.

What health problems might be associated with having a BCHE risk allele?

Increased risk for developing Alzheimer's disease—Having both the risk allele for the BCHE gene *and* the ApoE 4 gene can create a synergistic effect that increases your risk of developing Alzheimer's disease[2]. Having a BCHE risk allele doesn't mean that you will develop Alzheimer's, but it does warrant taking extra precautions to prevent the disease. Developing Alzheimer's is multifactorial and greatly depends on your environment and lifestyle.

I have one or more risk allele(s) in the BCHE gene. What should I talk to my doctor about doing so that I can reduce my health risks?

- *Exercise caution when taking drugs that are metabolized by the BCHE gene*—These drugs will be harder for your body to metabolize and break down (i.e., this includes various local anesthetics, certain recreational drugs such as cocaine and heroin, and short-acting muscle relaxants[1]). Talk to your prescribing doctor before discontinuing any medications.

  * Read the section titled, "Proven ways to reduce the risk of developing Alzheimer's disease" on page 157 for more information.

I have one or more risk allele(s) in the BCHE gene. What labs/testing should I consider to continually monitor my health?

- ✓ *Smell test*—Loss of sense of smell is one of the first signs of Alzheimer's. Therefore, testing your sense of smell is a great way to monitor your brain health.

- ✓ *Memory recall testing*

- ✓ *Vitamin D levels (blood test)*—Vitamin D is important for brain health. I prefer to see vitamin D level around 70 to 100 on lab work.

- ✓ *Homocysteine (blood work)*—High homocysteine is associated with an increased risk of developing Alzheimer's disease. I prefer homocysteine to be at or below 8 on blood work.

References:

1.) Kamendulis LM, Brzezinski MR, et al. Metabolism of cocaine and heroin is catalyzed by the same human liver carboxylesterases. J Pharmacol Exp Ther. 1996 Nov; 279(2):713-7.

2.) Wiebusch H, Poirier J, Sévigny P, Schappert K. Further evidence for a synergistic association between APOE epsilon4 and BCHE-K in confirmed Alzheimer's disease. Hum Genet. 1999;104(2):158–63.

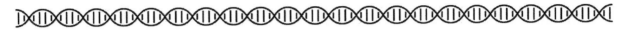

CLU gene
Clusterin gene

Names of CLU gene genetic variants (SNP identification)	rsnumber	Risk allele
CLU	rs11136000	Risk allele is C

What does the CLU gene do?

The CLU gene cleans up cellular debris and plays an important part in apoptosis (programmed cell death).

What health problems might be associated with having a CLU risk allele?

- *Increased risk of developing late-onset Alzheimer's disease*—There is a slightly increased risk of developing Alzheimer's disease if you have this risk allele. The increased risk is only 1.16 times more than if you did not have the risk allele[1]. Having CLU gene risk alleles doesn't mean that you'll develop Alzheimer's, but it does warrant taking extra precautions to prevent the disease. Developing Alzheimer's is multifactorial and greatly depends on your environment and lifestyle.

- *Fewer and weaker myelin sheaths around the neurons in the brain*—The myelin sheaths protect the brain and nervous system.

I have one or more risk allele(s) in the CLU gene. What should I talk to my doctor about doing so that I can reduce my health risks?

Christy L. Sutton D.C.

Read the section titled, "Proven ways to reduce the risk of developing Alzheimer's disease" on page 157 for more information.

I have one or more risk allele(s) in the CLU gene. What labs/testing should I consider to continually monitor my health?

✓ ***Smell test***—Loss of sense of smell is one of the first signs of Alzheimer's. Therefore, testing your sense of smell is a great way to monitor your brain health.

✓ ***Memory recall testing***

✓ ***Vitamin D levels (blood test)***—Vitamin D is important for brain health. I prefer to see vitamin D level around 70 to 100 on lab work.

✓ ***Homocysteine (blood work)***—High homocysteine is associated with an increased risk of developing Alzheimer's disease. I prefer homocysteine to be at or below 8 on blood work.

References:

1) Braskie M. N., Jahanshad N., Stein J. L., et al. (2011). Common Alzheimer's disease risk variant within the CLU gene affects white matter microstructure in young adults. J. Neurosci. 31 6764–6770 10.

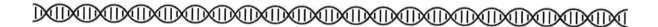

TF gene
Transferrin gene

Names of TF gene genetic variants (SNP identification)	rsnumber	Risk allele
TF	rs1049296	Risk allele is T

What does the TF gene do?

TF (transferrin) regulates iron so that it cannot freely cause damage throughout the body. TF's main role is to deliver iron to the body's tissues. It's essential for iron to be tightly regulated in the body because unbound iron that isn't tightly controlled can cause free radicals and damage to the body.

What health problems are associated with having a TF risk allele?

Increased risk for developing Alzheimer's disease apoptosis—Having a risk allele in the TF gene can increase your risk for developing Alzheimer's disease. Having a risk allele in *both* rs1049296 (TF) *and* rs1800562 (HFE) is associated with an increased risk of developing Alzheimer's, especially if you have high levels of iron on blood work[1]. Having chronically high iron levels can cause brain damage and neurodegeneration, including Alzheimer's disease[1,2,3]. If you have the risk allele for both rs1049296 (TF) and rs1800562 (HFE), you're at an increased risk of having chronically high iron levels. You can learn more about the HFE gene on page 376.

I have one or more risk allele(s) in the TF gene. What should I talk to my doctor about doing so that I can reduce my health risks?

- *Consider donating blood if blood tests indicate that your iron levels are high*—Donating blood will quickly remove the extra iron from your body. As long as your iron and ferritin levels aren't elevated, then having the risk allele for the TF gene is not generally considered hazardous to your health.

- *If iron levels high, then avoid eating a diet high in iron-rich foods such as red meat.*

*Read the section titled, "Proven ways to reduce the risk of developing Alzheimer's disease" on page 157 for more information.

I have one or more risk allele(s) in the TF gene. What labs/testing should I consider to continually monitor my health?

- ✓ *Monitor for high iron levels (blood work)*—Labs that measure iron include ferritin, transferrin, iron, TIBC, UIBC, hemoglobin and hematocrit.

- ✓ *Memory recall testing and sense of smell*—These measure for cognitive decline associated with Alzheimer's disease. One of the first signs of Alzheimer's is a decreased sense of smell. Therefore, testing your sense of smell is a great way to monitor your brain health.

References:

1.) Kauwe J. S. K., Bertelsen S., et al. Suggestive synergy between genetic variants in TF and HFE as risk factors for Alzheimer's disease. The American Journal of Medical Genetics, Part B: Neuropsychiatric Genetics. 2010;153(4):955–959.

Christy L. Sutton D.C.

2.) Wang Y, Xu S, Liu Z, Lai C, Xie Z, et al. Meta-Analysis on the Association Between the TF Gene rs1049296 and AD. Can J Neurol Sci. 2013;40:691–697.

3.) Yunlong Tao, YuWang, et al. Perturbed Iron Distribution in Alzheimer's Disease Serum, Cerebrospinal Fluid, and Selected Brain Regions: A Systematic Review and Meta-Analysis. Journal of Alzheimer's Disease 42 (2014) 679–690.

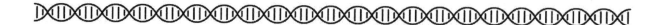

IDE gene
Insulin-degrading enzyme

Names of IDE gene genetic variants (SNP identification)	rsnumber	Risk allele
IDE	rs6583817	Risk allele is C

What does the IDE gene do?

The IDE gene, important for both your blood sugar and brain, produces a protein called insulin-degrading enzyme (IDE). IDE's function is to break down insulin, but it also breaks down a protein linked to Alzheimer's disease called amyloid beta (Aβ)[1,2].

What health problems are associated with having an IDE risk allele?

There is an increased risk of developing Alzheimer's disease if you have the C allele (risk allele). Mice with the C risk allele have shown to accumulate a larger amount of Alzheimer's-related plaques in their brains.

Having the T (non-risk) allele is associated with a *decreased* rate of developing Alzheimer's[1]. If you have the T (non-risk) allele for the IDE gene, your body produces more of the enzyme that breaks down the β-amyloid plaques that accumulate in the brain (and can lead to Alzheimer's). This means that you will break down the Alzheimer's plaques faster than a person with the T allele.

I have one or more risk allele(s) in the IDE gene. What should I talk to my doctor about doing so that I can reduce my health risks?

- *Intermittent fasting*—Intermittent fasting helps to break down plaquing associated with Alzheimer's and improves insulin sensitivity. Intermittent fasting involves reduced calorie intake or full fasting for 16–24 hours, followed by regular eating. Fasting is not safe for everyone and should be performed under the care of an experienced health care provider.

- **Ensure adequate zinc levels**—Zinc is a cofactor for the IDE enzyme. Therefore, if you're deficient in zinc, your IDE enzyme will have a harder time breaking down the β-amyloid Alzheimer's plaques in the brain. Foods naturally high in zinc include beef, oysters, cashews and spinach.

Read the section titled, "Proven ways to reduce the risk of developing Alzheimer's disease" on page 157 for more information.

I have one or more risk allele(s) in the IDE gene. What labs/testing should I consider to continually monitor my health?

- ✓ **Measure zinc levels:**

    - ➢ **Zinc taste test**—This involves putting liquid zinc in the mouth. If the zinc tastes like water, then it indicates a deficiency in zinc.

    - ➢ **Zinc blood test**

- ✓ **Monitor blood sugar levels through Hemoglobin A1C (blood test)**—This test will show your average blood sugar for the last three months.

- ✓ **C-peptide**—*This will monitor insulin levels.*

- ✓ **Memory recall testing and sense of smell**—These are measuring for cognitive decline associated with Alzheimer's disease. One of the first signs of Alzheimer's is a decreased sense of smell. Therefore, testing your sense of smell is a great way to monitor your brain health.

References:

1.) Carrasquillo MM, Belbin O, Zou F, et al. Concordant association of insulin degrading enzyme gene (IDE) variants with IDE mRNA, Abeta, and Alzheimer's disease. PLoS One. 2010;5:e8764.

2.) Kurochkin IV, Goto S (May 1994). "Alzheimer's beta-amyloid peptide specifically interacts with and is degraded by insulin degrading enzyme". FEBS Letters345 (1): 33–7.

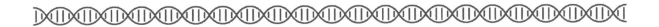

Christy L. Sutton D.C.

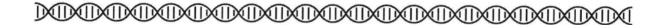

<u>Chapter 7</u>

Sleep

Mental Health

Mood

Anxiety

Stress

Substance Abuse and Focus

AANAT gene
Aralkylamine N-acetyltransferase gene

Names of AANAT gene genetic variants (SNP identification)	rsnumber	Risk allele
AANAT	rs11077820	Risk allele is T

What does the AANAT gene do?

The AANAT gene plays an important role in the body's ability to make melatonin by providing the instructions for the body to make the AANAT enzyme. The AANAT enzyme controls the night/day rhythm of melatonin production.

What health problems are associated with having an AANAT risk allele?

Inability to fall asleep or have a sound night's sleep—Having a risk alle in the AANAT gene could prevent you from creating adequate levels of melatonin, leading to a disruption in the sleep/wake cycle—mostly a disruption in the ability to fall asleep. Having a risk allele in the AANAT gene may contribute to falling asleep late and having a hard time waking up in the morning[1].

Picture credit[1]

I have one or more risk allele(s) in the AANAT gene. What should I talk to my doctor about doing so that I can reduce my health risks?

- *Consider supplementing with vitamin B-5, vitamin B-6 and tryptophan*—The AANAT enzyme requires vitamin B-5 and serotonin, so taking tryptophan and vitamin B-5 could be helpful. Vitamin B-6 in the activated form called P-5-P is necessary for the body to make serotonin, which is a precursor to making melatonin.

- **_Consider supplementing with melatonin_**—Because people with the AANAT risk allele may not naturally make as much melatonin as they normally would, taking melatonin might be all it takes to make up the difference between having a good or bad night of sleep.

  ➤ *What if supplementing with melatonin makes you feel horrible?* Some people take melatonin and feel wired rather than tired. If this applies to you, you need to understand if you have the MAOA genetic variants that lead to high levels of serotonin (Pg. 187).

  ➤ Taking melatonin while having a genetic predisposition toward high serotonin levels could lead to even higher serotonin levels, which can lead to feeling wired rather than tired.

- **_Eat a diet that maintains a stable blood sugar_**—Many people's sleep problems are a result of their blood sugar being too low or high throughout the day and night.

I have one or more risk allele(s) in the AANAT gene. What labs/testing should I consider to continually monitor my health?

✓ **_Adrenal testing_**—This will help ensure that your sleep problems are not related to adrenal issues. The inability to fall asleep is often caused by high cortisol levels rather than low melatonin. If adrenal tests show high cortisol in the evening, then try phosphatidylserine to help lower cortisol and help you fall asleep.

✓ **_Measure melatonin levels (blood or saliva test)_**

References:

1.) Picture retrieved from: https://en.wikipedia.org/wiki/Aralkylamine_N-acetyltransferase

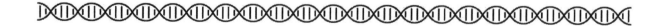

COMT genes
Catechol-O-methyltransferase genes

Names of COMT gene genetic variants (SNP identification)	rsnumber	Risk allele
COMT VI58M	rs4680	Risk allele = Worrier = A = slower COMT enzyme = higher levels of dopamine, epinephrine, norepinephrine and estrogen = potential for lower performance under stress, better memory, increased ability to concentrate[5] Warrior = G= faster COMT enzyme = lower levels of dopamine, epinephrine, norepinephrine and estrogen = potential for better performance under stress, worse memory, decreased ability to concentrate[5]
COMT	rs4633	Risk allele is T

What do the COMT genes do?

The COMT genes plays an important role in modulating stress and the stress response in the body. The COMT genes provide instructions for several COMT enzymes that degrade estrogen, neurotransmitter dopamine and the adrenal catecholamines (epinephrine and norepinephrine). The COMT enzyme is responsible for breaking down dopamine in the frontal lobe of the brain.

What health problems are associated with having a COMT risk allele?

Having a risk allele in a COMT gene can lead to high levels of dopamine, norepinephrine, epinephrine and estrogen. For this reason, having a COMT risk allele can be associated with an increased risk of developing certain health problems.

- *Anxiety*—High levels of dopamine, norepinephrine or epinephrine can cause a heightened stress response, which could manifest in feeling very anxious.

- *Early onset antisocial behaviors*

Christy L. Sutton D.C.

- *Substance abuse*

- *Novelty-seeking personalities*

- *Drug addiction*

- *Hypertension*

- *Schizophrenia*—Dopamine is a neurotransmitter involved with the brain's ability to focus and pick out patterns. Too much dopamine could cause you to start picking out patterns that aren't there, as in schizophrenia. Too little dopamine could leave you oblivious and depressed.

- *Decreased ability to break down dopamine, epinephrine, norepinephrine and estrogen*—A more complete list of health conditions that can result from not properly breaking down dopamine, epinephrine, norepinephrine, and estrogen are included in the table below:

Health problems associated with an inability to break down Dopamine	Health problems associated with an inability to break down Epinephrine/Norepinephrine (Adrenalin)	Health problems associated with an inability to break down Estrogen
• Schizophrenia/Paranoia • Anxiety/Panic disorders • High cortisol levels • Nervousness • Sleeping problems • Bipolar disorder • ADHD (Attention Deficient Hyperactivity Disorder) • Depression • Alcoholism • Cancer • Increased stress response • High blood pressure/ hypertension	• Anxiety/Panic disorders • High cortisol levels • Nervousness • Sleeping problems • High blood pressure/ hypertension • Increased fracture risk • Increased risk of coronary artery events • Increased pain sensitivity such as fibromyalgia and RSD (Reflex Sympathetic Dystrophy) • Cancer • Increased stress response • Insomnia	• Breast cancer

Are you a worrier or a warrior?
COMT V158M (rs4680)

- **The "Worrier" genotype** = (A/A) genotype—Having the A allele for the COMT VI58M rs4680 is sometimes called the "worrier gene" because your COMT enzyme is less efficient, resulting in your having higher dopamine, epinephrine, norepinephrine and estrogen levels[4]. The higher dopamine level leads to a lower pain threshold, enhanced vulnerability to deal with stress, and an increased ability to focus—but you're more efficient at processing information[5,6]. Having the worrier gene is linked to major depressive disorders and suicide in some cases.

- **The "Warrior" genotype** = (G/G) genotype—Having the G allele for COMT VI58M rs4680 is sometimes called the "warrior gene" because your COMT enzyme is more efficient, resulting in your having lower dopamine, epinephrine, norepinephrine and estrogen levels. Lower dopamine levels can lead to a higher pain threshold and better stress reliance—but a moderate reduction in executive function[5,6]. If you have the (G/G) genotype for COMT VI58M, don't smoke marijuana. There is an increased chance of developing psychotic/schizophrenia in adulthood among people with GG genotype who used marijuana as an adolescent.

- **The "Goldilocks'" genotype** = (G/A) genotype—The "Goldilocks genotype" is a term I personally use to describe a person who inherited one "worrier" gene and one "warrior" gene. People with this genotype may have a more neutral balance of intelligence, drive, focus, emotional affect, happiness and success.

It's important to remember that much of our behavior is learned and doesn't only depend on the genes we received from our parents. How we're raised as a child and the environment that we're exposed to are essential factors in our level of empathy and our behavior.

 Christy L. Sutton D.C.

I have one or more risk allele(s) in the COMT gene. What should I talk to my doctor about doing so that I can reduce my health risks?

- *Protect your brain with proper nutrition*—Excess dopamine and chronic stress can damage the brain, particularly the prefrontal cortex. Nutrients that help protect the brain include:

  - ➤ *Consider supplementing with fish oil*—Fish oil can help protect the brain from the damage that stress can cause.

  - ➤ *Consider supplementing with Phosphatidylserine*—Phosphatidylserine has been shown to not only protect the brain, but also to lower stress-induced spikes in cortisol levels. In addition to combating mental stress, phosphatidylserine has been shown to combat exercise-induced stress and improve performance and recovery in golf and cycling[1,2]. Try taking it for your putting game and see if it makes a difference!

  - ➤ *Antioxidants*—High levels of stress can easily deplete vitamin C. Vitamins C, A, E, alpha lipoic acid, glutathione and CoQ10 are antioxidants that can protect the brain from damage. A diet high in fruits and veggies is high in antioxidants.

  - ➤ *Consider supplementing with B vitamins*—Stress depletes B vitamins, which are very important for a healthy brain and body. Ensure that a B-complex has adequate levels of vitamin B-6 in the form called P-5-P. Stress especially depletes vitamin B-6.

- *Ensure adequate levels of trace minerals*—Trace minerals are important for the COMT enzyme to function properly, but also for supporting a calm state of mind. The trace minerals *must include boron and magnesium*. Some people with COMT benefit from a trace mineral with lithium due to its calming effects. Boron-enriched diets have been shown to reduce prostate, cervical and lung cancer because boron-containing compounds interfere with the physiology and reproduction of cancer cells[3]. Foods naturally high in boron include chickpeas, almonds, beans, vegetables, bananas, walnuts and avocados. Anyone drinking reverse osmosis water needs to take extra trace minerals to replace the minerals removed from the water.

- *Practice aerobic exercise at or below your target heart rate*—While exercise is a good stress reliever and is also essential for health, certain types of exercise can be stress-inducing. Some of these exercises include extreme sports, aerobic exercise and aerobic exercise that is above your target heart range. These activities can increase your body's stress response, which can cause an excessive amount of dopamine, norepinephrine and epinephrine if you have COMT risk alleles. It's important to monitor heart rate and blood pressure, as high levels of norepinephrine and epinephrine can increase both. I recommend that you exercise with a heart rate monitor to ensure you're not overtaxing your body. Talk to your doctor before starting any new exercise programs.

- *Minimize exposure to estrogenic hormones*

  - ➢ *Don't drink out of plastic bottles/don't microwave food in plastic—* Plastics produce chemicals that can cause an estrogen-like reaction in the body. Even BPA-free plastics are a problem. The excess estrogenic chemicals build up faster in people with COMT risk alleles, and can increases the risk of devloping breast and uterine cancer.

  - ➢ *Consider supplementing with Diindolylmethane (DIM)—If estrogen levels are high,* DIM is a compound from cruciferous vegetables that can help detoxify estrogens.

- *Avoid caffeine and smoking*—Caffeine and smoking increase dopamine levels, which can already be too high with certain COMT genotypes.

- *Take caution is using amphetamine-based drugs*—Amphetamine-based drugs can ramp up dopamine, norepinephrine and epinephrine. These drugs are often used to treat narcolepsy, ADD and ADHD.

- *Use calming essential oils*—Smell can have very powerful effects on the brain. The right calming smells can quickly decrease a stress response.

- *Ensure the methylation cycle is working efficiently to prevent SAH from building up*—The COMT enzyme is inhibited by S-adenosylhomocysteine (SAH), a byproduct of the methylation cycles that builds up when someone is deficient in methylated B vitamins. Therefore, keeping SAH and homocysteine levels low by taking an activated B vitamin is important. SAH and homocysteine levels often increase with stress.

- *Exercise caution when using dopamine-increasing drugs such as Wellbutrin and L-dopa*—Contact your prescribing physician before changing or stopping any drugs.

Christy L. Sutton D.C.

- ***Monitor and reduce stress***—Stress can initiate a viscous cycle that is hard to break for anyone with a risk allele in the COMT gene. Meditation, long relaxing walks and massages can keep your body's stress level from getting too high, which can prevent you from developing health problems. Staying calm will reduce your potential for health problems related to having a COMT risk allele because you'll have lower levels of norepinephrine, epinephrine and dopamine. Lower levels of stress and proper stress-handling techniques will reduce your potential for health problems related to having a COMT risk allele.

- ***Eat a diet high in vegetables, fruit, good fats and protein***—This can help keep your blood sugar stable, reducing your overall stress level.

I have one or more risk allele(s) in the COMT gene. What labs/testing should I consider to continually monitor my health?

- ✓ ***Comprehensive hormonal testing, including adrenal hormones***—This test monitors for potential hormone imbalances and stress hormones.

- ✓ ***Nutreval Plasma by Genova Diagnostics (blood and urine test)***—The Nutreval test measures metabolites that reflect how good dopamine, epinephrine and norepinephrine are being broken down in your body. This test also measures the levels of vitamin, minerals and good fats, which are important for a healthy brain.

- ✓ ***Routine breast cancer screenings***

- ✓ ***Methylation profile***—This test measures SAMe, SAH and homocysteine levels. Low SAMe, high SAH and high homocysteine inhibit the COMT enzyme—further decreasing your body's ability to break down dopamine, norepinephrine, epinephrine and estrogen.

- ✓ ***Monitor blood pressure and heart rate***—Having a COMT risk allele can increase dopamine, epinephrine and norepinephrine levels, which can increase blood pressure and heart rate.

  - ➢ ***The Ragland's test***—This blood pressure test requires your blood pressure to be tested both laying down and immediately after standing up. If your blood pressure doesn't go up at least 10 points when going from laying to standing, that indicates adrenal weakness.

✓ **Neurotransmitter testing**—There are various ways to measure neurotransmitters, but due to the inability for most neurotransmitters to cross the blood brain barrier, there isn't a good way to measure the levels of neurotransmitters affecting the brain. While there is value in testing neurotransmitter levels, if you don't know where to start, the best place is with a test called the Braverman assessment.

  ➢ **The Braverman assessment**—This simple question-and-answer test was designed by the Psychiatrist Eric Braverman and attempts to analyze the levels of dopamine, serotonin, GABA and acetylcholine that are actually affecting the brain. The Braverman assessment can be found in Dr. Braverman's book titled, "The Edge Effect."

References:

1.) Kingsley MI, Miller M, Kilduff LP, McEneny J, et al. (January 2006). "Effects of phosphatidylserine on exercise capacity during cycling in active males". Medicine and Science in Sports and Exercise 38 (1): 64–71.

2.) Jäger R, Purpura M, Geiss K-R, et al. (December 2007). "The effect of phosphatidylserine on golf performance". International Society of Sports Nutrition 4 (1): 23.

3.) Scorei, Romulus, Popa, Radu. "Boron-Containing Compounds as Preventive and Chemotherapeutic Agents for Cancer". Anti-cancer agents in medicinal chemistry 10(4): 346-351.

4.) Fallon, James. (2014) The Psychopath Inside. New York, New York. Penguin group. (pg 53).

5.) Stein DJ, Newman TK, Savitz J, Ramesar R. Warriors versus worriers: the role of COMT gene variants. CNS Spectr. 2006 Oct;11(10):745-8.

6.) Mier D, Kirsch P, Meyer-Lindenberg A. Neural substrates of pleiotropic action of genetic variation in COMT: a meta-analysis. Mol Psychiatry. 2010 Sep;15(9):918-27.

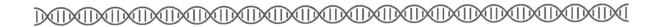

MAOA & MAOB genes

Monoamine oxidase A Monoamine Oxidase B genes

Names of MAOA and MAOB gene genetic variants (SNP identification)	rsnumber	Risk allele
MAOA C42794T	rs909525	Risk allele is C = Warrior gene = slower enzyme= higher levels of serotonin, dopamine and norepinephrine = high stress response + more aggressive behavior Normal allele is T = enzyme works at normal rate = lower levels of serotonin, dopamine and norepinephrine = lower stress response + less aggressive behavior
MAOA R297R/G492T	rs6323	Risk allele is T = Warrior gene = slower enzyme = higher levels of serotonin, dopamine and norepinephrine= decreased chance of depression + high stress response + more aggressive behavior Normal allele is G = faster enzyme = lower levels of serotonin, dopamine and norepinephrine = increased risk for depression = increased chance of depression + lower stress response + less aggressive behavior
MAOB A118723G	rs1799836	Risk allele is C = higher levels of dopamine and histamines

What do the MAO-A and MAO-B genes do?

MAOA and MAOB genes can only be passed down from the mother because they are only on the X-chromosome. Men will only have one copy of this gene, because they only have one X chromosome, whereas women will have two copies of the gene because they have two X chromosomes.

- **The MAOA gene**—This gene provides the body's instructions for making the MAO-A enzyme, which is involved in the metabolism of monoamines like serotonin, norepinephrine and dopamine.

- **The MAOB gene**—This gene provides the body's instructions for making the MAOB enzyme, which is mainly involved in the metabolism of the *dopamine neurotransmitter and allergy-inducing histamines.*

What does having the MAOA warrior gene mean?

Having the MAOA warrior gene is much different than having the COMT warrior gene.

The MAOA "warrior gene" is associated with *higher* levels of dopamine, serotonin and norepinephrine. The COMT "warrior gene" is associated with *lower* levels of dopamine, epinephrine, norepinephrine and estrogen.

The MAOA warrior gene is associated with aggressive behavior, a stronger stress response and a possible lack of empathy[8]. The combination of being aggressive and lacking empathy can be beneficial for a warrior going into battle.

A study from Caltech found that people with the MAOA warrior gene tend to make better financial decisions under pressure rather than freezing in a stressful situation[11].

About 30 percent of Caucasians have the MAOA warrior gene 11. The percentage is much higher among Africans, Chinese, and the indigenous Maori people of New Zealand[11].

What health problems are associated with having an MAOA or MAOB risk allele?

Most health problems associated with the MAOA or MAOB risk alleles are because the MAO enzymes are too slow or too fast at breaking down serotonin, dopamine and norepinephrine. This can lead to abnormally high low levels of serotonin, dopamine and norepinephrine.

- **Slower MAO enzyme**—If you have the genotype that causes the MAO enzyme to work slower, then you are said to have the *"warrior gene."* The warrior gene is associate with having a slower MAOA enzyme, which leads to higher levels of dopamine, serotonin and norepinephrine. These higher levels tend to create more aggressive behavior, a more intense stress response and a potential lack of empathy[8]. Below is a list of some health problems associated with having a risk allele that causes the MAO enzyme to work at a much slower rate, as in

Christy L. Sutton D.C.

people with the genotypes MAOA C42794T (rs909525-C allele) and MAOA (rs6323-T allele).

- ➢ Schizophrenia[5, 6]
- ➢ Alcoholism[1, 11]
- ➢ Nicotine dependence in women[1]
- ➢ Panic disorders[2]
- ➢ Obsessive compulsive disorder[3, 11]
- ➢ Bipolar disorder[4]
- ➢ Novelty-seeking personality
- ➢ Sleep disorders
- ➢ Fibromyalgia
- ➢ Allergies (allergies are more common with MAO-B risk alleles)
- ➢ Psychopathic disorders
- ➢ Antisocial personality disorder in women[7]
- ➢ Aggressive behavior[8,11]
- ➢ ADHD in females[9]
- ➢ Social phobia[11]
- ➢ Hypertension[11]
- ➢ Difficulty experiencing and expressing love[11]
- ➢ Allergies (this is only with the risk allele for the MAOB gene)

- **Faster MAO enzyme**—If you have a risk allele that causes the MAO enzyme to break down serotonin, dopamine and norepinephrine too quickly, as in people with the genotype MAOA (rs6323-G allele), you're at an increased risk for low levels of serotonin, dopamine, and norepinephrine. This can lead to depression.

  - ➢ **Depression**—Having the G allele for the MAOA (rs6323) can lead to an MAO-A enzyme that works at a faster rate than normal, which can lead to depression due to having lower levels of serotonin, dopamine and norepinephrine[10].

It's important to remember that much of our behavior is learned, and doesn't only depend on the genes that we received from our parents. How we are raised as a child and the environment that you're exposed to are essential factors in your levels of empathy and behavior.

The Warrior Genes (COMT and MAO Genes) and Stress

Stress activates the sympathetic nervous system, the part of the nervous system that triggers the fight or flight response. The sympathetic nervous system is what makes you want to fight or run away when confronted with a stressful situation. When this system is activated, it causes increased production of dopamine, epinephrine and norepinephrine.

One way to prevent overstimulation of the sympathetic nervous system is to promote the "rest and digest" part of our nervous system, called the parasympathetic nervous system (PNS).

Ways to decrease your "fight or flight" response and increase your "rest and digest" response including:

- Meditation

- Massage

- A chiropractic adjustment of the occiput or sacrum

- Deep breathing

- Be in nature

- Light exercise

- Maintain a stable blood sugar

- Live below your means

- Laugh

- Focus on the positive

- Make time to be thankful

A genetic combination that can make you more sensitive to stress

Below is a list of genotypes that can lead to higher levels of dopamine, norepinephrine, epinephrine, and serotonin. The higher levels of these substances is what can lead to sensitivity to stress.

- COMT V158M (rs4680- A allele)
- MAOA C42794T (rs909525-C allele)
- MAOA (rs6323- T allele).
- MAOB A118723G (rs1799836- C allele)

Christy L. Sutton D.C.

I have one or more risk allele(s) in the MAOA or MAOB genes. What should I talk to my doctor about doing so that I can reduce my health risks?

- **Consider supplementing with a quality vitamin B-complex**—The B complex should contain all of the B vitamins and plenty of vitamins B-2, B-5, and B-6. Taking a high-quality B- complex with the activated form of vitamin B-2 (Riboflavin 5-Phosphate), vitamin B6 (Pyridoxal-5-Phosphate) and vitamin B5 (pantothenic acid) is very important.

  - ➤ **Vitamin B-2**—The MAO-A and MAO-B enzyme requires vitamin B-2. Taking Vitamin B-2 will ensure that the MAO-A enzyme is functioning at the highest level possible and breaking down serotonin, dopamine and norepinephrine at the highest rates possible.

  - ➤ **Vitamins B6 and B5**—Both are important for helping the body metabolize extra serotonin.

- **Ensure you aren't low in zinc or progesterone**—Zinc and progesterone increase the MAO enzyme efficiency and synthesis, which can help counter the lower level of MAO enzyme activity seen with the genotypes MAOA C42794T (rs909525-C allele) and MAOA (rs6323-T allele). Being deficient in zinc can lead to low levels of progesterone.

- **Monitor and reduce stress**—Stress can initiate a viscous cycle that is hard to break for anyone with a risk allele in the COMT gene. Meditation, long relaxing walks and massages can keep your body's stress level from getting too high, which can protect you from developing health problems related to having a risk allele in the MAOA or MAOB genes. Lower levels of stress and proper stress-handling techniques will reduce the potential for health problems related to having a MAOA or MAOB risk allele.

- **Protect your brain with proper nutrition**—Excess dopamine and chronic stress can be damaging to the brain, particularly to the prefrontal cortex. Nutrients that help protect the brain include:

  - ➤ **Fish oil**—Fish oil can help protect the brain from the damage that stress can cause.

> ***Phosphatidylserine***—Phosphatidylserine has shown to not only protect the brain, but also to lower stress-induced spikes in cortisol levels. In addition to combating mental stress, phosphatidylserine has been shown to combat exercise-induced stress and improve performance and recovery in golf and cycling[12,13]. Try taking it for your putting game and see if it makes a difference!

> ***Antioxidants***—High levels of stress can easily deplete vitamin C. Vitamins C, A, E, alpha lipoic acid, glutatheione, and CoQ10 are antioxidants that can protect the brain from damage. A diet high in fruits and veggies is high in antioxidants.

- ***Participate in aerobic exercise at or below your target heart rate***—While exercise is a good stress reliever and is essential for health, certain types of exercise can be stress-inducing—including extreme sports, aerobic exercise and aerobic exercise that is above the target heart range. These activities can increase the body's stress response, which can cause an excessive amount of dopamine, norepinephrine and epinephrine in someone with MAOA or MAOB gene risk alleles. It's important to monitor heart rate and blood pressure because high levels of norepinephrine and epinephrine can increase both. I recommend that you exercise with a heart rate monitor to ensure that you're not overtaxing your body. Talk to your doctor before starting a new exercise program.

- ***Avoid caffeine and smoking***—Caffeine and smoking increase dopamine levels, which can get too high with certain MAOA and MAOB risk alleles.

- ***Practice caution is using amphetamine-based drugs***—Amphetamine-based drugs can ramp up dopamine, norepinephrine and epinephrine. These drugs are often used to treat narcolepsy, ADD and ADHD. Contact your prescribing physician before changing or stopping any drugs.

- ***Calming essential oils***—Smell can have very powerful effects on the brain. The right calming smells can quickly decrease a stress response.

- ***Exercise caution when using dopamine- and serotonin-increasing drugs***—Contact your prescribing physician before stopping any drugs.

- ***Eat a diet high in vegetables, fruit, good fats and protein***—This can help to keep your blood sugar stable, which can reduce the body's overall stress level.

Christy L. Sutton D.C.

I have one or more risk allele(s) in the MAOA or MAOB gene. What labs/testing should I consider to continually monitor my health?

There are functional tests anyone with MAO mutations should consider. These tests should be performed by a qualified and trained health care provider.

✓ ***Nutreval Plasma by Genova Diagnostics (blood and urine test)***—The Nutreval test measures metabolites that reflect how your body is breaking down dopamine, epinephrine and norepinephrine. The test also measures the levels of vitamins, minerals and good fats, which are important for a healthy brain.

✓ ***Monitor blood pressure and heart rate***—If you have an MAOA or MAOB risk allele, that can increase dopamine, epinephrine and norepinephrine levels, which can increase blood pressure and heart rate.

  ➢ ***The Ragland's test***—This blood pressure test requires blood pressure to be tested when laying and immediately after standing up. If blood pressure does not go up at least 10 points when going from laying to standing, then that indicates adrenal weakness.

✓ ***Neurotransmitter testing***—There are various ways to measure neurotransmitters, but due to the inability for most neurotransmitters to cross the blood brain barrier, there is not a good way to measure the levels of neurotransmitters affecting the brain. While there is value in testing neurotransmitter levels, if you don't know where to start, start with a test called the Braverman assessment.

  ➢ The Braverman assessment—This simple question-and-answer test was designed by psychiatrist Eric Braverman and attempts to analyze the levels of dopamine, serotonin, GABA and acetylcholine that are actually affecting the brain. The Braverman assessment can be found in Dr. Braverman's book titled, "The Edge Effect."

All Convicted Psychopaths Have the MAOA "Warrior" Gene + Childhood Trauma

"Real nurture can overcome a lousy hand
of cards dealt by nature"
— James Fallon

What does it take to become a psychopath?

Dr. James Fallon, a neuroscientist and professor of psychiatry, wrote a very good book titled, "The Psychopath Inside." The book identifies three genetic and environmental factors for becoming a psychopath, including:

1.) *Having the MAO "warrior" genes that lead to a slower MAO-A enzyme, and thus to naturally higher levels of serotonin, dopamine and norepinephrine*—Serotonin is a major neurotransmitter in mood disorders and psychopathy. People who have the MAOA "warrior genes" can have chronically high levels of serotonin. As a result, the parts of their brain that respond to serotonin become desensitized to serotonin and effectively those parts can get turned off. The "turning off" of the serotonin parts of the brain begins in utero, especially in the 2nd and 3rd trimesters. Fetuses that inherit the MAOA warrior genes develop brains in a high serotonin environment. The high serotonin levels that a fetus is exposed to during the 2nd and 3rd trimesters are a significant part of what leads to developing a brain that doesn't respond to serotonin appropriately. It's the brain's inappropriate response to serotonin that ultimately leads to the altered moods and emotions that can been seen in people with the MAOA warrior genes.

Why are men more likely to be psychopaths than women? It's well known that men are more likely to become psychopaths than women. It's thought that the reason is because the MAOA gene is only on the X chromosome. Men only have one X chromosome, and therefore, only have one copy of the MAOA gene, whereas women have two copies of the MAOA gene. In this case the second X chromosome that women have can function as a "spare tire" to help balance their brain chemistry.

2.) **Abuse or exposure to severe trauma as a young child (abuse can be physical, emotional or sexual)**—Exposure to abuse is most damaging during the first three years of a child's life. Abuse during that time causes irreversible damage to the brain, particularly to the frontal lobe. Damage to the frontal lobe of the brain is always seen on the PET scans of convicted psychopaths. Dr. Fallon's research found that all convicted psychopaths had experienced abuse as a child, and many had lost one or more of their biological parents[11].

3.) **Damage to certain parts of the brain**—Dr. Fallon found that certain parts of the brain are damaged in psychopaths. The brain damage is a result of being exposed to high levels of serotonin in utero and experiencing abuse as a young child. The parts of the brain that were damaged in psychopaths include:

- **The frontal lobe (orbital cortex)**—The orbital cortex of the frontal lobe processes ethics, morality and impulsivity. This part of the brain does not develop if there is abuse during the early years of life. This means that young children who are abused will develop brains that are less capable of making ethical, moral and controlled decisions.

- **The amygdala**—The amygdala was found to be shrunken in psychopaths. The amygdala is a part of the brain called the limbic system and is important for regulation of emotions. People with a shrunken amygdala are more likely to be considered hot-headed, or quick to anger.

- **The insula**—The insula is part of the brain's temporal lobe, and is important for self-awareness, perception and empathy. If this part of the brain is damaged, there will be a lack of self-awareness and empathy. The insula is deep within the brain, so a very high-quality PET scan of the brain is required to pick up damage to the insula.

How to Raise a Healthy Child Who May Have Inherited Your 'Warrior Gene'

We can't change the genes that we pass on to our children. However, we can change the environment that we expose our children to. Passing on the warrior gene is not necessarily a bad thing if the child is raised in the correct environment. In fact, many of the smartest, most successful, most influential people in the world have the "warrior genes," which have given them a strong drive and ability to focus. There are some specific things that can and should be done to nurture a child with a warrior gene to help them thrive:

1.) ***Avoid stress while pregnant***—Stressors like maternal use of alcohol, illegal drugs, psychoactive medications, maternal anxiety and fear can alter the later behavior of a child[11].

2.) ***While pregnant, eat a diet to promote lower serotonin levels rather than high serotonin levels***—A diet high in protein, vegetables and healthy fats promotes lower serotonin levels, whereas a diet high in carbohydrates and sugar will increase serotonin levels. Therefore, while pregnant it's important to eat a diet that is low in sugar and high in protein, vegetables and healthy fats.

High serotonin levels during the early stages of fetal development can lead to a brain that doesn't respond to serotonin and is more likely to have mental problems. Serotonin is released early in fetal brain development; therefore, it's important to eating a diet that will promote lower serotonin levels throughout your entire pregnancy.

3.) ***Provide a loving, safe, nurturing and mentally stimulating environment for your child so that their brain will develop properly.***

4.) ***Ensure proper nutrition while pregnant:***

- Consider supplementing with a high-quality multivitamin/multimineral prior to and throughout the pregnancy and while breastfeeding.

- Consider supplementing with fish oil—The good fats in fish oil are essential for brain development in utero.

- Eat a healthy diet that is low in sugar, high in protein, high in healthy fats, and high in fruits and vegetables.

- Drink plenty of water.

- Don't drink alcohol—Alcohol can increase serotonin levels and is bad for fetal brain development.

5.) ***Exercise regularly while pregnant***—Walking 45 minutes a day while pregnant will go a long way toward giving birth to a child with a healthy, balanced brain.

6.) ***Take as long of a maternity leave as possible***—The first couple months of a baby's life are sometimes called the 4th trimester. It's a vulnerable time for a baby's brain development[11]. This is a time when a child needs to feel safe and loved in a low-stress environment[11]. While maternity leave can be a huge financial burden for many families, it's a huge investment in your child's future mental health.

References:

1.) Philibert R. A., Gunter T. D., Beach S. R., Brody G. H. & Madan A.MAOA methylation is associated with nicotine and alcohol dependence in women. American journal of medical genetics Part B, Neuropsychiatric genetics: the official publication of the International Society of Psychiatric Genetics 147B, 565–570 (2008).

2.) Reif, A., Richter, J. et al. MAOA and mechanisms of panic disorder revisited: from bench to molecular psychotherapy. Molecular Psychiatry (2014) 19, 122–128.

3.) Camarena B, Rinetti G, et al. Additional evidence that genetic variation of MAO-A gene supports a gender subtype in obsessive-compulsive disorder. Am J Med Genet. 2001 Apr 8;105(3):279–282.

4.) Preisig M, Bellivier F, et al. Association between bipolar disorder and monoamine oxidase A gene polymorphisms: results of a multicenter study. Am J Psychiatry.2000;157(6):948–55.

5.) Kim SK, Park HJ, Seok H, et al. Association study between monoamine oxidase A (MAOA) gene polymorphisms and schizophrenia: lack of association with schizophrenia and possible association with affective disturbances of schizophrenia. Mol Biol Rep (2014) 41:3457–64.

6.) Wei YL, Li CX, Li SB, et al. Association study of monoamine oxidase A/B genes and schizophrenia in Han Chinese. Behav Brain Funct. 2011;7:42.

7.) Philibert RA, Wernett P, Plume J, et al (Jul 2011). "Gene environment interactions with a novel variable Monoamine Oxidase A transcriptional enhancer are associated with antisocial personality disorder". Biological Psychology 87 (3): 366–71.

8.) Cases O, Seif I, Grimsby J, Gaspar P, et al. (Jun 1995). "Aggressive behavior and altered amounts of brain serotonin and norepinephrine in mice lacking MAOA". Science 268(5218): 1763–6.

9.) Biederman J, Kim JW, Doyle AE, et al. Sexually dimorphic effects of four genes (COMT, SLC6A2, MAOA, SLC6A4) in genetic associations of ADHD: a preliminary study. Am J Med Genet B Neuropsychiatr Genet. 2008;147B(8):1511–1518.

10.) Leuchter AF, Mccracken JT, et al.. Monoamine oxidase a and catechol-O-methyltransferase functional polymorphisms and the placebo response in major depressive disorder. J. Clin. Psychopharmacol. 2009;29(4):372–377.

11.) Fallon, James. (2014) The Psychopath Inside. New York, New York. Penguin group.

12.) Kingsley MI, Miller M, Kilduff LP, et al. (January 2006). "Effects of phosphatidylserine on exercise capacity during cycling in active males". Medicine and Science in Sports and Exercise 38 (1): 64–71.

13.) Jäger R, Purpura M, Geiss K-R, Weiß M, Baumeister J, et al. (December 2007). "The effect of phosphatidylserine on golf performance". International Society of Sports Nutrition 4 (1): 23.

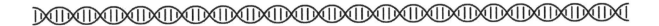

SLC6A2 gene

Solute carrier family 6 member 2 (AKA NET- norepinephrine transporter gene)

Names of SLC6A2 gene genetic variants (SNP identification)	rsnumber	Risk allele
SLC6A2 C10565T	rs3785143	Risk allele is T
SLC6A2 C41517T	rs11568324	Risk allele is T
SLC6A2 T32009C	rs3785152	Risk allele is T
SLC6A2 G47034T	rs1566652	Risk allele is T

What does the SLC6A2 gene do?

The SLC5A2 gene plays an important role in clearing dopamine from the prefrontal cortex, the area of our brain involved in personality, planning, inhibition of behaviors, abstract thinking, emotion and working (short-term) memory.

The SLCA2 gene provides the body's instructions to make a protein called SLC6A2—also known as norepinephrine transporter (NET). The protein SLCA2 is important for bringing dopamine and norepinephrine back into the cell so that it can no longer cause the nervous system to be stimulated and excited.

Christy L. Sutton D.C.

What health problems are associated with having an SLC6A2 risk allele?

- *Depression*

- *Orthostatic intolerance (POTS)*—Elevation of heart rate when standing, light-headedness, fatigue and passing out from going from a resting to standing position.

- *ADHD*[1,2]

  - Having the risk allele for rs3785143 and rs11568324—Associated with an increased risk of developing ADHD.

  - Having the risk allele for rs1566652 G allele—Associated with better response to treatment of ADHD with atomoxetine[3].

  - Having the risk allele for rs3785152 T allele—Associated with better response to treatment of ADHD with atomoxetine[3].

- *Panic disorders*[4]

I have one or more risk allele(s) in the SLC6A2 gene. What should I talk to my doctor about doing so that I can reduce my health risks?

- *Protect your brain with proper nutrition*—Excess dopamine and chronic stress can damage the brain, particularly the prefrontal cortex. Nutrients that help protect the brain include:

  - *Fish oil*—Fish oil can help protect the brain from the damage that stress can cause.

  - *Phosphatidylserine*—Phosphatidylserine has been shown to not only protect the brain, but also to lower stress-induced spikes in cortisol levels. In addition to combating mental stress, phosphatidylserine has been shown to reduce exercise-induced stress and improve performance and recovery in golf and cycling.

> *Antioxidants*—High levels of stress can easily deplete vitamin C. Vitamins C, A, E, alpha lipoic acid, glutathione, and CoQ10 are antioxidants that can protect the brain from damage. A diet high in fruits and veggies is high in antioxidants.

> *B-vitamins*—Stress depletes B vitamins, which are important for a healthy brain and body. Ensure the B-complex has adequate levels of vitamin B-6 in the form called P-5-P. Vitamin B-6 is especially depleted from stress.

- *Monitor and actively try to reduce stress levels*—Stress can cause high dopamine levels, which can exacerbate problems in people with the risk allele for the SLC6A3 gene. Some ways to reduce stress include walking, meditation, talk therapy, sleep and maintaining a stable blood sugar.

- *Participate in aerobic exercise at or below your target heart rate*—Exercise is important for brain health, especially the part of the brain affected by the SLC6A3 gene. While exercise is a good stress reliever and is essential for health, certain types of exercise can be stress-inducing, including extreme sports, aerobic exercise and aerobic exercise above the target heart range. These activities can increase the body's stress response, which can cause an excessive amount of dopamine. Talk to your doctor before starting a new exercise program.

- *Eat a diet high in vegetables, fruit, good fats and protein*—This provides essential nutrients while maintaining a stable blood sugar, which are both essential for brain health.

I have one or more risk allele(s) in the SLC6A2 gene. What labs/testing should I consider to continually monitor my health?

✓ *Monitor blood pressure and heart rate*—If you have an SLC6A2 risk allele, you're at an increased risk of having high dopamine levels, which can increase blood pressure and heart rate.

> *The Ragland's test*—This blood pressure test requires blood pressure to be tested when laying and immediately after standing up. If blood pressure does not go up at least 10 points when going from laying to standing, then that indicates adrenal weakness.

Christy L. Sutton D.C.

✓ **Adrenal testing**—This test monitors stress hormones such as cortisol. High levels of stress hormones can dramatically increase your dopamine levels, which can be hard on the brain, especially if you have a risk allele in the SLC6A2 gene and don't clear dopamine very well from the brain.

✓ **Neurotransmitter testing**—There are various ways to measure neurotransmitters, but due to the inability for most neurotransmitters to cross the blood brain barrier, there is not a good way to measure the levels of neurotransmitters affecting the brain. While there is value in testing neurotransmitter levels, if you don't know where to start, start with a test called the Braverman assessment.

➢ **The Braverman assessment**—This simple question-and-answer test was designed by psychiatrist Eric Braverman and attempts to analyze the levels of dopamine, serotonin, GABA and acetylcholine actually affecting the brain. The Braverman assessment can be found in Dr. Braverman's book titled, "The Edge Effect."

References:

1.) Tellioglu T, Robertson D (November 2001). "Genetic or acquired deficits in the norepinephrine transporter: current understanding of clinical implications". Expert Rev Mol Med 2001 (29): 1–10.

2.) Kim CH, Hahn MK, Joung Y, et al. (December 2006). "A polymorphism in the norepinephrine transporter gene alters promoter activity and is associated with attention-deficit hyperactivity disorder". Proc. Natl. Acad. Sci. U.S.A. 103 (50): 19164–9.

3.) Ramoz N1, Boni C, Downing AM, et al. A haplotype of the norepinephrine transporter (Net) gene Slc6a2 is associated with clinical response to atomoxetine in attention-deficit hyperactivity disorder (ADHD). Neuropsychopharmacology. 2009 Aug;34(9):2135-42.

4.) Esler M, Alvarenga M, Pier C, et al. (Jul 2006). "The neuronal noradrenaline transporter, anxiety and cardiovascular disease". Journal of Psychopharmacology 20 (4 Suppl): 60–6.

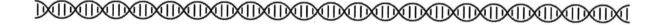

SLC6A3 gene

(Solute carrier family 6 member 2- AKA DAT- dopamine active transporter)

Names of SLC6A3 gene genetic variants (SNP identification)	rsnumber	Risk allele
SLC6A3 G37899A	rs27048	Risk allele is C
SLC6A3 G56022A	rs27072	Risk allele is C
SLC6A3 T26639C	rs464049	Risk allele is A

What does the SLC6A3 gene do?

The SLC6A3 gene is the blueprint for a protein called SLC6A3, which helps remove excessive dopamine from most of the brain. The frontal lobe is the only part of the brain from which SLC6A3 does not clear excess dopamine. The SLC6A2 gene may play a larger role in clearing excess dopamine from the frontal lobe[1].

What health problems are associated with the SLC6A3 gene?

The SLC6A3 gene plays a role in many dopamine-related disorders, such as:

- *ADHD*—Having the risk allele for SLC6A3 G37899A (rs27048) is associated with an increased risk of ADHD.

- *Schizophrenia*—Having the risk allele for SLC6A3 T26639C (rs464049) is associated with an increased risk of developing schizophrenia.

- *Bipolar disorder*

- *Clinical depression*

- *Alcoholism*

- *Parkinson's*

- *Tourette syndrome*

- *Substance abuse*

Christy L. Sutton D.C.

I have one or more risk allele(s) in the SLC6A3 gene. What should I talk to my doctor about doing so that I can reduce my health risks?

- **Protect your brain with proper nutrition**—Excess dopamine and chronic stress can be damaging to the brain, particularly to the prefrontal cortex. Nutrients that help protect the brain include:

  - ➤ **Fish oil**—Fish oil can help protect the brain from the damage that stress can cause.

  - ➤ **Phosphatidylserine**—Phosphatidylserine has been shown to not only protect the brain, but also lower stress-induced spikes in cortisol levels. In addition to combating mental stress, phosphatidylserine has been shown to combat exercise-induced stress and improve performance and recovery in golf and cycling[2,3].

  - ➤ **Antioxidants**—High levels of stress can easily deplete vitamin C. Vitamins C, A, E, alpha lipoic acid, glutathione, and CoQ10 are antioxidants that can protect the brain from damage. A diet high in fruits and veggies is high in antioxidants.

  - ➤ **B-vitamins**—Stress depletes B vitamins, which are important for a healthy brain and body. Ensure adequate levels of Vitamin B-6 in the form called P-5-P. Vitamin B-6 is especially depleted from stress.

- **Monitor and actively try to reduce stress levels**—Stress can cause high dopamine levels, which can exacerbate problems in people with the risk allele for the SLC6A3 gene. Some ways to reduce stress include walking, meditation, talk therapy, sleep and maintaining a stable blood sugar.

- **Participate in aerobic exercise at or below your target heart rate**—Exercise is important for brain health, especially the part of the brain affected by the SLC6A3 gene. While exercise is a good stress reliever and is essential for health, certain types of exercise can be stress-inducing. Some of those exercises include extreme sports, aerobic exercise and aerobic exercise that is above the target heart range. These activities can increase your body's stress response, which can cause an excessive amount of dopamine.

- **Eat a diet high in vegetables, fruit, good fats and protein**—This provides essential nutrients while maintaining a stable blood sugar, which are both essential for brain health.

I have one or more risk allele(s) in the SLC6A3 gene. What labs/testing should I consider to continually monitor my health?

✓ **Adrenal testing**—This test monitors stress hormone such as cortisol. High levels of stress hormones can dramatically increase your dopamine levels, which can be hard on the brain, especially if you have a risk allele in the SLC6A3 gene and don't clear dopamine very well from the brain.

✓ **Monitor blood pressure and heart rate**—If you have an SLC6A3 risk allele, you're at an increased risk of having high dopamine levels, which can increase blood pressure and heart rate.

    ➤ **The Ragland's test**—This blood pressure test requires blood pressure to be tested when laying down and immediately after standing up. If blood pressure doesn't go up at least 10 points when going from laying to standing, then that indicates adrenal weakness.

✓ **Neurotransmitter testing**—There are various ways to measure neurotransmitters, but due to the inability for most neurotransmitters to cross the blood brain barrier, there isn't a good way to measure the levels of neurotransmitters affecting the brain. While there is value in testing neurotransmitter levels, if you don't know where to start, start with a test called the Braverman assessment.

    ➤ **The Braverman assessment**—This simple question-and-answer test was designed by psychiatrist Eric Braverman. This test attempts to analyze the levels of dopamine, serotonin, GABA and acetylcholine that are actually affecting the brain. The Braverman assessment can be found in Dr. Braverman's book titled, "The Edge Effect."

Christy L. Sutton D.C.

The risks of smoking marijuana

Teenagers who smoke marijuana are at an increased risk of developing schizophrenia or other psychotic disorders as adults, especially if they have a family history of mental illness[1]. There are many genetic variants associated with an increased risk of schizophrenia and or other psychotic disorders. While you can't change your genes, you can change your environment.

References:

1.) MacDonald, Anna. Harvard Health Publications Teens who smoke pot at risk for later schizophrenia, psychosis. (2011. March 7TH). Retrieved from: http://www.health.harvard.edu/blog/teens-who-smoke-pot-at-risk-for-later-schizophrenia-psychosis-201103071676

References:

1.) Carboni E, Tanda GL, Frau R, Di Chiara G (1990). "Blockade of the noradrenaline carrier increases extracellular dopamine concentrations in the prefrontal cortex: evidence that dopamine is taken up in vivo by noradrenergic terminals". J. Neurochem. 55 (3): 1067–70.

2.) Kingsley MI, Miller M, Kilduff LP, et al. (January 2006). "Effects of phosphatidylserine on exercise capacity during cycling in active males". Medicine and Science in Sports and Exercise 38 (1): 64–71.

3.) Jäger R, Purpura M, Geiss K-R, Weiß M, et al. (December 2007). "The effect of phosphatidylserine on golf performance". International Society of Sports Nutrition 4 (1): 23.

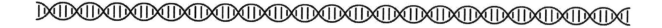

Personalized genetic report found at http://geneticdetoxification.com

GAD1 gene
Glutamate decarboxylase 1 gene

Names of GAD1 gene genetic variants (SNP identification)	rsnumber	Risk allele
GAD1 C10180T	rs2241165	Risk allele is C
GAD1 C14541T	rs3828275	Risk allele is T
GAD1 C2627A	rs12185692	Risk allele is A
GAD1 C34281T	rs701492	Risk allele is T
GAD1 G25509C	rs769407	Risk allele is C
GAD1 G39901A	rs3791850	Risk allele is A
GAD1 G3992T	rs3791878	Risk allele is T
GAD1 G5276A	rs3749034	Risk allele is A
GAD1 T21922C	rs2058725	Risk allele is C
GAD1 T30473C	rs3791851	Risk allele is C

What does the GAD1 gene do?

The GAD1 gene helps prevent anxiety. The GAD1 gene provides the body with the blueprint to make the GAD1 enzyme, which converts the excitatory and anxiety-producing neurotransmitter called glutamate into the calming neurotransmitter called GABA.

There is another gene called GAD2 that is sometimes confused with GAD1 due to their similarity in appearance. GAD1 is only in the brain, whereas GAD2 is found in the brain and pancreas. For this reason, GAD2 is also associated with diabetes, whereas GAD1 is not be associated with diabetes.

What health problems might be associated with having a GAD1 risk allele?

A GAD1 risk allele can lead to an increased anxiety level due to low levels of the calming neurotransmitter GABA and high levels of the excitatory neurotransmitter glutamate[2]. Some health problems associated with having a risk allele in the GAD1 gene include:

- *Major depression*[1]

Christy L. Sutton D.C.

- *Generalized anxiety disorder[1,2]/Panic disorder[1]/Agoraphobia[1]/Social phobia[1]/Neuroticism[1]*

- *Schizophrenia, bipolar disorder and panic disorders*—Having a risk allele for GAD1 G5276A (rs3749034) is associated with an increased risk for developing schizophrenia, bipolar disorder and panic disorders.

- *Increased risk of developing a heroin dependence*—Having the risk allele(s) for GAD1 rs1978340, rs3791878, and rs11542313 are largely associated with an increased risk of heroin dependence[3]. The increased chance of heroin dependence is likely a self-medicating mechanism that results from an attempt to manage low levels of the calming neurotransmitter GABA.

- *Post traumatic seizures*—Having the risk allele for GAD1 C14541T (rs3828275) is associated with an increased risk of developing post-traumatic seizures[4].

Simply having the risk alleles for the GAD1 gene doesn't mean that you'll definitely develop the associated health problems. It's important to remember that our daily habits and environment play a large role in mental health and mental illnesses.

I have one or more risk allele(s) in the GAD1 gene. What should I talk to my doctor about doing so that I can reduce my health risks?

- *Consider GABA or L-theanine supplementation if anxiety levels are high*— These can sometimes help decrease or prevent anxiety.

- *Avoid MSG and MSG-like chemicals in food*—Eating a diet high in MSG or free from glutamic acid can increase symptoms like anxiety, diarrhea, increased heart rate and headaches after consuming MSG. MSG causes on over-excitatory response in the nervous system. Read more about MSG on page 120.

- *Ensure high-quality sleep*—Adequate sleep is essential for brain health.

- *Find out if gluten is a problem*—People with celiac disease are known to produce antibodies to the GAD protein. If you produce antibodies to the GAD protein, that could compound the health problems related to having a GAD1 risk allele.

- **_Practice stress monitoring and stress-reducing activities_**—Stress can increase the health problems related to having a GAD1 risk allele because stress can increase the amount of glutamate that the body makes. Walking, meditation, prayer, talk therapy, sleep, maintaining a stable blood sugar and aerobic exercise can be helpful in controlling stress levels.

- **_Participate in aerobic exercise at or below your target heart rate_**—Aerobic exercise can be a great way to lower stress. However, exercise that is above your target heart range can add more stress to the body. Talk to your doctor before beginning a new exercise program.

- **_Protect your brain with proper nutrition_**—High levels of glutamate and chronic stress can be damaging to the brain, particularly to the prefrontal cortex. Nutrients that help protect the brain include:

  - **_Fish oil_**—Fish oil can help protect the brain from damage caused by stress.

  - **_Phosphatidylserine_**—Phosphatidylserine has shown to not only protect the brain, but also to lower stress-induced spikes in cortisol levels. In addition to combating mental stress, phosphatidylserine has shown to combat exercise-induced stress and improve performance and recovery in golf and cycling.

  - **_Antioxidants_**—High levels of stress can easily deplete vitamin C. Vitamins C, A, E, alpha lipoic acid, glutathtione, and CoQ10 are antioxidants that can protect the brain from damage. A diet high in fruits and veggies is high in antioxidants.

  - **_B-vitamins_**—Stress depletes B vitamins, which are important for a healthy brain and body. Ensure adequate levels of vitamin B-6 in the form called P-5-P. Vitamin B-6 is especially depleted from stress.

- **_Eat a diet high in vegetables, fruit, good fats and protein_**—This will help provide essential nutrients while maintaining a stable blood sugar, which are both essential for brain health.

Christy L. Sutton D.C.

I have one or more risk allele(s) in the GAD1 gene. What labs/testing should I consider to continually monitor my health?

- ✓ **Neurotransmitter testing**—There are various ways to measure neurotransmitters, but due to the inability for most neurotransmitters to cross the blood brain barrier, there is not a good way to measure the levels of neurotransmitters affecting the brain. While there is value in testing neurotransmitter levels, if you don't know where to start, start with a test called the Braverman assessment.

  - ➤ **The Braverman assessment**—This simple question-and-answer test was designed by psychiatrist Eric Braverman. This test attempts to analyze the levels of dopamine, serotonin, GABA and acetylcholine that are actually affecting the brain. The Braverman assessment can be found in Dr. Braverman's book titled, "The Edge Effect."

- ✓ **Consider testing for celiac disease**—Celiac disease can lead to additional anxiety and damage to the part of the brain that makes GABA.

References:

1.) Neale MC, Bukszar J, van den Oord EJ, et al. Association between glutamic acid decarboxylase genes and anxiety disorders, major depression, and neuroticism. 2006 Aug;11(8):752-62. Epub 2006 May 23.

2.) Weber H1, Scholz CJ, Domschke K, , et al. Gender differences in associations of glutamate decarboxylase 1 gene (GAD1) variants with panic disorder. PLoS One. 2012;7(5):e37651.

3.) Wu W1, Zhu YS, Li SB. Polymorphisms in the glutamate decarboxylase 1 gene associated with heroin dependence. Biochem Biophys Res Commun. 2012 May 25;422(1):91-6.

4.) Darrah SD1, Miller MA, Ren D, et al. Genetic variability in glutamic acid decarboxylase genes: associations with post-traumatic seizures after severe TBI. Epilepsy Res. 2013 Feb;103(2-3):180-94.

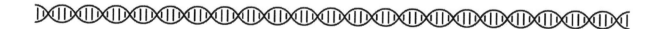

GCH1 gene
GTP cyclohydrolase 1 gene

Names of GCH1 gene genetic variants (SNP identification)	rsnumber	Risk allele
GCH1	rs2878169	Risk allele is T

What does the GCH1 gene do?

The GCH1 gene is the blueprint for the GTPCH (GTP cyclohydrolase I) enzyme, which is the rate-limiting step in the production of tetrahydrobiopterin (BH4). BH4 is a chemical that plays an important role in blood circulation, synthesis of amino acids, synthesis of dopamine, synthesis of serotonin, synthesis pain-regulating catecholamines, and synthesis of nitric oxide. High levels of BH4 are known to increase pain.

What health problems are associated with having a GCH1 risk allele?

Low levels of BH4—Having a risk allele in the GCH1 gene can lead to lower levels of BH4, which can have many other health effects:

- *Lower pain levels*[1]—High levels of BH4 can lead to higher levels of pain. While BH4 is necessary for health, you can have too much of a good thing.

- *Decreased serotonin and dopamine production*—Low serotonin levels can result in depression and sleep disturbances, while low dopamine can cause fatigue, lack of focus, and depression.

- *Lower levels of nitric oxide, which can lead to:*

  ➢ Fatigue
  ➢ Decreased circulation
  ➢ Decrease workout stamina
  ➢ Erectile dysfunction or decreased libido
  ➢ Irritability, depression, anxiety
  ➢ Neurodegenerative diseases
  ➢ Difficulty sleeping
  ➢ High blood pressure/ hypertension
  ➢ Heart attack
  ➢ Asthma
  ➢ Strokes

Christy L. Sutton D.C.

> ➤ Pregnancy-induced hypertension and separation of the placenta (placenta abruption)

Having a risk allele in the GCH1 gene can cause BH4 deficiency. Other genes covered in this book that indirectly affect BH4 levels include the MTHFR A1298C, the NOS1 gene, the NOS2 gene, the NOS3 gene and the DHFR gene.

I have one or more risk allele(s) in the GCH1 gene. What should I talk to my doctor about doing so that I can reduce my health risks?

- *Exercise*—Exercise is one of the best ways to promote brain health and naturally increase production of neurotransmitters and nitric oxide.

- *Consider taking a complete B-complex with all the B vitamins in the active form*—This can help support normal BH4 levels and brain health.

- *Monitor and reduce inflammation*—Some of the best ways to reduce inflammation include supplementing with turmeric and fish oil and eating a low-sugar diet. It's also important to remove chronic inflammation triggers such as food allergies, chronic infections, stress and high levels of toxins.

I have one or more risk allele(s) in the GCH1 gene. What labs/testing should I consider to continually monitor my health?

- ✓ *Nitric oxide (salivary test)*—This can help determine if your nitric oxide levels are too low. Low nitric oxide levels can be aside effect of having a GCH1 risk allele and can lead to circulatory problems.

- ✓ *Inflammatory markers including CRP and homocysteine (blood test).*

- ✓ *Calcium score test*—This test is used to check for heart disease in an early stage and to determine how severe it is. It monitors for buildup of calcium in plaque on the walls of the arteries in the heart. This test does emit a low level of radiation, so antioxidants should be increased prior to and after this test.

References:

1.) Tegeder I, Costigan M, Griffin RS, et al. GTP cyclohydrolase and tetrahydrobiopterin regulate pain sensitivity and persistence. Nat Med. 2006;12(11):1269–77.

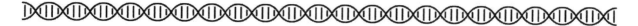

Personalized genetic report found at http://geneticdetoxification.com

DRD1, DRD2, DRD3, DRD4 genes
Dopamine receptor 1, 2, 3, and 4 genes

Names of DRD1, DRD2, DRD3, DRD4 gene genetic variants (SNP identification)	rsnumber	Risk allele
DRD1 T5262C	rs265981	Risk allele is G
DRD1 G6014A	rs4532	Risk allele is T
DRD2 A61820G—Increased risk of developing schizophrenia[7]	rs1079727	Risk allele T
DRD1 C7464T	rs686	Risk allele is A
DRD2 G54716A	rs1079597	Risk allele is T
DRD2 G65466T	rs2283265	Risk allele is C
DRD2 G67314T— Increased risk for alcoholism	rs1076560	Risk allele is A
DRD3 C26625T— Associated with autism spectrum disorder	rs167771	Risk allele is G
DRD4 C8887A— Increased risk for schizophrenia	rs11246226	Risk allele is A

What do the DRD1, DRD2, DRD3, and DRD4 genes do?

The DRD1, DRD2, DRD3, and DRD4 genes are important for the body to make dopamine receptors—what dopamine binds to so that it can stimulate the nervous system. Without dopamine receptors, dopamine will have no effect on the brain and body. The D1 dopamine receptors (made by the DRD1 gene) are the most abundant dopamine receptors in the central nervous system.

What health problems might be associated with having a DRD1, DRD2, DRD3, and DRD4 risk allele?

Having the risk alleles for the DRD1, DRD2, DRD3 or DRD4 genes can alter the ability for dopamine receptors to bind to dopamine, thus creating abnormal responses in the brain and body. Abnormal responses to dopamine have been implicated in a variety of neuropsychiatric disorders, including:

- Social phobia, Tourette's syndrome, Parkinson's, schizophrenia, ADHD and drug and alcohol dependence[2,3,4,5,6].

- Simply having the risk alleles for the DRD1, DRD2, DRD3 and DRD4 genes doesn't mean that you'll definitely develop health problems associated with the gene. It's important to remember that your daily habits and environment play a large role in mental health and mental illnesses.

I have one or more risk allele(s) in the DRD1, DRD2, DRD3 and DRD4 genes. What should I talk to my doctor about doing so that I can reduce my health risks?

Promote a healthy nervous system through exercise, a healthy diet, blood sugar regulation, stress reduction, smart nutrition, avoid environmental toxins, and adequate intake of good fats to help keep the brain healthy.

I have one or more risk allele(s) in the DRD1, DRD2, DRD3, and DRD4 genes. What labs/testing should I consider to continually monitor my health?

There are no specific tests for the dopamine receptors, but certain tests can provide a level of insight into your overall health, including:

- ✓ **Neurotransmitter testing**—There are various ways to measure neurotransmitters, but due to the inability for most neurotransmitters to cross the blood brain barrier, there isn't a good way to measure the levels of neurotransmitters affecting the brain. While there is value in testing neurotransmitter levels, if you don't know where to start, start with a test called the Braverman assessment.

  - ➤ **The Braverman assessment**—This simple question-and-answer test was designed by psychiatrist Eric Braverman. This test attempts to analyze the levels of dopamine, serotonin, GABA and acetylcholine that are actually affecting the brain. The Braverman assessment can be found in Dr. Braverman's book titled, "The Edge Effect."

- ✓ **Adrenal testing**—Adrenal testing can reveal if cortisol levels are high. Chronically high cortisol levels can be damaging to the brain. The reduced response to dopamine can lead to an increase in cortisol levels.

Boys and autism

Why do boys get autism more than girls? We do not entirely understand why, but a genetic combination could play a role in answering that question.

There is a genetic combination implicated in autism spectrum disorder in families where only males are affected[8]. Having the exact genotype listed below is associated with an increased risk of autism spectrum disorder in boys.

- **DRD1 T5262C (rs265981) (C, C)**
- **DRD1 G6014A (rs4532) (A, A,)**
- **DRD1 C7464T (rs686). (T, T)**

Having this genetic combination is associated with more severe social interaction problems and greater difficulties with nonverbal communication. If your son has this genetic combination, he won't absolutely develop autism. Developing autism is much more complicated and multi-factorial than just this genetic combination.

There are many things that we can do to improve our health. In general, it's helpful to focus on what can be changed rather than what we cannot change. This doesn't mean that ignorance is bliss. It's important to be aware of potential health problems so that you can make informed health decisions.

References:

1) Hettinger JA, Liu X, et al. A DRD1 haplotype is associated with risk for autism spectrum disorders in male-only affected sib-pair families. Am J Med Genet B Neuropsychiatr Genet. 2008;147B:628–636.

2.) Schneier FR, Liebowitz MR, et al. (2000). "Low dopamine D(2) receptor binding potential in social phobia". Am J Psychiatry 157 (3): 457–459.

3.) Kienast T, Heinz A (2006). "Dopamine and the diseased brain". CNS Neurol Disord Drug Targets 5(1): 109–31.

4.) Fuxe K, Manger P, Genedani S, Agnati L (2006). "The nigrostriatal DA pathway and Parkinson's disease". J. Neural Transm. Suppl. Journal of Neural Transmission. Supplementa 70 (70): 71–83.

5.) Faraone SV, Khan SA (2006). "Candidate gene studies of attention-deficit/hyperactivity disorder". J Clin Psychiatry. 67 Suppl 8: 13–20.

6.) Hummel M, Unterwald EM (2002). "D1 dopamine receptor: a putative neurochemical and behavioral link to cocaine action". J. Cell. Physiol. 191 (1): 17–27.

7.) Glatt SJ, Faraone SV, Lasky-Su JA, et al. Family-based association testing strongly implicates DRD2 as a risk gene for schizophrenia in Han Chinese from Taiwan.Mol Psychiatry. 2009;14(9):885–893.

8.) Hettinger J. A., Liu X., Schwartz C. E., et al. (2008). A DRD1 haplotype is associated with risk for autism spectrum disorders in male-only affected sib-pair families. Am. J. Med. Genet. B Neuropsychiatr. Genet. 147B, 628–636.

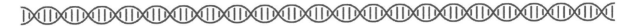

Christy L. Sutton D.C.

ANKK1 gene

Ankyrin repeat and kinase domain containing 1 gene

Names of ANKK1 gene genetic variants (SNP identification)	rsnumber	Risk allele
ANKK1	rs1800497	Risk allele is A

What does the ANKK1 gene do?

The ANKK1 gene can influence the dopamine D2 receptor (DRD2) gene, as well as the response that dopamine has on the brain.

What health problems might be associated with having an ANKK1 risk allele?

Having this risk allele in the ANKK1 gene is associated with a reduced number of dopamine-binding sites in the brain[1], which can lead to a reduced response to dopamine. This can cause the following symptoms:

- *Slower to learn from mistakes that provided negative stimulus/being a slow learner*

- *Poor ability to concentrate*

- *Depression*

- *Increased risk of developing addictive behaviors, including smoking, cocaine use, alcoholism and overeating[1,2]*

I have one or more risk allele(s) in the ANKK1 gene. What should I talk to my doctor about doing so that I can reduce my health risks?

- *Exercise*—Exercise is one of the best ways to promote brain health and naturally increase neurotransmitter production.

- *Consider nutritional support to increase dopamine:*

> ***Vitamin B-6 in the activated form called pyridoxal-5-phosphat (P-5-P)***
> —Vitamin B-6 is required for dopamine production

> ***Tyrosine***

> ***Rhodiola***

- ***Monitor cortisol levels***—A reduced response to dopamine, as seen with ANKK1 risk alleles, can lead to an increase in cortisol levels. Chronically high cortisol levels can be damaging to the brain. If you have high cortisol levels, phosphatidylserine supplementation can help protect your brain.

- ***Promote a healthy nervous system***—The best way to promote a healthy nervous system is through exercise, a healthy diet, good sleep and blood sugar regulation.

- ***Consider supplementing with fish oil***—The good fats found in fish oil can protect the brain and promote mental health.

I have one or more risk allele(s) in the ANKK1 gene. What labs/testing should I consider to continually monitor my health?

There are no specific tests for the dopamine receptors, but there are tests that can provide a level of insight into your overall health, including:

✓ ***Neurotransmitter testing***—There are various ways to measure neurotransmitters, but due to the inability for most neurotransmitters to cross the blood brain barrier, there isn't a good way to measure the levels of neurotransmitters affecting the brain. While there is value in testing neurotransmitter levels, if you don't know where to start, start with a test called the Braverman assessment.

> ***The Braverman assessment***—This simple question-and-answer test was designed by psychiatrist Eric Braverman. This test attempts to analyze the levels of dopamine, serotonin, GABA and acetylcholine that are actually affecting the brain. The Braverman assessment can be found in Dr. Braverman's book titled, "The Edge Effect."

Christy L. Sutton D.C.

✓ **_Adrenal testing_**—Adrenal testing can reveal if your cortisol levels are too high. Chronically high cortisol levels can be damaging to the brain. A reduced response to dopamine can lead to an increase in cortisol levels.

References:

1.) Pohjalainen T, Rinne JO, Någren K, , et al. The A1 allele of the human D2 dopamine receptor gene predicts low D2 receptor availability in healthy volunteers. Mol Psychiatry. 1998;3:256–60.

2.) Klein TA1, Neumann J, Reuter M, Hennig J, et al. Genetically determined differences in learning from errors Science. 2007 Dec 7;318(5856):1642-5.

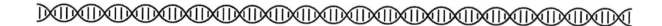

Personalized genetic report found at http://geneticdetoxification.com

ANK3
Ankyrin 3 gene

Names of ANK3 gene Genetic variants (SNP identification)	rsnumber	Risk allele
ANK3 C666301A	rs11599164	Risk allele is T
ANK3 G318473A	rs10994336	Risk allele is T
ANK3 T197902C	rs1938526	Risk allele is G
ANK3 T62085337C	rs10761482	Risk allele is C
ANK3 G658454A	rs9804190	Risk allele is T

What does the ANK3 gene do?

The Ankyrin 3 gene (ANK3 gene) produces the Ankyrin G protein that plays an integral role in regulating neuronal activity and brain health[1].

What health problems are associated with having an ANK3 risk allele?

- *Post-traumatic Stress Disorder (PTSD)*[1]

- *Schizophrenia*[3]—Having the risk allele for ANK3 rs10761482 is associated with a high occurrence of schizophrenia[5]

- *Cardiac arrhythmia* (*palpitations, pounding in chest, dizziness, fainting, shortness of breath, chest pain, fatigue*)[4]

- *Intellectual disability*

- *Bipolar disorder*—Having the risk allele for ANK3 rs10994336 is linked to an increased risk of bipolar disorder. The (C, T) genotype is associated with a 1.45x increased chance of developing bipolar disorder, and the (T, T) genotype is associated with a 2.9x increased chance of developing bipolar disorder[2].

Simply having the risk alleles for the ANK3 doesn't mean that you'll definitely develop health problems associated with the gene. It's important to remember that your daily habits and environment play a large role in mental health and mental illnesses.

Christy L. Sutton D.C.

I have one or more risk allele(s) in the ANK3 gene. What should I talk to my doctor about doing so that I can reduce my health risks?

Ensure quality sleep, avoid stress, exercise regularly, eat a healthy diet with plenty of protein and good fats for the brain, avoid environmental toxins, and consider supplementing with a high-quality B-complex.

I have one or more risk allele(s) in the ANK3 gene. What labs/testing should I consider to continually monitor my health?

Because the health problems associated with high-risk ANK3 genes are largely stress-related, monitoring stress and promoting general health are your best options.

- ✓ *Monitor blood pressure and heart rate*—If you experience any symptoms of a cardiac arrhythmia, immediately go to your doctor to see if you need further heart testing.

- ✓ *Adrenal testing*—Adrenal testing can reveal if cortisol levels are too high. Chronically high cortisol levels can be damaging to the brain.

- ✓ *Nutreval by Genova Diagnostic's (blood and urine)*—This lab tests your levels of antioxidants, vitamins, minerals, heavy metals, toxins and amino acids. The Nutreval test provides a valuable and overarching look at how your environment is affecting your overall health.

- ✓ *Neurotransmitter testing*—There are various ways to measure neurotransmitters, but due to the inability for most neurotransmitters to cross the blood brain barrier, there isn't a good way to measure the levels of neurotransmitters affecting the brain. While there is value in testing neurotransmitter levels, if you don't know where to start, start with a test called the Braverman assessment.

  - ➢ *The Braverman assessment*—This simple question-and-answer test was designed by psychiatrist Eric Braverman. It attempts to analyze the levels of dopamine, serotonin, GABA and acetylcholine that are actually affecting the brain. The Braverman assessment can be found in Dr. Braverman's book titled, "The Edge Effect."

References:

1.) Logue MW, Solovieff N, Leussis MP, et al. The ankyrin-3 gene is associated with post-Traumatic stress disorder and externalizing comorbidity. Psychoneuroendocrinology(2013) 38:2249–5710.

2.) Retrieved from: http://snpedia.com/index.php/Rs10994336

3.) Iqbal, Zafar; Vandeweyer, Geert; van der Voet, et al. (2013). "Homozygous and heterozygous disruptions of ANK3: at the crossroads of neurodevelopmental and psychiatric disorders". Human Molecular Genetics.

4.) Mohler PJ, Rivolta I, Napolitano C, LeMaillet G, et al. (December 2004). "Nav1.5 E1053K mutation causing Brugada syndrome blocks binding to ankyrin-G and expression of Nav1.5 on the surface of cardiomyocytes". Proc. Natl. Acad. Sci. U.S.A.101 (50): 17533–8.

5.) Yuan A, et al. ANK3 as a risk gene for schizophrenia: new data in Han Chinese and meta analysis. Am J Med Genet B Neuropsychiatr Genet. 2012;159B:997–1005.

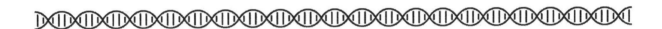

CACNA1C gene

Calcium Channel, Voltage-dependent, L Type, Alpha-1C Subunit gene

Names of CACNA1C gene genetic variants (SNP identification)	rsnumber	Risk allele
CACNA1C A2729632G	rs216013	Risk allele is G
CACNA1C C271442T	rs2159100	Risk allele is T
CACNA1C G115699A	rs1006737	Risk allele is A
CACNA1C T709021C	rs2302729	Risk allele is T

What does the CACNA1C gene do?

The CACNA1C gene provides instructions for making calcium channels, which ultimately play a pivotal role in exciting a nerve and generating electrical signals throughout the brain and body.

What health problems are associated with having a CACNA1C risk allele?

A large-scale genetic analysis conducted revealed the possibility that CACNA1C is associated with bipolar disorder, and subsequently also with schizophrenia[1,2,3].

Christy L. Sutton D.C.

I have one or more risk allele(s) in the CACNA1C gene. What should I talk to my doctor about doing so that I can reduce my health risks?

Support brain health—The best way to support brain health is with regular exercise, high-quality sleep, monitoring and moderating stress in your life, eating a healthy diet, and keeping your brain active through social activity and learning new things.
A healthy diet should include ample amounts of healthy fats, protein, vegetables and fruits. Eating a diet that maintains a stable blood sugar is essential for brain health. Avoid environmental toxins that can disrupt brain health.

I have one or more risk allele(s) in the CACNA1C gene. What labs/testing should I consider to continually monitor my health?

- ✓ *Nutreval Plasma by Genova Diagnostics (blood and urine test)*—The Nutreval test measures metabolites that reflect the levels of dopamine, serotonin, epinephrine and norepinephrine that are being metabolized in the body. This is important because abnormal levels can lead to mental disruption. This test also measures the body's good fats, which are important for a healthy brain. In addition, this lab tests your levels of antioxidants, vitamins, minerals, heavy metals, toxins and amino acids.

- ✓ *Neurotransmitter testing*—There are various ways to measure neurotransmitters, but due to the inability for most neurotransmitters to cross the blood brain barrier, there isn't a good way to measure the levels of neurotransmitters affecting the brain. While there is value in testing neurotransmitter levels, if you don't know where to start, start with a test called the Braverman assessment.

  - ➢ *The Braverman assessment*—This simple question and answer test was designed by psychiatrist Eric Braverman. This test attempts to analyze the levels of dopamine, serotonin, GABA and acetylcholine that are actually affecting the brain. The Braverman assessment can be found in Dr. Braverman's book titled, "The Edge Effect."

- ✓ *Cholesterol, triglycerides, blood pressure and C-reactive protein (blood test)*—Having a risk allele in the CACNA1C gene has been associated with an increased risk for cardiovascular events. These labs monitor blood markers that are important for cardiovascular health.

References:

1.) Green EK, Grozeva D, Jones I, Jones L, et al. (October 2010). "The bipolar disorder risk allele at CACNA1C also confers risk of recurrent major depression and of schizophrenia". Mol. Psychiatry 15(10): 1016–22.

2.) Curtis D, Vine AE, McQuillin A, , et al. (February 2011). "Case-case genome-wide association analysis shows markers differentially associated with schizophrenia and bipolar disorder and implicates calcium channel genes".Psychiatr. Genet. 21 (1): 1–4.

3.) Ferreira MA, O'Donovan MC, Meng YA et al. (September 2008). "Collaborative genome-wide association analysis supports a role for ANK3 and CACNA1C in bipolar disorder". Nat. Genet. 40 (9): 1056 -8.

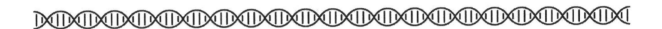

Christy L. Sutton D.C.

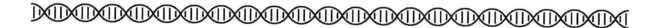

For more information on genes related to brain health, consult the following pages:

Cancer-associated genes:
- SOD2 Pg. 247
- CAT Pg. 251
- NQO1 Pg. 255

Detoxification genes:

- **Methylation Phase II detox genes**
  - MTHFR Pg. 87
  - MTHFD1L Pg. 94
  - MTRR Pg.101
  - MTR Pg. 99
  - MAT1A Pg. 109
  - CBS Pg. 118
  - BHMT Pg. 116

Vitamin and mineral metabolism genes:
- NBPF3 Pg. 366
- VDR Pg. 368
- GC Pg. 370
- SLC30A8 Pg. 374

Immune health genes:
- IL6 Pg. 261
- Celiac genes Pg. 270
- LRP6 Pg. 299
- TLR4 Pg. 304

Cardiovascular health genes:
- CETP. Pg. 351
- NOS1, NOS2, and NOS3 Pg. 358
- LDLR Pg. 353
- OLR1 Pg. 355

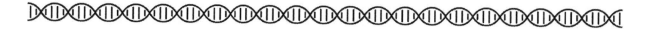

 Personalized genetic report found at http://geneticdetoxification.com

Part 3

Genes Associated with Cancer

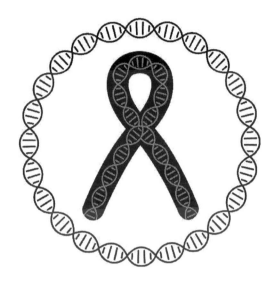

Cancer can be caused by damage to the DNA. Avoiding DNA-damaging activities and having high antioxidant levels is a great way to prevent cancer. Some people are genetically predisposed toward developing cancer because they've inherited genes that prevent them from being able to properly prevent DNA damage and repair damaged DNA.

In this section, you'll learn if you may have inherited some of the genetic changes that may make you more vulnerable to developing cancer, and what you can do to help protect yourself by modifying your environment.

"23andMe" does not sequence all the genes that are associated with cancer. If you are interested in doing more comprehensive genetic testing for cancer, then you should consider doing follow-up genetic testing with your doctor, or through one of the many available direct-to-consumer companies that specializes in doing hereditary cancer genetic testing. It is important to work with your doctor to both prevent cancer and diagnose it in the early stages.

Christy L. Sutton D.C.

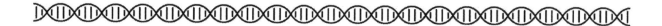

Chapter 8

DNA Damage and Cancer

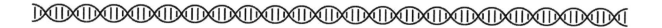

Personalized genetic report found at http://geneticdetoxification.com

BRCA1 and BRCA2
Breast cancer 1 and 2 genes

Names of BRCA1 and BRCA2 genetic variants (SNP identification)	rsnumber	Risk allele
BRCA1 Q356R *	rs1799950	Risk allele is C
BRCA1 S1140G	rs2227945	Risk allele is C
BRCA1 K1183R	rs16942	Risk allele is C
BRCA2 N372H *	rs144848	Risk allele is C
BRCA2 T1915M	rs4987117	Risk allele is T
BRCA2 R2034C	rs1799954	Risk allele is T
BRCA2 S2835P	rs11571746	Risk allele is C
BRCA2 E2856A	rs11571747	Risk allele is C
BRCA2 I2944F	rs4987047,	Risk allele is T
BRCA2 K3326stop	rs11571833	Risk allele is T
BRCA2 I3412V	rs1801426	Risk allele is G

Each risk allele represents an independently minor, but cumulatively significant, increased risk for breast cancer. This means that the more risk alleles you have in the BRCA1 and BRCA2 genes, the higher your risk for breast cancer.

*The above chart of genetic SNPs for BRCA1 and BRCA2 is **not** a complete list. If you are concerned about having risk alleles for the BRCA1 and BRCA2 genes, then you should consider having more thorough genetic testing performed through either your doctor or through a direct-to-consumer company like "color", which specialized in hereditary cancer screenings. It is important to work with your doctor to understand your risk for cancer, and help you decrease your risk of developing cancer.*

What do the BRCA1 and BRCA1 genes do?

BRCA1 and BRCA2 genes suppress tumor formation in the body by playing a role in DNA repair, and eliminating damaged cells if DNA cannot be repaired. The BRCA1 and BRCA2 genes are important for preventing breast, ovarian, and other cancers.

Christy L. Sutton D.C.

What health problems might be associated with having BRCA1 or BRCA2 risk alleles?

- *Women*

  - ➤ ***Women with abnormal BRCA1 and BRCA2 genes have an increased risk for developing breast cancer***—BRCA1 and BRCA2 genes have been described as "breast cancer susceptibility genes". Having many problematic genetic changes in BRCA1 and BRCA2 can result in an increased risk of developing breast cancer. This increased risk of developing breast cancer is due to accumulating more DNA damage and unhealthier breast cells.

    Hereditary BRCA1 and BRCA2 genetic changes account for about 60% of _inherited_ breast cancer and are the only known causes of hereditary breast and ovarian cancer syndrome[1]. _However, most people who develop breast cancer do not inherit an abnormal breast cancer gene and have no family history of the disease_[2]. Therefore, it is essential for every woman to actively work on decreasing her risk of developing breast cancer through practicing healthy daily diet and lifestyle choices.

    You can read ore about how to prevent breast cancer on pages 229-234.

  - ➤ ***Women with an abnormal BRCA1 or BRCA2 gene have an increased risk of developing ovarian, colon, and pancreatic cancers, as well as melanoma***[2].

- *Men*

  - ➤ ***Men who have an abnormal BRCA2 gene have an increased risk of developing breast and prostate cancer***[2].

  - ➤ ***Men with an abnormal BRCA1 gene have a slightly higher risk of prostate cancer***[2].

I have one or more risk allele(s) in the BRAC1 and/or BRAC2 genes. What should I talk to my doctor about doing so that I can reduce my health risks?

To protect yourself from developing cancer, it is necessary to know what factors increase and decrease your risk for developing cancer.

- **Factors that have been shown to *increase* your risk of developing breast cancer, or cancer in general, includes:**

  - *Previous radiation exposure to the breast tissue.*

  - *Taking oral contraceptives.*

  - *Late pregnancy, never being pregnant, or never breastfeeding.*

  - *Being overweight, especially after menopause*—If you have a body mass index over 25, then you are at a higher risk of developing breast cancer, especially if you are post-menopausal or have a personal history of having breast cancer (recurrence). Being overweight increases the risk of developing breast cancer because fat cells make estrogen; extra fat cells means more estrogen in the body, which can make hormone-receptor-positive breast cancers develop and grow[6.]

  - *Early menstrual cycle.*

  - *Being sedentary.*

  - *Being diabetic, or having high insulin levels*-- Postmenopausal women 50 years or older who have type 2 diabetes have about a 20-27 percent increased risk of breast cancer[11.] High insulin levels increase the risk of breast cancer because insulin stimulated the growth of breast cells[12.]

  - *Drinking alcohol*—Increased alcohol consumption is directly correlated with an increased risk of breast cancer. The more that you drink the higher your risk for developing breast cancer.

  - *Smoking*—Smoking and heavy second-hand smoke have been linked to an increased risk of developing breast cancer.

  - *Using hormone replacement therapy*—The hormones that have been shown to increase breast cancer include estrogen, especially estradiol, and

Christy L. Sutton D.C.

synthetic progesterone (progestin). Because the female hormone estrogen stimulates breast cell growth, exposure to estrogen over long periods of time, without any breaks, can increase the risk of breast cancer[6.]

➤ *Family or personal history of breast cancer*—The risk of developing breast cancer is higher if a first-degree relative has had breast cancer (mother, sister, daughter).

➤ *Personal history of certain non-cancerous breast diseases*—Some non-cancerous breast diseases such as atypical hyperplasia or lobular carcinoma are associated with a higher risk of developing breast cancer.

➤ *Routine mammograms*—While mammograms are helpful at diagnosing breast cancer, they <u>do</u> emit cancer causing radiation. You can help reduce the risk of damage from a mammogram by dramatically increasing your antioxidant intake *before and after* having a mammogram. If you are planning to have a mammogram, then you might consider paying extra for the 3-D mammogram. 3-D mammograms provide a clearer image and makes it easier to detect breast cancer. However, mammograms can still miss 20% of breast cancers that are simply not visible using this technique[5]. Other important tools for detecting breast cancer include a monthly breast self-exam, an annual clinical breast examination, ultrasound, and MRI[5]. Finding breast cancer early reduces your risk of dying from the disease by 25-30% or more[3.]

❖ *Cancer-preventing antioxidants that should be considered before and after a mammogram include:*

  ○ Glutathione cream used topically on the breast tissue.
  ○ Vitamin C, Vitamin A, beta carotene, and Vitamin E.
  ○ Vitamin D
  ○ Glucoraphanin
  ○ N-Acetyl cysteine
  ○ Alpha-lipoic acid

➤ *Having dense breast.*

> **Increased age, especially being over 50 years old**—Below is a chart that displays women's risk for developing breast cancer based on their age[4].

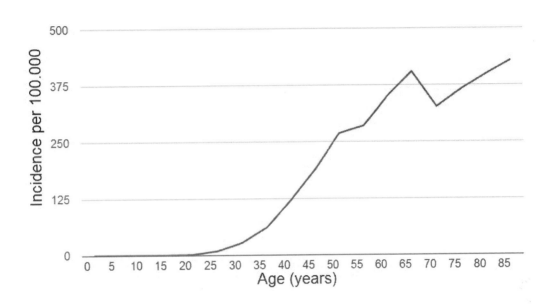

- **Factors that have been shown to naturally _decrease_ your risk of developing breast cancer, or cancer in general, includes:**

  > **Exercise**— Research shows a link between exercising regularly at a moderate or intense level for 4 to 7 hours per week, and a lower risk of breast cancer by 10-20 percent [6-10]. All ages of women experienced a decreased risk of breast cancer with regular exercise, but the most significant decreased risk is seen in post-menopausal women[7-10]. Exercise can also prevent the recurrence of breast cancer if you have already been diagnosed. Exercise consumes and controls blood sugar and limits blood levels of insulin growth factor, a hormone that can affect how breast cells grow and behave[6]. People who exercise regularly tend to be healthier and are more likely to maintain a healthy weight[6].

  > **Ensure you are not deficient in zinc**—Zinc is required for the BRCA1 and BRCA2 proteins to function properly in repairing DNA damage. Therefore, being low in zinc can further diminish your body's ability to suppressor cancer formation.

  > **Eat organic**—Eating food grown without pesticides may protect against unhealthy cell changes associated with pesticides. This is especially important if you have a risk allele in the PON1 gene found on page 132.

Christy L. Sutton D.C.

➤ **Avoid alcohol**—Compared to women who don't drink at all, women who have three alcoholic drinks per week have a 15% higher risk of breast cancer[6]. Experts estimate that the risk of breast cancer goes up another 10% for each additional drink a woman regularly has each day[6]. Research consistently shows that drinking alcohol can increase levels of estrogen and other hormones associated with hormone-receptor-positive breast cancer[6]. Alcohol also may increase breast cancer risk by damaging DNA in cells.

➤ **Maintain a healthy blood sugar and insulin levels**—If diet and exercise are not sufficient for naturally lowering your blood sugar, then nutritional supplementation may help, however, you cannot supplement your way out of an unhealthy diet and lack of exercise. Some nutritional supplements that have been proven to help lower blood sugar include:

   ❖ **Gymnema**—This is an herb that has been shown to improve blood sugar levels by promoting the health and regeneration of the insulin producing cells in the pancreas[13,14]. If you have problems with sugar craving, then sucking on a gymnema tablet prior to eating the sugar can help reduce the sugar cravings.
   ❖ **Rutin**[18]
   ❖ **Bitter Melon**—Some research has indicated that bitter melon either repairs damaged pancreatic beta cells or prevents their death[14].
   ❖ **Quercitin**[19,20]
   ❖ **Resveratrol**— A randomized trial with type 2 diabetic subjects found that the fasting blood glucose, HbA1c, total cholesterol, triglyceride, and low-density lipoprotein concentrations were significantly reduced in the resveratrol group (250 mg/day for three months) compared with those in the control group[16].
   ❖ **Curcumin**[14]
   ❖ **Silymarin**— A randomized double-blind clinical trial also demonstrated a beneficial effect of silymarin (200 mg/day) on high blood sugar levels as shown by a significant decrease in HbA1c at four months after treatment[15,17].
   ❖ **Berberine**[14]
   ❖ **Alpha-lipoic acid**—Research indicates that alpha-lipoic acid lowers blood sugar levels by improving insulin sensitivity.

➤ **Avoid antiperspirant**—Antiperspirant prevent sweating. Sweating, especially in the armpits, is necessary for elimination of toxins around the breast tissue. The connection between antiperspirant and breast cancer is not well studies or established, but the connection between decreased ability to detoxify and an increased risk of breast cancer is well established. Therefore, to increase the body's ability to detoxify it would be wise to not wear antiperspirant.

➢ *Maintain high antioxidant levels*—Antioxidants protect you from DNA damage and cancer. Foods high in antioxidants include fruits, vegetables and green tea. Some antioxidants that can be taken in supplemental form include vitamin C, vitamin E, vitamin A, alpha-lipoic acid, and glucoraphanin. Glutathione is an important antioxidant that is poorly absorbed when taken in supplemental form. However, you can use glutathione creams that are absorbed trans dermally or consider taking nutritional supplementation that can naturally boost your levels—this would include NAC, selenium, and silymarin.

➢ *Maintain high levels of vitamin D*— Research suggests that women with low levels of vitamin D have a higher risk of breast cancer[21]. Vitamin D may play a role in controlling normal breast cell growth and may be able to stop breast cancer cells from growing[21].

➢ *Ensure your body is detoxifying adequately*—You can learn more about how your detox pathways are functioning in the section on detoxification found in part I of this book (pg. 19-140).

➢ *Minimize exposure to estrogenic hormones:*

    ❖ *Avoid excessive estrogen exposure*—Estrogen can be given as a hormone in birth control and hormone replacement therapy. However, many chemicals in our environment act like estrogen in the body (i.e. soy, BPA plastics, pesticides, nail polish, nail polish remover, stearalkonium chloride, and certain creams and cosmetics with parabens).

    ❖ *Don't drink out of plastic bottles or microwave food in plastic*— Plastics contain chemicals that can cause an estrogen-like reaction in the body.

    ❖ *Increase consumption of cruciferous vegetables*—Broccoli, cabbage, cauliflower, Brussel sprouts and watercress. Cruciferous vegetables are high in substances that detoxify estrogen and can reduce cancer risk.

    ❖ *DIM in supplemental form*—Diindolylmethane (DIM) is naturally occurring in cruciferous vegetables, but can also be taken in a supplemental form to help your body remove extra estrogen and reduce cancer risk.

> ***Toss the chemicals***—Try to substitute chemicals that are known to be toxic with nontoxic options. For example, you can clean with baking soda and vinegar rather than toxic cleaning products. This can help to decrease your overall toxicity exposure and level. Many household chemicals are known to be cancer causing and dangerous to your health.

> ***If you can breastfeed, then do***— Breastfeeding has been associated with a decreased risk of breast cancer.

> ***Ensure you are not iodine deficient***—Iodine and iodine-rich seaweed has been shown to inhibit breast tumor development.

> ***Support a healthy lymphatic system***—Having a healthy lymphatic system is essential for preventing breast cancer. Ways to naturally promote a healthy lymphatic system include:

> ❖ Exercise, especially cardiovascular exercise.
> ❖ Drinking plenty of water.
> ❖ Lymphatic brushing.
> ❖ Lymphatic massages.

I have one or more BRCA1 or BRCA2 risk alleles. What labs/testing should I consider to continually monitor my health?

✓ ***Breast examination***— Finding breast cancer early reduces your risk of dying from the disease by 25-30% or more[3]. Examinations to diagnose cancer include a monthly breast self-exam, an annual clinical breast examination, ultrasound, MRI, and mammograms.

✓ ***Routine cancer screenings***—All applicable tests should be performed regularly: colonoscopy, EGD (upper endoscopy of the stomach), skin exam, thyroid exam, prostate exam, Pap smear, and routine blood work.

✓ ***Monitor estrogen levels, especially estradiol.***

✓ ***Vitamin D levels (blood test)***—Vitamin D is important for preventing cancer. I prefer to see vitamin D level around 70 to 100 on lab work.

✓ ***Nutreval by Genova Diagnostic's (blood and urine)***—This lab test monitors your levels of antioxidants, vitamins, minerals, heavy metals, toxins and amino acids. The Nutreval test provides a valuable and overarching look at how your environment is affecting your overall health.

✓ **Measure zinc levels**—Zinc is necessary for the BRCA1 and BRCA2 proteins to function properly in preventing cancer. Ways to monitor zinc levels include.

  o **Zinc taste test**—This is an easy and accurate test that involves putting some liquid zinc in the mouth. If the zinc tastes like water, then it indicates a deficiency.

  o **Zinc blood test**

✓ **Monitor blood sugar levels—Elevated blood sugar and insulin are associated with an increased risk of breast cancer. Labs to consider having to monitor blood glucose levels include:**

  ➤ **Hemoglobin A1C**—This will tell you what your blood sugar has been on average for the previous three months.

  ➤ **C-peptide**—This will tell you the level of insulin your body is making.

  ➤ **Fasting blood glucose**—This will tell you what your blood sugar is at the time of the blood draw.

✓ **DNA oxidative damage test**—This test indicates DNA damage by measuring Urinary 8-hydroxy-2'-deoxyguanosine (8-OHdG), an excellent biomarker of oxidative stress and a risk factor for a variety of diseases, including cancer.

✓ **Monitor Iodine levels**.

✓ **Ivygene**—This is a blood test that measures for circulating tumor DNA (ctDNA), and can identify if cancer is present in very early stages[22].

References:

1.) Pruthi S, Gostout BS, Lindor NM. Identification and Management of Women With BRCA Mutations or Hereditary Predisposition for Breast and Ovarian Cancer. Mayo Clin Proc. 2010;85:1111–1120.

2.) Retrieved from: http://www.breastcancer.org/risk/factors/genetics

3.) Retrieved from: http://www.breastcancer.org/symptoms/slideshows/mammograms

4.) Retrieved from: https://commons.wikimedia.org/wiki/File:Breast_cancer_incidence_by_age_in_women_in_the_UK_2006-2008.png

Christy L. Sutton D.C.

5.) Retrieved from: http://www.breastcancer.org/symptoms/slideshows/mammograms?slide=8

6.) Retrieved from: http://www.breastcancer.org/risk/factors/slideshows/can-control

7.) Eliassen AH, Hankinson SE, Rosner B, et al. Physical activity and risk of breast cancer among postmenopausal women. Arch Intern Med. 170(19):1758-64, 2010.

8.) Wu Y, Zhang D, Kang S. Physical activity and risk of breast cancer: a meta-analysis of prospective studies. Breast Cancer Res Treat. 137(3):869-82, 2013.

9.) Hildebrand JS, Gapstur SM, et al. Recreational physical activity and leisure-time sitting in relation to postmenopausal breast cancer risk. Cancer Epidemiol Biomarkers Prev. 22(10):1906-12, 2013.

10.) Moore SC, Lee I-M, Weiderpass E, et al. Association of leisure-time physical activity with risk of 26 types of cancer in 1.44 million adults. JAMA Intern Med. 176(6):816-25, 2016.

11.) P. Boyle, M. Boniol, A. Koechlin, C. Robertson, et al. "Diabetes and breast cancer risk: a meta-analysis.," Br. J. Cancer, vol. 107, no. 9, pp. 1608–17, Oct. 2012.

12.) Retrieved from: https://www.sciencedaily.com/releases/2009/01/090109173207.htm

13.) Baskaran K, Kizar Ahamath B, Radha Shanmugasundaram K, Shanmugasundaram ER. Antidiabetic effect of a leaf extract from Gymnema sylvestre in non-insulin-dependent diabetes mellitus patients. J Ethnopharmacol. 1990 Oct; 30(3):295-300.

14.) Retrieved from: https://www.ncbi.nlm.nih.gov/pmc/articles/PMC4637477/

15.) Retrieved from :https://www.ncbi.nlm.nih.gov/pmc/articles/PMC4637477/

16.) Bhatt JK, Thomas S, Nanjan MJ. Resveratrol supplementation improves glycemic control in type 2 diabetes mellitus. Nutr Res. 2012 Jul; 32(7):537-41.

17.) Huseini H. F., Larijani B., et al. The efficacy of Silybum marianum (L.) Gaertn. (silymarin) in the treatment of type II diabetes: a randomized, double-blind, placebo-controlled, clinical trial. Phytotherapy Research. 2006;20(12):1036–1039.

18.) Mainzen Prince P. S., Kamalakkannan N. Rutin improves glucose homeostasis in streptozotocin diabetic tissues by altering glycolytic and gluconeogenic enzymes. Journal of Biochemical and Molecular Toxicology. 2006;20(2):96–102.

19.) Kim J.-H., Kang M.-J., et al. Quercetin attenuates fasting and postprandial hyperglycemia in animal models of diabetes mellitus. Nutrition Research and Practice. 2011;5(2):107–111.

20.) Brown A. R., Covington M., et al. The total chemical synthesis of monocyte chemotactic protein-1 (MCP-1) Journal of Peptide Science. 1996;2(1):40–46.

21.) Retrieved from: http://www.breastcancer.org/risk/factors/low_vit_d

22.) Retrieved from: https://www.ivygenelabs.com/

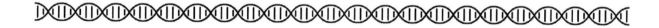

Personalized genetic report found at http://geneticdetoxification.com

TRPM7 gene
Transient receptor potential cation channel

Names of TRPM7 gene genetic variants (SNP identification)	rsnumber	Risk allele
TRPM7	rs8042919	Risk allele is A

What does the TRPM7 gene do?

This gene maintains adequate levels of magnesium in the body.

What health problems are associated with having a TRPM7 risk allele?

Increased risk of developing colon cancer—The increased risk for developing colon cancer is secondary to magnesium/calcium ratios being off, or from being magnesium-deficient.

I have one or more risk allele(s) in the TRPM7 gene. What should I talk to my doctor about doing so that I can reduce my health risks?

> *Consider increasing magnesium intake*—Higher magnesium intake can decrease your risk of developing colon cancer. If you have the A risk allele, you might need a larger amount of magnesium than people with the G allele. Having adequate magnesium is the most important thing you can do if you have the TRPM7 risk allele.

> *Other ways to prevent colon cancer*:

>> *Exercise*—30 minutes of exercise a day can drastically decrease your risk of colon cancer.

>> *Don't smoke or drink*—Both increase your colon cancer risk.

>> *Clean up your diet*—Eat a diet high in fiber, raw fruits, and raw vegetables, but low in red and processed meats.

>> *Consider supplementing with extra vitamin B-9 in the methyl-activated form*—This is especially important if you have any of the risk alleles for the vitamin B-9 genes (pg 86-96, 379-380). Extra vitamin B-9 has shown to lower colon cancer risk.

Christy L. Sutton D.C.

➢ **Consider supplementing with probiotics**—Probiotics are important for a healthy intestinal lining.

➢ **Consider supplementing with vitamin D**—Low vitamin D will increase your colon cancer risk. This is especially important if you have the risk allele in the vitamin D genes (pg 369-371).

➢ **Consider supplementing with Glucoraphanin**—This promotes phase II detox pathways. Glucoraphanin converts into Sulforaphane, which is found to be an effective long-acting indirect antioxidant and significant inducer of phase II detoxification enzymes. The anti-oxidant effects of glucoraphanin are significantly longer lasting than vitamins C, E, and A. Because they assist in maintaining health throughout adult life, phytonutrients, such as glucoraphanin, are considered "lifespan essentials." Glucoraphanin is believed to play an important role in maintaining healthy gastrointestinal flora; healthy cellular life cycles; immune, eye, and cardiovascular health; and a normal response to inflammation.

Are you getting enough magnesium?

The best way to know if you're getting enough magnesium is to take magnesium to bowel tolerance.

This means that you slowly increase magnesium intake until it causes loose stools. Once you develop loose stools from the magnesium, then you slowly decrease the magnesium until you're taking the maximum amount without having loose stools.

I have one or more risk allele(s) in the TRPM7 gene. What labs/testing should I consider to continually monitor my health?

✓ **Magnesium bowel tolerance test**—This test entails taking magnesium to the point that it causes loose stools, and then backing off to the highest level possible without having diarrhea.

✓ **RBC-Magnesium (blood test)** —This is the most accurate way to monitor magnesium levels.

✓ **Colonoscopy**—There is an increased risk of developing colon cancer in people that have both a risk allele for the TRPM7 gene and who are low in magnesium. Routine colonoscopies can help to identify and remove cancerous polyps from the colon.

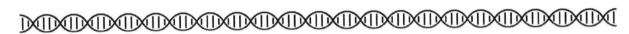

RAD50 gene

DNA repair protein RAD50 gene

Names of RAD50 gene genetic variants (SNP identification)	rsnumber	Risk allele
RAD50	rs2040704	Risk allele is G
RAD50	rs2240032	Risk allele is T

What does the RAD50 gene do?

The RAD50 gene is essential for repairing damaged DNA, and thus for preventing DNA damage.

What health problems might be associated with having a RAD50 risk allele?

Increased risk for developing cancer due to a decreased ability to repair damaged DNA.

I have one or more risk allele(s) in the RAD50 gene. What should I talk to my doctor about doing so that I can reduce my health risks?

- **Avoid DNA damage**—Many things are known to increase DNA damage and inhibit your ability to properly heal from DNA damage. Some ways to protect yourself from DNA damage include:

  ➢ **Limit radiation exposure**—This includes exposure to X-rays, mammograms, CT, overexposure to sunlight and flying. Radiation exposure causes significant DNA damage, increasing cancer risk.

Christy L. Sutton D.C.

> *Antioxidants*—Having high antioxidant levels will neutralize harmful free radicals and prevent DNA damage. Some of the most important antioxidants include glutathione, Vitamin A, Vitamin E, Vitamin C, glutathione, glucoraphanin, and alpha-lipoic acid. It's especially important to have high antioxidant levels when exposed to DNA-damaging radiation from X-rays, mammograms, CT or even flying.

> *Ensure adequate sleep*—Sleep deprivation is associated with DNA damage, especially in the brain[1].

> *Monitor and protect yourself from stress*—Stress is known to damage DNA and cause serious damage to the body.

> *Eat a healthy diet filled with high quality protein, vegetables, fruits and healthy fats*—Vegetables and fruits are high in antioxidants, which will help prevent DNA damage. Don't cook olive oil at a high temperature because it can cause DNA-damaging free radicals. The best fats to cook with are butter and coconut oil.

> *Maintain a healthy weight*—Obesity is associated with a higher level of DNA damage, and thus an increased cancer risk [1.]

> *Avoid toxins, pesticides and other cancer-inducing chemicals*—Eating organic foods, drinking purified water and avoiding using toxic chemicals in or around your home can greatly decrease overall toxic exposure.

- *Participate in regular aerobic exercise*—Walking for 45 minutes a day is one of the best exercises for longevity. It helps reduce stress, keep the blood flowing and maintain a healthy blood sugar.

- *Ensure adequate levels of vitamin D*—Low vitamin D levels can increase your cancer risk. I prefer to see vitamin D level around 70 to 100 on lab work.

- *Consider supplementing with glucoraphanin*—This promotes phase II detox pathways. Glucoraphanin converts into Sulforaphane, which is found to be an effective long-acting indirect antioxidant and significant inducer of phase II detoxification enzymes. The antioxidant effects of glucoraphanin are significantly longer lasting than vitamins C, E, and A. Because they assist in maintaining health throughout adult life, phytonutrients, such as glucoraphanin, are considered "lifespan essentials." Glucoraphanin is believed to play an important role in maintaining healthy gastrointestinal flora; healthy cellular life cycles; immune, eye, and cardiovascular health; and a normal response to inflammation.

I have one or more risk allele(s) in the RAD50 gene. What labs/testing should I consider to continually monitor my health?

✓ **Routine cancer screenings**—All appropriate tests should be performed regularly: colonoscopy; EGD (upper endoscopy of the stomach); Pap smear, routine blood work; and a skin, thyroid, and prostate/breast exam.

✓ **Measuring antioxidant levels**—Antioxidants protect the body from DNA damage.

> **Nutreval by Genova Diagnostic's (blood and urine)**—This test measures your levels of antioxidants, vitamins, minerals, heavy metals, toxins and amino acids. The Nutreval test provides a valuable and overarching look at how your environment affects your overall health.

✓ **DNA oxidative damage test**—This test indicates DNA damage by measuring Urinary 8-hydroxy-2'-deoxyguanosine (8-OHdG), an excellent biomarker of oxidative stress and a risk factor for a variety of diseases, including cancer.

✓ **Ivygene**—This is a blood test that measures for circulating tumor DNA (ctDNA), and can identify if cancer is present in very early stages[2].

References:

1.) Tenorio NM, Ribeiro DA, Alvarenga TA, et al. The influence of sleep deprivation and obesity on DNA damage in female Zucker rats. Clinics (Sao Paulo) (2013); 68:385–389

2.) Retrieved from: https://www.ivygenelabs.com/

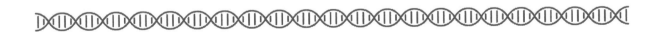

Christy L. Sutton D.C.

TFAM gene

Mitochondrial transcription factor A gene

Names of TFAM gene genetic variants (SNP identification)	rsnumber	Risk allele
TFAM	rs1937	Risk allele is C

What does the TFAM gene do?

TFAM helps maintain mitochondrial DNA integrity[1].

What health problems might be associated with having a TFAM risk allele?

Increased cancer risk.

I have one or more risk allele(s) in the TFAM gene. What should I talk to my doctor about doing so that I can reduce my health risks?

- *Avoid DNA damage*—Many things are known to increase DNA damage and inhibit your ability to properly heal from DNA damage. Some ways to protect yourself from DNA damage include:

    - *Limit radiation exposure*—This includes exposure to X-rays, mammograms, CT, and overexposure to sunlight and flying. Radiation exposure causes significant DNA damage, increasing your cancer risk.

    - *Antioxidants*—Having high antioxidant levels neutralizes harmful free radicals and prevents DNA damage from occurring. Some of the most important antioxidants include glutathione, vitamin A, vitamin E, vitamin C, glutathione, glucoraphanin, and alpha-lipoic acid. It's especially important to have high antioxidant levels when exposed to DNA-damaging radiation from X-rays, mammograms, CT or flying.

    - *Ensure adequate sleep*—Sleep deprivation is associated with DNA damage, especially in the brain[2].

    - *Monitor and protect yourself from stress*—Stress is known to damage DNA and cause serious damage to the body.

> ➤ ***Eat a healthy diet filled with high-quality protein, vegetables, fruits and healthy fats***—Vegetables and fruits are high in antioxidants, which prevents DNA damage. Don't cook olive oil at a high temperature because it can lead to DNA-damaging free radicals. The best fats to cook with are butter and coconut oil.

> ➤ ***Maintain a healthy weight***—Obesity is associated with a higher level of DNA damage, and thus an increased cancer risk[2].

> ➤ ***Avoid toxins, pesticides and other cancer-inducing chemicals***—Eating organic foods, drinking purified water and avoiding using toxic chemicals in or around your home can greatly decrease overall toxic exposure.

- ***Participate in regular aerobic exercise***—Walking for 45 minutes a day is one of the best exercises for longevity. It helps reduce stress, keep the blood flowing and maintain a healthy blood sugar.

- ***Ensure adequate levels of vitamin D***—Low levels of vitamin D can increase your cancer risk. I prefer to see vitamin D level around 70 to 100 on lab work.

- ***Consider supplementing with glucoraphanin***—This promotes phase II detox pathways. Glucoraphanin converts into Sulforaphane, which is found to be an effective long-acting indirect antioxidant and significant inducer of phase II detoxification enzymes. The anti-oxidant effects of glucoraphanin are significantly longer lasting than vitamins C, E, and A. Because they assist in maintaining health throughout adult life, phytonutrients, such as glucoraphanin, are considered "lifespan essentials." Glucoraphanin is believed to play an important role in maintaining healthy gastrointestinal flora; healthy cellular life cycles; immune, eye, and cardiovascular health; and a normal response to inflammation.

I have one or more risk allele(s) in the TFAM gene. What labs/testing should I consider to continually monitor my health?

- ✓ ***Routine cancer screenings***—All appropriate tests should be performed regularly: colonoscopy; EGD (upper endoscopy of the stomach); Pap smear, routine blood work; and a skin, thyroid, and prostate/breast exam.

Christy L. Sutton D.C.

✓ ***Measure antioxidant levels***—Antioxidants protect the body from DNA damage. DNA damage significantly increases your cancer risk.

> ➤ ***Nutreval by Genova Diagnostic's (blood and urine)*** —This test measures your levels of antioxidants, vitamins, minerals, heavy metals, toxins and amino acids. It provides a valuable and overarching look at how your environment affects your overall health.

✓ ***DNA oxidative damage test***—This test indicates DNA damage by measuring Urinary 8-hydroxy-2'-deoxyguanosine (8-OHdG), an excellent biomarker of oxidative stress and a risk factor for a variety of diseases, including cancer.

References:

1.) Zhang Q, Yu JT, Wang P, et al. Mitochondrial transcription factor A (TFAM) polymorphisms and risk of late-onset Alzheimer's disease in Han Chinese. Brain Res. 2011;1368:355–360

2.) Tenorio NM, Ribeiro DA, Alvarenga TA, et al. The influence of sleep deprivation and obesity on DNA damage in female Zucker rats. Clinics (Sao Paulo) (2013);68:385–389

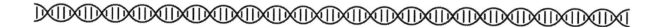

ADA gene
Adenosine deaminase gene

Names of ADH gene genetic variants (SNP identification)	rsnumber	Risk allele
ADA C10783T	rs6031692	A

What does the ADA gene do?

The ADA gene is necessary for the body to properly deal with and heal from DNA damage. This gene protects the body from cancer by converting a toxic byproduct from DNA damage into a nontoxic substance.

Specifically, the ADA enzyme, which is made from the ADA gene, converts a toxic substance (called deoxyadenosine) into a substance that is nontoxic to the immune system (called deoxyinosine). The toxic substance deoxyadenosine can cause damage to the immune system, specifically the part of the immune system called the lymphocytes, which are important for combating viral infections.

What health problems could result from having this risk allele in the ADA gene?

- *Possible increased risk of developing cancer*—This is due to a decreased ability to metabolize the toxic byproducts of DNA damage into a less-toxic form.

- *Possible immune system problems*—This refers specifically with viral infections, and with the part of the immune system called lymphocytes.

I have a risk allele for the ADA gene. What should I talk to my doctor about doing so that I can reduce my health risks?

- *Avoid DNA damage*—Many things are known to increase DNA damage and inhibit your ability to properly heal from DNA damage. Some ways to protect yourself from DNA damage include:

  - *Limit radiation exposure*—This includes exposure to X-rays, mammograms, CT, overexposure to sunlight and flying. Radiation exposure causes significant DNA damage, increasing your cancer risk.

  - *Antioxidants*—Having high antioxidant levels neutralizes harmful free radicals and prevents DNA damage from occurring. Some of the most important antioxidants include glutathione, vitamin A, vitamin E, vitamin C and alpha-lipoic acid. It's especially important to have high antioxidant levels when exposed to DNA-damaging radiation from X-rays, mammograms, CT or flying.

  - *Ensure adequate sleep*—Sleep deprivation is associated with DNA damage, especially in the brain[1].

  - *Monitor and protect yourself from stress*—Stress is known to damage DNA and cause serious damage to the body.

  - *Eat a healthy diet filled with high quality protein, vegetables, fruits and healthy fats*—Vegetables and fruits are high in antioxidants, which prevent DNA damage. Don't cook olive oil at a high temperature because it can lead to DNA-damaging free radicals. The best fats to cook with are butter and coconut oil.

> **Maintain a healthy weight**—Obesity is associated with a higher level of DNA damage, and thus an increased cancer risk[1].

> **Avoid toxins, pesticide, and other cancer-inducing chemicals**—Eating organic foods, drinking purified water and avoiding using toxic chemicals in or around your home can greatly decrease overall toxic exposure.

- **Participate in regular aerobic exercise**—Walking for 45 minutes a day is one of the best exercises for longevity. It helps reduce stress, keep the blood flowing and maintain a healthy blood sugar.

- **Support a healthy immune system**—Some natural ways to support the immune system and decrease your cancer risk include supplementing with vitamin C, zinc, probiotics and vitamin D.

- **Consider supplementing with glucoraphanin**—This promotes phase II detox pathways. Glucoraphanin converts into Sulforaphane, which is found to be an effective long-acting indirect antioxidant and significant inducer of phase II detoxification enzymes. The anti-oxidant effects of glucoraphanin are significantly longer lasting than vitamins C, E, and A. Because they assist in maintaining health throughout adult life, phytonutrients, such as glucoraphanin, are considered "lifespan essentials." Glucoraphanin is believed to play an important role in maintaining healthy gastrointestinal flora; healthy cellular life cycles; immune, eye, and cardiovascular health; and a normal response to inflammation.

I have one or more risk allele(s) in the ADA gene. What labs/testing should I consider to continually monitor my health?

✓ **Routine cancer screenings**—All appropriate tests should be performed regularly: colonoscopy; EGD (upper endoscopy of the stomach); Pap smear, routine blood work; and a skin, thyroid, and prostate/breast exam.

✓ **Measure antioxidant levels**—Antioxidants protect the body from DNA damage. The Nutreval test from Genova Diagnostics measures antioxidant levels.

✓ **DNA oxidative damage test**—This test indicates DNA damage by measuring Urinary 8-hydroxy-2'-deoxyguanosine (8-OHdG), an excellent biomarker of oxidative stress and a risk factor for a variety of diseases, including cancer.

References:

1.) Tenorio NM, Ribeiro DA, Alvarenga TA, et al. The influence of sleep deprivation and obesity on DNA damage in female Zucker rats. Clinics (Sao Paulo) (2013);68:385–389

SOD2 gene
Superoxide dismutase gene

Names of SOD2 gene genetic variants (SNP identification)	rsnumber	Risk allele
SOD2 A16V	rs4880	Risk allele is G

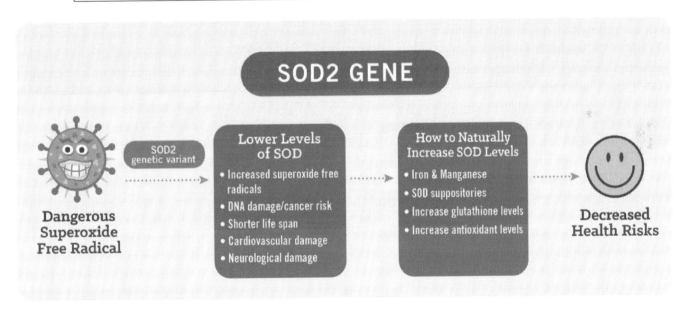

What does the SOD2 gene do?

The SOD2 gene is essential for the body to make the essential antioxidant superoxide dismutase (SOD). SOD neutralizes toxic superoxide free radicals. Superoxide free radicals cause cell damage that can lead to cancer and inflammation, which is why the ability for SOD to neutralize these free radicals is so important at preventing cancer

Christy L. Sutton D.C.

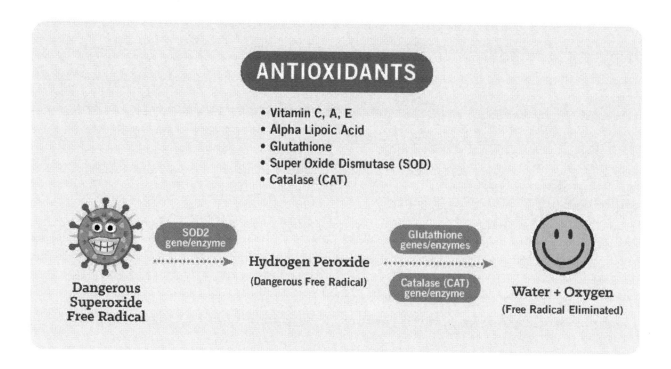

What health problems might be associated with having a SOD2 risk allele?

- *Low SOD levels*—As a result, you'll have a higher level of DNA-damaging free radicals.

- *Increased risk cardiovascular problems*—This includes idiopathic cardiomyopathy (IDC) and atherosclerosis.

- *Increased risk for neurological problems*—These include sporadic motor neuron disease and neurodegenerative disorders like ALS.

- *Increased cancer risk*—Mice with one risk allele for the SOD2 gene showed an increased cancer risk[1].

- *Shorter life span*[2]—Having the risk allele for the SOD2 gene can lead to lower levels of the antioxidant SOD. Low levels of the antioxidant SOD can lead to a shorter life span, whereas increased levels of the antioxidant SOD may lead to a longer life span.

I have one or more risk allele(s) in the SOD2 gene. What should I talk to my doctor about doing so that I can reduce my health risks?

- *Increase antioxidant levels*—If you have risk alleles for the SOD2 gene, the key is antioxidants, antioxidant, antioxidants. Having a high number of antioxidants will help protect you from some of the side effects associated with having the SOD2 risk alleles.

  - ➤ *Eat a diet high in fruits and veggies*—This is a great way to increase antioxidant levels.

  - ➤ *Consider supplementing with additional antioxidants*—These include vitamin C, vitamin E, vitamin A, vitamin D, alpha-lipoic acid, glutathione, glucoraphanin, and SOD.

- *Support high SOD and glutathione levels*—One way to accomplish this is to use a cream or suppository that contains both SOD and glutathione. SOD and glutathione are generally not absorbed well into the digestive system, so taking them orally can have a limited effect. Therefore, the best option to bypass having high-risk SOD is regular use of the SOD/glutathione cream or suppository. You can read more about glutathione on page 57.

- *Ensure you aren't deficient in iron and manganese*—Iron and manganese are necessary for the SOD enzyme to function. Without adequate levels of these minerals, the SOD enzyme won't efficiently remove DNA-damaging free radicals. Don't take iron if you're not iron-deficient because too much iron can cause damage and inflammation.

- **Limit radiation exposure**—This includes exposure to X-rays, mammograms, CT, overexposure to sunlight and flying. These things dramatically increase the number of damaging free radicals in the body.

- *Minimize exposure to environmental triggers that deplete SOD and increase damaging free radicals*—This includes exposure to toxins, heavy metals, chemicals, radiation, stress and sleep deprivation.

- *Support high catalase and glutathione levels*—Catalase and glutathione are important for the body to remove the hydrogen peroxide that SOD creates. The catalase and glutathione genes are found on pages 57 and 251.

Christy L. Sutton D.C.

- **Drink plenty of water**—Dehydration increases free radical production.

- **Consider supplementing with glucoraphanin**—This promotes phase II detox pathways. Glucoraphanin converts into Sulforaphane, which is found to be an effective long-acting indirect antioxidant and significant inducer of phase II detoxification enzymes. The antioxidant effects of glucoraphanin are significantly longer lasting than vitamins C, E, and A. Because they assist in maintaining health throughout adult life, phytonutrients, such as glucoraphanin, are considered "lifespan essentials." Glucoraphanin is believed to play an important role in maintaining healthy gastrointestinal flora; healthy cellular life cycles; immune, eye, and cardiovascular health; and a normal response to inflammation.

I have one or more risk allele(s) in the SOD2 gene. What labs/testing should I consider to continually monitor my health?

- ✓ **Monitor for deficiencies in iron and manganese**—The Nutreval test from Genova Diagnostics measures for manganese deficiencies. This tests your ferritin, hemoglobin, hematocrit and serum iron.

- ✓ **Measure glutathione levels**—Increasing SOD levels without increasing glutathione levels can create more free radicals because the hydrogen peroxide that SOD makes isn't neutralized by glutathione. The test also measures glutathione levels.

- ✓ **Oxidative stress test**—This test measures the amount of oxidative stress and antioxidant reserves. Antioxidants like catalase, SOD and glutathione neutralize free radicals that cause oxidative stress and DNA damage. High oxidative stress, high levels of free radicals, high levels of DNA damage and low levels of antioxidants can increase your cancer risk.

References:

1.) Van Remmen H. et al. Life-long reduction in MnSOD activity results in increased DNA damage and higher incidence of cancer but does not accelerate aging. Physiological genomics 16, 29–37 (2003).

2.) Soerensen M., Christensen K., Stevnsner T., Christiansen L. The Mn-superoxide dismutase single nucleotide polymorphism rs4880 and the glutathione peroxidase 1 single nucleotide polymorphism rs1050450 are associated with aging and longevity in the oldest old. Mech. Ageing Dev. 2009;130:308–314.

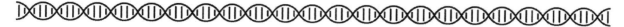

CAT genes
Catalase genes

Names of CAT gene genetic variants (SNP identification)	rsnumber	Risk allele
CAT A12175G	rs480575	Risk allele is G
CAT C21068T	rs2300181	Risk allele is T
CAT	rs769217	Risk allele is C

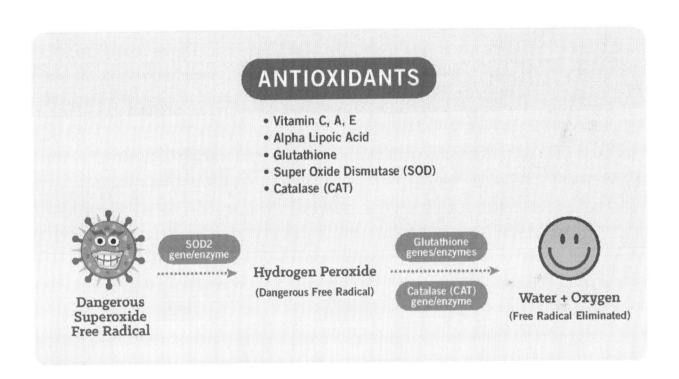

What does the CAT gene do?

The CAT gene provides the body's instructions to make catalase, an enzyme that serves as a key antioxidant in the body's defense against oxidative stress (cancer-causing stress).

- Catalase converts hydrogen peroxide to water, thereby mitigating hydrogen peroxide's toxic effects

- Catalase also helps detoxify alcohol

Christy L. Sutton D.C.

What health problems are associated with having a CAT risk allele?

The catalase enzyme, made from the CAT gene, helps protect the body from dangerous cancer-causing free radicals. Many chronic diseases are associated with high levels of free radicals.

Some health conditions that are associated with high levels of free radicals and with having insufficient catalase (due to having a risk allele in the CAT gene) include:

- *Graying of hair due to insufficient catalase activity, which leads to high levels of hydrogen peroxide[1]*

- *Diabetes*

- *Alzheimer's disease*

- *Lupus*

- *Rheumatoid arthritis*

- *Cancer*

- *Decreased ability to metabolize alcohol*

- *Periodontal disease*—Being homozygous (+/+) for CAT SNPs can increase your risk of developing acatalasemia, a disorder that can increase your risk of periodontal disease.

I have one or more risk allele(s) in the CAT gene. What should I talk to my doctor about doing so that I can reduce my health risks?

- *Catalase suppositories*—Catalase is similar to other antioxidants, like SOD and glutathione, in that they are difficult to absorb through the digestive tract. Suppositories that contain catalase can bypass the stomach and be directly absorbed into the body.

- *Avoid alcohol*—The CAT gene plays a minor role in alcohol detoxification.

- *Ensure you're not iron-deficient*—Iron is necessary for catalase to function. Don't take iron if you're not iron-deficient because too much iron can cause damage and inflammation.

- *Increase antioxidant levels*—If you have risk alleles for the SOD2 gene, the key is antioxidants, antioxidants, antioxidants. Having a high number of antioxidants will help protect you from some of the side effects associated with having the SOD2 risk alleles.

  - *Eat a diet high in fruits and veggies*—These are naturally high in antioxidants, many of which have not yet been discovered and isolated by science.

  - *Consider supplementing with additional antioxidants*—This includes vitamin C, vitamin E, vitamin A, vitamin D, alpha-lipoic acid, glutathione and SOD.

- *Limit radiation exposure*—This includes X-rays, mammograms, CT, overexposure to sunlight and flying. These things dramatically increase the number of damaging free radicals in the body, which increases your cancer risk.

- *Support high glutathione levels*—Catalase and glutathione are required for the body to remove the hydrogen peroxide that SOD creates. You can protect yourself the side effects of having a CAT risk allele (which leads to low catalase) by increasing your glutathione levels. Information on glutathione genes can be found on page 57.

- *Consider supplementing with glucoraphanin*—This promotes phase II detox pathways. Glucoraphanin converts into Sulforaphane, which is found to be an effective long-acting indirect antioxidant and significant inducer of phase II detoxification enzymes. The anti-oxidant effects of glucoraphanin are significantly longer lasting than vitamins C, E, and A. Because they assist in maintaining health throughout adult life, phytonutrients, such as glucoraphanin, are considered "lifespan essentials." Glucoraphanin is believed to play an important role in maintaining healthy gastrointestinal flora; healthy cellular life cycles; immune, eye, and cardiovascular health; and a normal response to inflammation.

                                        Christy L. Sutton D.C.

I have one or more risk allele(s) in the CAT gene. What labs/testing should I consider to continually monitor my health?

✓ ***Monitor for iron deficiencies (blood work)***—The catalase enzyme needs iron to function. The best tests to measure iron include ferritin, hemoglobin, hematocrit and serum iron.

✓ ***Measure antioxidant levels, including glutathione***—The Nutreval test from Genoa Diagnostics measures antioxidant levels. It doesn't measure catalase levels, but it will measure glutathione and many other antioxidants that are essential for health.

✓ ***Oxidative stress test***—This test measures the amount of oxidative stress and antioxidant reserves. Antioxidants like catalase, SOD and glutathione neutralize free radicals that cause oxidative stress and DNA damage. High oxidative stress, high levels of free radicals, high levels of DNA damage and low levels of antioxidants can increase your cancer risk.

Be on the alert for this cancer-causing genetic combo

Having multiple risk alleles in the SOD2, glutathione and catalase (CAT) genes can lead to high levels of DNA- damaging free radicals. High levels of free radicals can increase your cancer risk, the rate at which you age and your overall level of degeneration. The enzymes made by the glutathione, SOD2 and catalase genes are the most important enzymes of the cell antioxidant defense system[1].

Read more about SOD2 on pages 247-251.

References:

1.)Etienne Pigeolet, et al. Glutathione peroxidase, superoxide dismutase, and catalase inactivation by peroxides and oxygen derived free radicals. Mechanisms of Ageing and Development. Volume 51, Issue 3, 15 February 1990, Pages (283-297.

References:

1.) Schallreuter KU, Salem MMAEL, Hasse S, Rokos H. The redox—biochemistry of human hair pigmentation. Pigment Cell and Melanoma Research. 2011;24(1):51–62

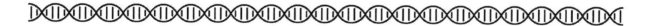

NQO1 gene

NAD(P)H dehydrogenase, quinone 1

Names of NQO1 gene genetic variants (SNP identification)	rsnumber	Risk allele
NQO1 C609T	rs1800566	Risk allele is A
NQO1 G13161A	rs689453	Risk allele is T

What does the NQO1 gene do?

The NQO1 gene helps remove tissue-damaging superoxide free radicals (DNA-damaging free radicals). The NQO1 gene also helps the body metabolize and remove xenobiotic (harmful foreign chemicals in the environment).

What health problems are associated with having an NQO1 risk allele?

- *Decreased ability to metabolize the antioxidant CoQ10 into the biologically available form of CoQ10 called ubiquinol*—Many health problems related to having one or more NQO1 risk alleles could be a side effect of not producing enough ubiquinol (activated form of CoQ10).

- *Tardive dyskinesia*—This is a movement disorder[1].

- *Sensitivity to benzene poisoning when exposed to benzene in petrochemicals*[1]—NQO1 C609T (rs1800566) (A, A) genotypes are 7.6 times more likely to get benzene poisoning[3]. Benzene is a carcinogen that is naturally found in petrochemicals like crude oil and gasoline.

- *Cancer*[1]

- *Alzheimer's disease*[1]

I have one or more risk allele(s) in the NQO1 gene. What should I talk to my doctor about doing so that I can reduce my health risks?

- *Exercise caution when taking blood thinners*—Blood thinners such as warfarin may inhibit this enzyme[2]. Therefore, anyone with movement disorders like tardive dyskinesia, combined with having this risk allele, should exercise

Christy L. Sutton D.C.

caution when taking blood thinners and consider supplementing with ubiquinol. Do not stop or change any medications without talking to your doctor.

- *Consider supplementing with CoQ10 in the ubiquinol form rather than the ubiquinone form*—Having the risk allele in the NQO1 gene can decrease your ability to metabolize CoQ10 into the biologically available form of CoQ10 called ubiquinol; therefore, people with NQO1 risk alleles should consider supplementing with ubiquinol.

- *Avoid exposure to benzene, crude oil and petrochemicals*—If you have the (A/A) genotype for NQO1 C609T, you are 7.6 times more likely to develop benzene poisoning due to having a decreased ability to remove any benzene you are exposed to[3]. Benzene is a carcinogen that is naturally found in crude oil and gasoline. Glutathione can help protect the body from benzene poising. Read more about glutathione on pages 57.

- *Consider supplementing with B vitamins and nutrients to increase glutathione levels.*

  - *Glutathione* can help protect the body from benzene poisoning. Ways to increase glutathione are included in the section on glutathione on pages 57.

  - *Vitamin B-3*—In the presence of vitamin B-3, the NQO1 enzyme can facilitate tumor suppression by blocking the degradation of p53 and p73, which are important tumor suppressors in the body.

  - *Vitamin B-2*—The NQO1 enzyme requires vitamin B-2 to function properly.

- *Consider supplementing with glucoraphanin*—This promotes phase II detox pathways. Glucoraphanin converts into Sulforaphane, which is found to be an effective long-acting indirect antioxidant and significant inducer of phase II detoxification enzymes. The anti-oxidant effects of glucoraphanin are significantly longer lasting than vitamins C, E, and A. Because they assist in maintaining health throughout adult life, phytonutrients, such as glucoraphanin, are considered "lifespan essentials." Glucoraphanin is believed to play an important role in maintaining healthy gastrointestinal flora; healthy cellular life cycles; immune, eye, and cardiovascular health; and a normal response to inflammation.

Read the section titled, "How can you reduce your risk of developing Alzheimer's disease" on Pg. 157.

I have one or more risk allele(s) in the NQO1 gene. What labs/testing should I consider to continually monitor my health?

- ✓ **Routine cancer screenings**—All appropriate tests should be performed regularly: colonoscopy; EGD (upper endoscopy of the stomach); Pap smear, routine blood work; and a skin, thyroid, and prostate/breast exam.

- ✓ **Nutreval by Genova Diagnostics (blood and urine test)**—This test measures antioxidant levels, including glutathione and CoQ10. It also measures your levels of vitamins, minerals, amino acids, heavy metals and some toxins. The Nutreval test provides a valuable and overarching look at how your environment affects your overall health.

- ✓ **Measure benzene levels**—This can be done through the Toxic Effects Core Profile by Genova Diagnostics (blood and urine). This profile provides more information on your carcinogen and toxin levels. It won't tell you exactly how well you're detoxifying, but it will tell you how many toxins are accumulating in your body, which is an indirect indicator of how well you're detoxifying.

- ✓ **Smell test**—Loss of sense of smell is one of the first signs of Alzheimer's. So testing your sense of smell is a great way to monitor your brain health.

- ✓ **Memory recall testing**—This would include trying to remember a series of numbers or names.

- ✓ **Vitamin D levels (blood test)**—Vitamin D is important for brain health. I prefer to see vitamin D level around 70 to 100 on lab work.
- ✓ **Homocysteine (blood work)**—High homocysteine is associated with an increased risk of developing Alzheimer's. I prefer homocysteine to be at or below 8 on blood work.

References:

1) NCBI. Retrieved from: http://www.ncbi.nlm.nih.gov/gene/1728

2.) Arlt VM, Stiborova M, et al. (Apr 2005). "Environmental pollutant and potent mutagen 3-nitrobenzanthrone forms DNA adducts after reduction by NAD(P)H: quinone oxidoreductase and conjugation by acetyltransferases and sulfotransferases in human hepatic cytosols".Cancer Research 65 (7): 2644.

Christy L. Sutton D.C.

3.) Rothman N, Smith MT, Hayes RB, et al. (Jul 1997). "Benzene poisoning, a risk factor for hematological malignancy, is associated with the NQO1 609C-->T mutation and rapid fractional excretion of chlorzoxazone". Cancer Research 57 (14): 2839–42.

4.) PhosphoSite Plus. Retrieved from: http://www.phosphosite.org/proteinAction.do?id=14721&showAllSites=true

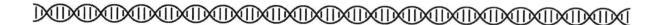

FOXE1 gene
Forkhead box protein E1 gene

Names of FOXE1 gene genetic variants (SNP identification)	rsnumber	Risk allele
FOXE1	rs10984009	Risk allele is A
FOXE1	rs1867277	Risk allele is A
FOXE1	rs28937575	Risk allele is A

What does the FOXE1 gene do?

The FOXE1 gene is essential for thyroid development.

What health problems are associated with having a FOXE1 risk allele?

- *Increased risk of thyroid cancer*[1]

- *Hypothyroidism, especially at a young age*—There is an increased risk of being born with hypothyroidism or of developing hypothyroidism at a very early age[1].

I have one or more risk allele(s) in the FOXE1 gene. What should I talk to my doctor about doing so that I can reduce my health risks?

- *Consider supplementing with iodine*—Being iodine-deficient can increase your thyroid cancer risk.

- *Avoid exposure to radiation, especially to the thyroid*—If you have to get a radiation-producing diagnostic image such as an X-ray, CT or mammogram, make sure your thyroid is always covered with a lead blanket for protection. In addition, consider increasing antioxidant intake prior to the images being taken.

- *Limit radiation exposure*—This includes X-rays, mammograms, CT, overexposure to sunlight and flying. These things will dramatically increase the number of cancer-causing free radicals in the body.

- *Consider supplementing with glucoraphanin*—This promotes phase II detox pathways. Glucoraphanin converts into Sulforaphane, which is found to be an effective long-acting indirect antioxidant and significant inducer of phase II detoxification enzymes. The anti-oxidant effects of glucoraphanin are significantly longer lasting than vitamins C, E, and A. Because they assist in maintaining health throughout adult life, phytonutrients, such as glucoraphanin, are considered "lifespan essentials." Glucoraphanin is believed to play an important role in maintaining healthy gastrointestinal flora; healthy cellular life cycles; immune, eye, and cardiovascular health; and a normal response to inflammation.

I have one or more risk allele(s) in the FOXE1 gene. What labs/testing should I consider to continually monitor my health?

- ✓ *Thyroid blood panels*—This should include TSH, free T4, reverse T3, T3 updake, T4, free T3, total T3, TPO antibodies and TGA antibodies.

- ✓ *Thyroid exams*—This is to determine if you have thyroid nodules.

- ✓ *Check iodine levels (blood and skin test)*—The iodine skin test involves putting iodine on the skin to see if the iodine is still present 24 hours later. If the iodine is not present or is greatly faded, that can mean your iodine levels may be low. The iodine skin test is not a perfect test—it should be followed up with a blood test to measure iodine levels.

- ✓ *Ivygene*—This is a blood test that measures for circulating tumor DNA (ctDNA), and can identify is cancer is present in very early stages[2].

References:

1.) Landa I, Ruiz-Llorente S, Montero-Conde C, et al. (2009) The variant rs1867277 in FOXE1 gene confers thyroid cancer susceptibility through the recruitment of USF1/USF2 transcription factors. PLoS Genet 5: e1000637

2.) Retrieved from: https://www.ivygenelabs.com/

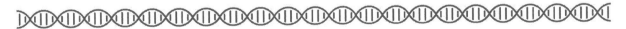

Christy L. Sutton D.C.

**If you have a risk allele for MPO or NQO1,
then use extra caution working around *petroleum products***

If you have risk alleles for the MPO or NQO1 genes, you should avoid exposure to oil products because you're at a higher risk for serious health problems, such as cancer, from benzene exposure. Benzene is in petroleum-based products such as oil, gasoline and petrochemicals.

MPO gene
Myeloperoxidase gene

Names of MPO gene genetic variants (SNP identification)	rsnumber	Risk allele
MPO A15067C	rs2071409	Risk allele is G
MPO C7900T	rs28730837	Risk allele is A

What does the MPO gene do?

The MPO gene is particularly important in a part of the immune system called neutrophils, which are white blood cells that help fight off bacteria.

What health problems are associated with having an MPO risk allele?

- *Increased risk of developing cancer*

- *Having the risk allele for MPO A15067C is associated with an increased risk for:*

    - *Kidney injury[1]*

    - *Benzene sensitivity*—Having this risk allele is associated with immune damage and toxicity when exposed to benzene[2].

I have one or more risk allele(s) in the MPO gene. What should I talk to my doctor about doing so that I can reduce my health risks?

- *Avoid exposure to benzene and other petrochemicals*—Avoid crude oil and coming into direct contact with oil.

- *Ensure you aren't iron-deficient*—MPO requires iron to function properly. Therefore, monitor and correct for any iron deficiencies.

- *Drink plenty of water*—This keeps your kidneys healthy and assists with detoxification.

- *Increase antioxidant levels*—High antioxidant levels decreases your cancer risk. Having high antioxidant levels neutralizes harmful free radicals and prevents cancer-causing DNA damage from occurring. Some of the most important antioxidants include glutathione, vitamin A, vitamin E, vitamin C, glucoraphanin, and alpha-lipoic acid.

- *Consider supplementing with Glucoraphanin*—This promotes phase II detox pathways. Glucoraphanin converts into Sulforaphane, which is found to be an effective long-acting indirect antioxidant and significant inducer of phase II detoxification enzymes. The anti-oxidant effects of glucoraphanin are significantly longer lasting than vitamins C, E, and A. Because they assist in maintaining health throughout adult life, phytonutrients, such as glucoraphanin, are considered "lifespan essentials." Glucoraphanin is believed to play an important role in maintaining healthy gastrointestinal flora; healthy cellular life cycles; immune, eye, and cardiovascular health; and a normal response to inflammation.

I have one or more risk allele(s) in the MPO gene. What labs/testing should I consider to continually monitor my health?

- ✓ *Monitor for iron deficiencies (blood work)*—The best tests to measure iron include ferritin, hemoglobin, hematocrit and serum iron.

- ✓ *Monitor kidney function (blood test)*—The most common labs for routinely monitoring the kidneys include creatinine and glomerular filtration rate (GFR).

Christy L. Sutton D.C.

- ✓ **Routine cancer screenings**—All appropriate tests should be performed regularly: colonoscopy; EGD (upper endoscopy of the stomach); Pap smear, routine blood work; and skin, thyroid, and prostate/breast exam.

- ✓ **Measure benzene levels, especially if you work around petroleum products**—This can be done through the Toxic Effects Core Profile by Genova Diagnostics (blood and urine). This profile lab test provides more information on your carcinogen and toxin levels. It won't tell you exactly how well you're detoxifying, but it will tell you how many toxins are accumulating in your body, which is an indirect indicator of how well you're detoxifying.

References:

1.) Acton, Ashton PhD. Issues in Kidney Disease Research and Treatment: 2013 Edition. pg 241.

2.) Shen, Min; Zhang, Luoping, et al. Polymorphisms in genes involved in innate immunity and susceptibility to benzene-induced hematotoxicity. (2011. June). Vol 43, No6. Retrieved from: http://superfund.berkeley.edu/pdf/354.pdf

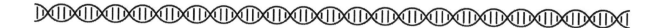

ESR2 gene
Estrogen receptor 2

Names of ESR2 gene genetic variants (SNP identification)	rsnumber	Risk allele
ESR2	rs2987983	Risk allele depends on diet and sex

What does the ESR2 gene do?

The ESR2 gene creates the instructions for the body to make the estrogen receptor beta (ER-β), which is a receptor that binds to estrogen.

What health problems are associated with having an ESR2 risk allele?

To eat soy or not? The answer depends on your sex and genotype.

- *Men*

  - If you're a male with a G allele, you may benefit from eating soy. Men with the G allele have an increased risk of developing prostate cancer, but they may have a decreased risk of developing prostate cancer when they eat isoflavone-rich foods such as soy[1].

  - If you're a male with an A allele, you may benefit from avoiding soy. Men with the A allele are at a lower risk of prostate cancer, but an increased risk of developing prostate cancer when they eat a diet high in isoflavone-rich food (soy)[1].

- *Women*

  - There is less research showing if women gain any benefit from avoiding soy. Because high estrogen can be associated with an increased breast cancer risk, I recommend women avoid soy regardless of their genotype. Soy is naturally high in estrogen-like substances. I believe all women should be cautious about estrogen exposure, including eating soy.

I have one or more risk allele(s) in the ESR2 gene. What should I talk to my doctor about doing so that I can reduce my health risks?

- Men with the **G** allele *may* benefit from eating a diet that ***includes*** soy.

- Men with the **A** allele *may* benefit from eating a diet ***excluding*** soy.

I have one or more risk allele(s) in the ESR2 gene. What labs/testing should I consider to continually monitor my health?

- ✓ ***Monitor estrogen levels***—It's important to monitor all three estrogens (estradiol, estrone and estriol). Estradiol is the strongest form of estrogen— it is 12 times stronger then estrone, and 80 times stronger than estriol. Estradiol may be the most likely estrogen to cause cell proliferation and cancer.

✓ **Routine cancer screenings**—All appropriate tests should be performed regularly: colonoscopy; EGD (upper endoscopy of the stomach); Pap smear, routine blood work; and skin, thyroid, and prostate/breast exams.

References:

1.) Hedelin M, Balter KA, Chang ET, Bellocco R, et al. Dietary intake of phytoestrogens, estrogen receptor-beta polymorphisms and the risk of prostate cancer. Prostate.2006;66(14):1512–20.

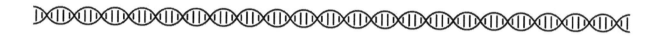

FCGR2A gene
Low affinity immunoglobulin gamma Fc region receptor II-a gene

Names of FCGR2A gene genetic variants (SNP identification)	rsnumber	Risk allele
FCGR2A	rs1801274	Risk allele is A

What does FCGR2A gene do?

The FCGR2A gene assists in the immune system's ability to target and clean up debris and helps prevent DNA from being damaged.

What health problems are associated with having an FCGR2A risk allele?

Increased risk of developing cancer—Having the risk allele in the FCG2A gene decreases the body's ability to recover from DNA damage, leading to an increased risk of developing cancer.

I have one or more risk allele(s) in the FCGR2A gene. What should I talk to my doctor about doing so that I can reduce my health risks?

- *Avoid DNA damage*—Many things are known to increase DNA damage and inhibit your ability to properly heal from DNA damage. Some ways to protect yourself from DNA damage include:

> ➢ *Limit radiation exposure*—This includes exposure to X-rays, mammograms, CT, overexposure to sunlight and flying. Radiation exposure causes significant DNA damage, increasing your cancer risk.

> ➢ *Consider increasing antioxidants levels*—Having high antioxidant levels neutralizes harmful free radicals and prevents DNA damage. Some of the most important antioxidants include glutathione, vitamin A, vitamin E, vitamin C and alpha-lipoic acid. It's especially important to have high antioxidant levels when exposed to DNA-damaging radiation from X-rays, mammograms, CT or flying.

> ➢ *Ensure adequate sleep*—Sleep deprivation is associated with DNA damage, especially in the brain[1].

> ➢ *Monitor and protect yourself from stress*—Stress is known to damage DNA and cause serious damage to the body.

> ➢ *Eat a healthy diet filled with high-quality protein, vegetables, fruits and healthy fats*—Vegetables and fruits are high in antioxidants, which will help prevent DNA damage. Don't cook olive oil at a high temperature because it can lead to DNA-damaging free radicals. The best fats to cook with are butter and coconut oil.

> ➢ *Maintain a healthy weight*—Obesity is associated with a higher level of DNA damage, and thus an increased cancer risk[1].

> ➢ *Avoid toxins, pesticides and other cancer-inducing chemicals*— Eating organic foods, drinking purified water, and avoiding using toxic chemicals in and around your home can greatly decrease overall toxic exposure.

- *Participate in regular aerobic exercise*—Walking for 45 minutes a day has been found to be one of the best exercises for longevity. One reason is because it helps reduce stress, keeps the blood flowing and maintains a healthy blood sugar.

- *Ensure adequate levels of vitamin D*—Low vitamin D levels can increase your cancer risk. I prefer to see vitamin D level around 70 to 100 on lab work.

Christy L. Sutton D.C.

- **Consider supplementing with Glucoraphanin**—This promotes phase II detox pathways. Glucoraphanin converts into Sulforaphane, which is found to be an effective long-acting indirect antioxidant and significant inducer of phase II detoxification enzymes. The anti-oxidant effects of glucoraphanin are significantly longer lasting than vitamins C, E, and A. Because they assist in maintaining health throughout adult life, phytonutrients, such as glucoraphanin, are considered "lifespan essentials." Glucoraphanin is believed to play an important role in maintaining healthy gastrointestinal flora; healthy cellular life cycles; immune, eye, and cardiovascular health; and a normal response to inflammation.

I have one or more risk allele(s) in the FCGR2A gene. What labs/testing should I consider to continually monitor my health?

- ✓ **Routine cancer screenings**—All appropriate tests should be performed regularly: colonoscopy; EGD (upper endoscopy of the stomach); Pap smear, routine blood work; and a skin, thyroid, and prostate/breast exam.

- ✓ **Measuring antioxidant levels**—Antioxidants protect the body from DNA damage and developing cancer. If antioxidant levels are low, you're at an increased risk for developing cancer

  - ➤ **Nutreval by Genova Diagnostics (blood and urine)**—This test measures your levels of antioxidants, vitamins, minerals, heavy metals, toxins and amino acids. The Nutreval test provides a valuable and overarching look at how your environment is affecting your overall health.

- ✓ **DNA oxidative damage test**—This test monitors DNA damage by measuring Urinary 8-hydroxy-2'-deoxyguanosine (8-OHdG), an excellent biomarker of oxidative stress and a risk factor for a variety of diseases, including cancer.

- ✓ **Ivygene**—This is a blood test that measures for circulating tumor DNA (ctDNA), and can identify if cancer is present in very early stages[2].

References:

1.) Tenorio NM, Ribeiro DA, Alvarenga TA, et al. The influence of sleep deprivation and obesity on DNA damage in female Zucker rats. Clinics (Sao Paulo) (2013);68:385–389

2.) Retrieved from: https://www.ivygenelabs.com/

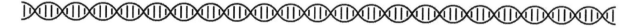

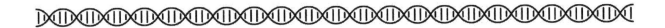

For more information on cancer-associated genes covered in this book, consult the following pages:

Detox genes

- Phase I detox genes (CYP genes) Pg. 21-51
- Phase II detox genes Pg. 55-124
  - ➢ Glutathione genes Pg. 57
  - ➢ Methylation genes Pg. 81-124
  - ➢ Sulfation genes Pg. 76-80
  - ➢ Glucuronidation genes Pg. 71-75
  - ➢ Acetylation genes Pg. 66-70

Immune health genes:

- Celiac genes Pg. 270
- IL-5 gene Pg. 288
- IL6 gene Pg. 291
- TNF gene Pg. 306

Mental health genes:

- COMT gene Pg. 181

Vitamin and mineral genes:

- VDR gene Pg. 368
- GC gene Pg. 370
- BCMO1 gene Pg. 371

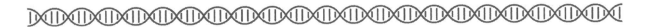

Christy L. Sutton D.C.

Part 4

Immunity-Related Genes

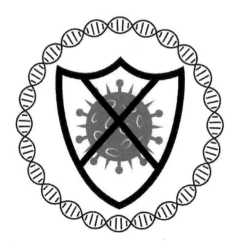

Our immune system is our defense against a deadly army of potential pathogenic bacteria, viruses and parasites. Without a healthy immune system, our lives would be short-lived due to infection. However, in many cases the immune system behaves in a misguided fashion and begins attacking things that aren't dangerous pathogens, such as in autoimmune diseases, allergies and sensitivities.

Some genetic variants can lead to an overactive immune system— this can predispose you to developing an autoimmune disease, allergies, sensitivities or inflammatory disorders. In this section you'll learn about some inherited genetic variants that may increase your risk for immune health problems, such as autoimmune disorders, allergies, inflammatory disorders and celiac disease—and how to prevent your genetic predisposed risk from becoming a lifelong health problem.

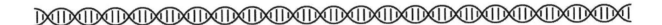

Chapter 9
Celiac Disease
Autoimmune
Inflammation Genes

What You Need to Know About Celiac Disease

What is celiac disease?

Celiac disease is not an allergy or sensitivity to gluten. It is an autoimmune disease triggered by eating gluten. This means that if someone with celiac disease eats gluten, their immune system will start attacking and destroying their body. The autoimmune disease process that occurs in someone with celiac disease is triggered by eating gluten and can cause irreversible damage. The average person has signs and symptoms of celiac disease for 11 years before being diagnosed.

Can my genes tell me if I have celiac disease?

No. Many people wonder if they have celiac disease based on their genetic testing. Your genes cannot tell you if you have celiac disease. Genetic testing can tell you if you're at a high risk, or genetically predisposed, to developing celiac disease, but it cannot tell you if you've developed celiac disease. There are some genetic variants (risk alleles) associated with celiac disease listed in this section, but they won't tell you if you've developed celiac disease. Genetic testing for celiac disease is a valuable way to rule out celiac disease, but should not be used to diagnose celiac disease.

The gold standard for celiac genetic testing cannot be done through "23andMe" genetic testing. This standard looks at the entire HLADQ2 and HLADQ8 genes rather than just a small part of the gene. The "23andMe" testing only looks at small parts of the gene rather than the entire gene.

Anyone who looks at your "23andMe" results and tells you that you have celiac disease or gluten sensitivity is misguided and incorrect. I believe that the best genetic testing for celiac disease is a combination of genetic testing that looks at *both* the "23andMe" genetic information *and* the full HLADQ2 and HLADQ8 genetic testing. However, even if genetic testing tells you that you're predisposed to developing celiac disease, it will never be able to diagnose you with either celiac disease or gluten sensitivity.

If I have the celiac genes, does that mean I will develop celiac disease?

No. Not everyone who has the celiac genes will develop celiac disease or other disease processes with exposure to gluten. The HLADQ2 risk alleles are present in more than 90 percent of individuals affected with celiac disease. The HLA-DQ2 and HLA-DQ8 are present in almost all celiac disease patients, but these genes are present in only about 50 percent of patients with gluten sensitivity[2].

Celiac disease is not just a digestive disease. People with celiac disease can have almost *any* symptom, including, but not limited to:

- Abdominal pain[4]
- Addison's disease[5]
- ADD/ADHD[6]
- ALS-like symptoms[7]
- Alopecia areata (patchy hair loss)[5]
- Anemia[5]
- Any autoimmune disease[7,8]
- Asthma[9]
- Behavioral problems
- Cancer[10]
- Cerebellar atrophy/balance problems[8]
- Chronic fatigue[11,12]
- Chronic sinusitis/sneezing
- Delayed menstruation[13]
- Delivery of child with low birth weight[5]
- Dental/enamel defects
- Depression[14]
- Diabetes[15,16]
- Diarrhea/digestive disorders
- Dizziness[8]
- Early menopause[13]
- Epilepsy
- Excessive weight loss or weight gain
- Fibromyalgia
- Gas/bloating
- IBS[5,17]
- Infertility[5,13]
- Joint pain/inflammation
- Multiple sclerosis[8]
- Liver problems[5]
- Malnourishment
- Mental illnesses
- Migraines[8,18,19]
- Muscle pain/muscle cramps[8]
- Neurodegenerative disorders[20]
- Obesity[21]
- Osteoporosis/osteo-penia[5,22]
- Numbness/tingling[8]
- Poor balance[8]
- Recurrent miscarriages[13]
- Rheumatoid arthritis[7]
- Short stature/delayed puberty
- Skin rashes[5]
- Thyroid disorders[5,23]
- Reoccurring mouth ulcers[5]

Interestingly, two-thirds of people with celiac disease had their symptoms manifest as neurological problems *without* having intestinal or digestive problems[3].

How do I know if I have celiac disease?

It's important to remember that you can have problems with gluten and not have celiac disease. Gluten sensitivity and wheat allergies are two examples of gluten problems that aren't celiac disease.

Tests that *can* tell you if you have celiac disease include:

Christy L. Sutton D.C.

- **Intestinal biopsy**—This rather invasive test doesn't work if you're avoiding gluten. It includes an endoscopy and having a small part of the small intestine biopsied. The sample is then analyzed to look for intestinal damage that disappears after avoiding gluten.

- **Celiac disease autoimmune antibodies (blood test)**—These tests don't work if you're avoiding gluten. It's important to have both the IgG and the IgA antibodies tested.

  ➢ **Anti-tissue transglutaminase antibodies (Anti-tTG) (IgG and IgA)**

  ➢ **Deamidated Gliadin Peptide Antibodies (Anti-DGP) (IgG and IgA)**

  ➢ **Anti-Endomysial Antibodies (anti-EMA)-(IgG and IgA)**

- **Food elimination test**—For this test you avoid gluten 100 percent for at least one month to see if symptoms improve. If symptoms improve while off gluten, but then reappear once gluten is reintroduced, it's best to permanently remove gluten from your diet, regardless of whether lab and genetic tests indicate otherwise. This test is very *sensitive* but less *specific*. If you feel better while not eating gluten for a month, you still don't know if you have celiac disease, gluten sensitivity or a wheat allergy. All you know is that you feel better without gluten and should probably avoid it.

What ancestral lines are most likely to carry the celiac disease genes?

Studies show that celiac disease occurs in all parts of the world but is most highly prevalent in people with ancestral lines from Ireland, Finland and northern Italy. People who live in northern India have a rather high prevalence of celiac genes. Interestingly, Germans with celiac genes are less likely to develop celiac disease than people of other European ancestries. It's unknown exactly why Germans have a decreased risk of developing celiac disease if they have celiac genes, but it's thought that they have some protective measure.

Is it possible to benefit from a gluten-free diet even if I don't have celiac disease?

Yes. Anyone with gluten sensitivity, wheat and/or barley allergies, or high inflammation levels could benefit from a gluten-free diet. The nutritional value of gluten is easy to replace in a balanced diet. There is no nutrient in gluten that cannot be found elsewhere in a well-balanced diet, and a daily multi-vitamin and mineral supplement.

How many people actually have gluten problems?

It's believed that 1 in 133 Americans have celiac disease. Screening studies predict that approximately one percent of the U.S. population has celiac disease, yet only 10 percent of affected individuals have been diagnosed thus far[24]. *This means that nine out of 10 people who have celiac are undiagnosed*. It's important to keep in mind that these numbers only reflect celiac disease and not those with gluten sensitivity or wheat allergies, which are growing rapidly in numbers. It's unknown what percent of people with gluten sensitivity and wheat allergies are undiagnosed.

Combined, wheat allergy, gluten sensitivity, and celiac disease are known to affect about 10 percent of the general population[25]. *This means that one in 10 people either has celiac, is gluten-sensitive or is wheat-allergic[1,25]*. Gluten sensitivity and wheat allergies are more like allergic reactions that are characterized by your body creating antibodies to either gluten or wheat. Unlike celiac disease, gluten sensitivity and wheat allergies are not autoimmune diseases, but can be triggers for autoimmune diseases, and can either lead to or occur in tandem with celiac disease.

If my doctor tells me that I don't have a problem with gluten, but I feel better when I'm off gluten, what could that mean?

It's possible to have incorrect lab results and/or for doctors to be wrong. If you feel better off of gluten, then you should avoid it. It might be helpful to take a high-quality multivitamin mineral to ensure that you have no nutritional deficiencies from avoiding gluten. It may also be beneficial to take a supplement with extra fiber if avoiding grains.

HLA risk alleles are indicators of autoimmune issues. The more HLA risk alleles you have, the more likely you are to develop autoimmune issues. HLA is instrumental in the immune system's ability to differentiate friend from foe, which is essential for preventing autoimmune issues.

Christy L. Sutton D.C.

Genetic variants associated with an increased risk of developing celiac disease and/or gluten sensitivity

Names of celiac gene genetic variants (SNP identification)	rsnumber	Risk allele
HLA	rs2858331	Risk allele is G
*HLA-DQA1—Associated with an increased risk of developing autoimmune diseases like lupus, in addition to celiac disease	rs2187668*	Risk allele is T
HLA-DQA2	rs9275224	Risk allele is A
HLA-DQ2.2 haplotype intergenic	rs7775228	Risk allele is C
HLA-DQ2.2 haplotype intergenic	rs2395182	Risk allele is T
*HLA-DQ8 intergenic	rs7454108*	Risk allele is C
CTLA4- increased risk for thyroid problems	rs231775	Risk allele is G
SH2B3	rs3184504	Risk allele is T

What do the HLA genes do?

The HLA genes help your body regulate the immune system so that it can distinguish between an invading pathogen (bacteria, virus or parasite) and your body's own tissues. In other words, the HLA genes are important for preventing autoimmune disorders by helping your immune system differentiate between friend and foe.

What health problems are associated with having a HLA risk allele?

Having an HLA risk allele is associated with an increased risk of developing:

- Autoimmune disorders
- Inflammatory disorders
- Lupus
- Celiac disease
- Multiple sclerosis

- Crohn's disease
- Hashimoto's thyroiditis
- Addison's disease
- Type 1 diabetes

SNPs with an * are currently used in "23andMe" Celiac Disease Genetic health Risk Report.

I have one or more risk allele(s) in the HLA gene. What should I talk to my doctor about doing so that I can reduce my health risks?

- *Remove chronic inflammation triggers*—Things that can trigger inflammation include infections, processed foods, food allergies, gluten, chemical toxicities, heavy metal toxicities and chronic stress.

- *Consider a trial period of avoiding gluten*—If you have health problems, do a month-long trial of eating 100 percent gluten-free. If your health improves while off gluten, then you should remain gluten-free.

- *Support a tolerant immune system to decrease autoimmune disease risk*— Some simple things have been shown to improve immune tolerance and potentially decrease your autoimmune disease risk include:

  - Vitamin D[26, 27]
  - Turmeric
  - Fish oil
  - Probiotics
  - Glutathione

- *Consider supplementing with digestive enzymes that help break down gluten*—The digestive enzyme DPPV-IV can decrease the effects of gluten exposure should you be accidently exposed.

I have one or more risk allele(s) in the HLA gene. What labs/testing should I consider to continually monitor my health?

✓ *Labs to rule out celiac disease and gluten sensitivity*

✓ *Vitamin D (blood test)*—Vitamin D is often low in people with autoimmune diseases. Low vitamin D can increase your risk of developing an autoimmune disease.

✓ *Monitor inflammation (blood test)*—Labs that monitor inflammation include CRP, ESR and homocysteine.

✓ *Calprotectin (stool test)*—Measuring calprotectin levels provides a clear idea of how much inflammation is occurring in your digestive system.

✓ *Autoimmune antibodies (blood test)*—Some common autoimmune antibodies include ANA, TPO and TPG.

✓ *Calcium score test*—This test is used to check for heart disease in an early stage and to determine how severe it is. It monitors for buildup of calcium in plaque on the walls of the arteries in the heart. This test does emit a low level of

Christy L. Sutton D.C.

radiation, so antioxidants should be greatly increased before and after this test is performed. This test is relevant due to fact that high levels of inflammation can lead to increased plaquing of the arteries.

✓ **Cyrex Lab's Panel 5**—This test can help you determine if you have developed an autoimmune disease. People that have celiac disease and gluten sensitivity are more likely to develop autoimmune diseases, especially if they continue to eat gluten.

References:

1.) Celiac disease. Centers for Disease Control and Prevention (2012) 'Basic Statistics'.

2.) Sapone A, Bai JC, Ciacii C, et al. Spectrum of gluten-related disorders: consensus on new nomenclature and classification. Mucosal Biology Research Center and Center for Celiac Research, University of Maryland School of Medicine, Baltimore, MD 21201, USA. BMC Med. 2012 Feb 7;10:13.

3.) M Hadjivassiliou, R A Grünewald and G A B Davies-Jones. Gluten sensitivity as a neurological illness. J Neurol Nurosurg Psychiatry, 2007: 72:560-563.

4.) Sanders DS, Hopper AD, Azmy IA, et al. Association of adult celiac disease with surgical abdominal pain: a case-control study in patients referred to secondary care. Ann Surg 2005;242:201-7.

5.) Andrew D Hopper, Marios Hadjivassiliou, et al. Adult coeliac disease. BMJ 2007; 335 (Published 13 September 2007).

6.) Niederhofer H, Pittschieler K. A preliminary investigation of ADHD symptoms in persons with celiac disease. J Atten Disord. 2006;10:200–204.7.) Turner MR, et al. A case of Celiac disease mimicking amytrophic lateral sclerosis. Neurology. 2007; 3:581- 584.

8.) M Hadjivassiliou, R A Grünewald and G A B Davies-Jones. Gluten sensitivity as a neurological illness. J Neurol Nurosurg Psychiatry, 2007: 72:560-563.

9.) Shewry PR1, Tatham AS2. Identification of the IgE-binding epitope in omega-5 gliadin, a major allegen in wheat dependent exercise-induced anaphylaxia. J Biol Chem. 2004 Mar 26; 279(13):1235-40.

10.) Brottveit M, Lundin KE. Cancer risk in coeliac disease. Tidsskr Nor Laegeforen. 2008;128(20):2312–5.

11.) Siniscalchi M1, Iovino P, Tortora R, Forestiero S Fatigue in adult Celiac disease. Aliment Pharmacol Ther. 2005 Sep1;22(5)489-94.

12.) Sanders DS, Evans KE, Hadjivassiliou M. Fatigue in primary care. Test for coeliac disease first? BMJ. 2010 Nov 2;341:c5161.

13.) Soni S1, Badawy SZ. Celiac disease and its effect on human reproduction: a review.J Reprod Med. 2010 Jan-Feb;55(1-2)3-8.

14.) Hallert C, Aström J.Psychic disturbances in adult Celiac disease. II. Psychological findings. Scand J Gastroenterol. 1982 Jan; 17(1):21-4.

15.) Martin Füchtenbusch, Anette-G. Ziegler, Elimination of dietary gluten and development of type 1 diabets in high risk subjects. Rev Diabet Stud. 2004 Spring; 1(1):39-41.

16.) Galicka-Latała D1, Zwolińska-Wcisło MThe role of Celiac disease and type 1 diabetes coexistence. Is celiac disease responsible for diabeteic status? Przegl Lek. 2009;66(4):170-5.

17.) Sanders DS, Carter MJ, Hurlstone DP, Pearce A, Ward AM, McAlindon ME, A Association of adult coeliac disease with irritable bowel syndrome: a case-control study in patients fulfilling ROME II criteria referred to secondary care. . Lancet. 2001 Nov 3;358(9292):1504-8.

18.) D'Amico D1, Rigamonti A, Spina L, et al. Migraine, Celiac disease, and cerebral calcification: a new case. Headache. 2005 Oct;45(9):1263-7.

19.). Gabrielli M1, Cremonini F, Fiore G,Association between migraine and celiac disease: results from a preliminary case-control and therapeutic study. Am J Gastroenterol. 2003 Mar; 98(3):625-9.

20.) De Vivo G1, Gentile V.Transglutaminase- catalyzed post-translational modifications of proteins in the nervous system and their possible involvement in neurodegenerative disease. CNS Neurol Disord Drug Targets.2008 Oct;7(4):370-5.

21.) Venkatasubramani, Narayanan; et al.†Obesity in Pediatric Celiac disease. J Pediatri Gastroenterol Nutr. 2010 May 12.

22.) Zofková I1. Celiac disease and its relation to bone metabolism. Cas Lek Cesk. 2009; 148(6):246-8.

23.) da Silva Kotze LM1, Nisihara RM, et al.Thyroid disorders in Brazilian patients with celiac disease. J of Clinical Gastroenterology. 2006 Jan; 40 (1): 33-6.

24.) Ehren J, Morón B, Martin E, et al. A food-grade enzyme preparation with modest gluten detoxification properties. PLoS One. 2009 Jul 21;4(7):e6313.

25.) Sapone A, Lammers KM, Mazzarella G, et al.. Differential mucosal IL-17 expression in two gliadin-induced disorders: gluten sensitivity and the autoimmune enteropathy celiac disease. Int Arch Allergy Immunol. 2010;152:75–80.

26.) Kivity S, Agmon-Levin N, Zisappl M, Shapira Y, Nagy EV, Dankó K, et al. Vitamin D and autoimmune thyroid diseases. Cell Mol Immunol. 2011;8:243–7.

27.) Chaudhary S1, Dutta D2, et al. Vitamin D supplementation reduces thyroid peroxidase antibody levels in patients with autoimmune thyroid disease: An open-labeled randomized controlled trial. Indian J Endocrinol Metab. 2016 May-Jun;20(3):391-8.

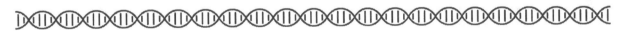

GGH gene
Gamma-glutamyl hydrolase gene

Names of GGH gene Genetic variants (SNP identification)	rsnumber	Risk allele
GGH C15472T	rs3780127	Risk allele is A
GGH C23421T	rs1031552	Risk allele is A
GGH C6699T	rs3780126	Risk allele is A
GGH G13894A	rs4617146	Risk allele is T
GGH G174A	rs11786893	Risk allele is T
GGH G91A	rs11545077	Risk allele is T

Christy L. Sutton D.C.

What health problems are associated with having a GGH risk allele?

There is a vague connection between GGH genetic variants and abnormal homocysteine levels, as well as between GGH genetic variants and tropical sprue (celiac disease).

I have one or more risk allele(s) in the GGH gene. What should I talk to my doctor about doing so that I can reduce my health risks?

- *Consider supporting a lower homocysteine levels*—Lowering homocysteine requires the methyl activated form of vitamin B-9 (Quatrefolic acid or L-5-MTHF), vitamin B-12 (methylcobalamin) and vitamin B-6 (P-5-P).

- *Heal your digestive system*—Support a healthy digestive lining and consider avoiding gluten, especially if having any symptoms of celiac disease or if you have celiac genes. Consider increasing your glutamine intake to help heal your digestive lining. Foods high in glutamine include beef, chicken, fish, eggs, cabbage, nuts, beans and beets.

I have one or more risk allele(s) in the GGH gene. What labs/testing should I consider to continually monitor my health?

- ✓ *Homocysteine (blood test)*— I prefer homocysteine to be at or below 8 on blood work.

- ✓ *Labs to rule out celiac disease and gluten sensitivity*

- ✓ *Vitamin D (blood test)*—Vitamin D is often low in autoimmune diseases. Low vitamin D can increase your risk of developing an autoimmune disease.

- ✓ *Monitor inflammation (blood work)*—Labs that monitor inflammation include CRP, ESR and homocysteine.

- ✓ *Calprotectin (stool test)*—Measuring calprotectin levels provides a clear idea of how much inflammation is occurring in your digestive system.

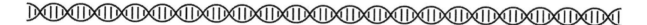

IFIH1 gene
Interferon-induced helicase C domain containing protein 1 gene

Names of IFIH1 gene genetic variants (SNP identification)	rsnumber	Risk allele
IFIH1	rs1990760	Risk allele is T

What does the IFIH1 gene do?

The IFIH1 gene plays a role in activating the immune system, especially in response to viral infections, by activating type 1 interferon. The IFIH1 gene may play a role in preventing cancer by enhancing the body's cancer killing cells (natural killer cell), inhibiting cancer cell growth, and the controlled cell death (apoptosis) in several tumor cell lines[5].

What health problems are associated with having an IFIH1 risk allele?

- *Increased risk for developing autoimmune diseases, including:*

  - Multiple sclerosis (MS)[1]
  - Graves' disease[2]
  - Type 1 diabetes[3]

I have one or more risk allele(s) in the IFIH1 gene. What should I talk to my doctor about doing so that I can reduce my health risks?

- *Remove environmental triggers that can lead to chronic inflammation and autoimmune diseases*—Environmental triggers of inflammation can include infections, processed foods, gluten, chemical toxicities, heavy metal toxicities, chronic stress and food allergies.

- *Consider supporting a tolerant immune system to decrease autoimmune disease risk*—Some simple things have been shown to improve immune tolerance and potentially decrease your autoimmune disease risk include:

  - Vitamins C and D
  - Probiotics
  - Antioxidants, such as glutathione
  - Rule out food allergies and celiac disease—These can be common autoimmune disease triggers

Christy L. Sutton D.C.

- *Monitor and control inflammation*—Natural ways to lower inflammation can include taking turmeric, fish oil, and following an anti-inflammatory diet low in sugar and grains and high in fruit, vegetables and fish.

I have one or more risk allele(s) in the IFIH1 gene. What labs/testing should I consider to continually monitor my health?

✓ *Perform regular blood work to measure inflammation levels throughout the body*—Labs that monitor inflammation in the body include CRP, ESR and homocysteine.

✓ *Vitamin D levels (blood test)*—A low vitamin D level can increase your autoimmune disease risk. Correcting a vitamin D deficiency can help improve MS[5] symptoms. One study found that children born to mothers who were vitamin D-deficient while pregnant had a 90 percent higher risk of developing MS when compared with those whose mothers had adequate vitamin D[4] during pregnancy. I prefer to see vitamin D level around 70 to 100 on lab work.

✓ *Consider testing for celiac disease, gluten sensitivity, and food allergies*—These can be triggers for autoimmune diseases.

✓ *Cyrex Lab's Panel 5 (blood test)*—This test can help you determine if you have developed an autoimmune disease. Cyrex Panel 5 analyses your blood to determine if you are creating antibodies against your own body, which is indicative of an autoimmune disease.

References:

1.) Couturier N, Gourraud PA, Cournu-Rebeix , et al. IFIH1-GCA-KCNH7 locus is not associated with genetic susceptibility to multiple sclerosis.Eur J Hum Genet. 2009;17:844–7.

2.) Zhao ZF, Cui B, Chen HY, Wang S, Li I. The A946T polymorphism in the interferon induced helicase gene does not confer susceptibility to Graves' disease in Chinese population. Endocrine. 2007;32:143–7.

3.) Jermendy A, Szatmari I, Laine AP, Lukacs K, , et al. (2010) The interferon-induced helicase IFIH1 Ala946Thr polymorphism is associated with type 1 diabetes in both the high-incidence Finnish and the medium-incidence Hungarian populations. Diabetologia 53: 98–102.

4.) Brazier, Yvette. (2016, March 7th). Could low vitamin D levels in pregnancy mean a risk for MS in offspring? Retrieved from URL: http://www.medicalnewstoday.com/articles/307516.php.

5.) Correale J, Ysrraelit MC, Gaitan MI.. Immunomodulatory effects of vitamin D in multiple sclerosis. Brain(2009) 132(Pt 5):1146–60.10.1093/brain/awp033.

Personalized genetic report found at http://geneticdetoxification.com

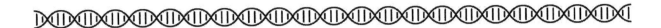

4q27 region gene

Names of 4q27 gene genetic variants (SNP identification)	rsnumber	Risk allele
4q27	rs6822844	Risk allele is T

What health problems are associated with having a 4q27 region risk allele?

- *Increased risk for developing an autoimmune disease*[1]—Some autoimmune diseases associated with having the risk allele in this gene include:

  - ➢ Rheumatoid arthritis
  - ➢ IBS
  - ➢ Crohn's disease
  - ➢ Ulcerative colitis

  - ➢ Celiac disease
  - ➢ Type 1 diabetes
  - ➢ Psoriatic arthritis
  - ➢ Lupus

Having this risk allele doesn't mean that you'll definitely develop an autoimmune disease. Developing an autoimmune disease is multifactorial and largely depends on your environment.

I have one or more risk allele(s) in the 4q27 Region gene. What should I talk to my doctor about doing so that I can reduce my health risks?

- *Remove environmental triggers that can lead to chronic inflammation and autoimmune diseases*—Environmental triggers of inflammation include infections, processed foods, gluten, chemical toxicities, heavy metal toxicities, chronic stress and food allergies.

- *Consider supporting a tolerant immune system to decrease autoimmune disease risk*—Some simple things have been shown to improve immune tolerance and potentially decrease your autoimmune disease risk include:
  - ➢ Vitamins C and D
  - ➢ Probiotics
  - ➢ Antioxidants, such as glutathione
  - ➢ Rule out food allergies and celiac disease—These can be common autoimmune disease triggers

Christy L. Sutton D.C.

- *Monitor and control inflammation*—Natural ways to lower inflammation can include taking turmeric, fish oil, and following an anti-inflammatory diet low in sugar and grains and high in fruit, vegetables and fish.

I have one or more risk allele(s) in the 4q27 Region gene. What labs/testing should I consider to continually monitor my health?

✓ *Perform regular blood work to measure inflammation levels throughout the body*—Labs that can monitor inflammation in the body include CRP, ESR and homocysteine.

✓ *Vitamin D levels (blood test)*—A low Vitamin D can increase your autoimmune disease risk. I prefer to see vitamin D level around 70 to 100 on lab work.

✓ *Consider testing for celiac disease and food allergies*—These can be autoimmune disease triggers.

✓ *Calprotectin (stool test)*—This test is especially important if you have digestive issues. Measuring calprotectin levels provides a clear idea of how much inflammation exists in your digestive system. Many associated with the 4q27 region risk allele lead to high inflammation levels in the digestive system.

✓ *Cyrex Lab's Panel 5 (blood test)*—This test can help you determine if you have developed an autoimmune disease. Cyrex Panel 5 analyses your blood to determine if you are creating antibodies against your own body.

References:

1.) Maiti AK, Kim-Howard X, Viswanathan P, et al. Confirmation of an association between rs6822844 at the IL2-IL21 region and multiple autoimmune diseases: evidence of a general susceptibility locus. Arthritis Rheum (2010) 62:323–910.1002/art.27222.

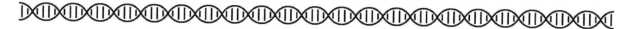

ATG16L1 gene
Autophagy-related protein 16-1

Names of ATG16L1 gene genetic variants (SNP identification)	rsnumber	Risk allele
ATG16L1	rs10210302	Risk allele is T
ATG16L1	rs2241880	Risk allele is G

What does the ATG16L1 gene do?

The ATG16L1 gene is significant in apoptosis, the controlled cell death that is essential for removing unhealthy cells so that new healthy cells can grow and thrive. This gene also helps the immune system destroy bacteria and viruses.

What health problems are associated with having an ATG16L1 risk allele?

- *Crohn's disease*
- *Ulcerative colitis*
- *Increased inflammation levels*

I have one or more risk allele(s) in the ATG16L1 gene. What should I talk to my doctor about doing so that I can reduce my health risks?

- ***Remove environmental triggers that can lead to chronic inflammation and autoimmune diseases***—Environmental triggers of inflammation include infections, processed foods, gluten, chemical toxicities, heavy metal toxicities, chronic stress and food allergies.

- ***Consider supporting a tolerant immune system to decrease autoimmune disease risk***—Some simple things have been shown to improve immune tolerance and potentially decrease your autoimmune disease risk include:

  - Vitamins C and D
  - Probiotics
  - Antioxidants, such as glutathione
  - Rule out food allergies and celiac disease—These can be common autoimmune disease triggers

- ***Monitor and control inflammation***—Natural ways to lower inflammation can include taking turmeric, fish oil, and following an anti-inflammatory diet low in sugar and grains and high in fruit, vegetables and fish.

Christy L. Sutton D.C.

I have one or more risk allele(s) in the ATG16L1 gene. What labs/testing should I consider to continually monitor my health?

✓ ***Perform regular blood work to measure inflammation levels throughout the body***—Labs that monitor inflammation in the body include CRP, ESR and homocysteine.

✓ ***Vitamin D levels (blood test)***—A low Vitamin D level can increase your autoimmune disease risk. I prefer to see vitamin D level around 70 to 100 on lab work.

✓ ***Consider testing for celiac disease, gluten sensitivity, and food allergies***—These be autoimmune disease triggers.

✓ ***Cyrex Lab's Panel 5 (blood test)***—This test can help you determine if you have developed an autoimmune disease. Cyrex Panel 5 analyses your blood to determine if you are creating antibodies against your own body, which is indicative of an autoimmune disease

---

A genetic combo that increases your Crohn's risk 20-fold[1]

Having this exact genotype significantly increases your risk of developing Crohn's disease.

- ATG16L1 (rS2241880) (G, G,)
- IBD5 (rs6596075) (C, C)
- NOD2 (rs17221417) (G, G,)

References:

1.) Wellcome Trust Case Control Consortium Genome-wide association study of 14,000 cases of seven common diseases and 3,000 shared controls. Nature 2007; 447:661–678.

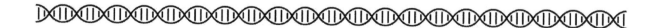

Personalized genetic report found at http://geneticdetoxification.com

CFH gene
Complement factor H

Names of CFH gene genetic variants (SNP identification)	rsnumber	Risk allele
CFH	rs6677604	Risk allele is A

What does the CFH gene do?

The CFH gene helps initiate the immune system's process to remove pathogens from the body.

What health problems are associated with having a CFH risk allele?

- *Increased risk of a kidney disease known as IgA nephropathy*
- *Lupus*

I have one or more risk allele(s) in the CFH gene. What should I talk to my doctor about doing so that I can reduce my health risks?

- *Avoid dehydration*—This is very hard on the kidneys.

- *Remove environmental triggers that can lead to chronic inflammation and autoimmune disease*—Environmental triggers of inflammation include infections, processed foods, gluten, chemical toxicities, heavy metal toxicities, chronic stress and food allergies.

- *Consider supporting a tolerant immune system to decrease autoimmune disease risk*—Some simple things have been shown to improve immune tolerance and potentially decrease your autoimmune disease risk include:

  - Vitamins C and D
  - Probiotics
  - Antioxidants, such as glutathione
  - Rule out food allergies and celiac disease—These can be common autoimmune disease triggers

- *Monitor and control inflammation*—Natural ways to lower inflammation can include taking turmeric, fish oil, and following an anti-inflammatory diet low in sugar and grains and high in fruit, vegetables and fish.

Christy L. Sutton D.C.

I have one or more risk allele(s) in the CFH gene. What labs/testing should I consider to continually monitor my health?

- ✓ *Monitor kidney function with BUN, creatinine and GFR blood tests.*

- ✓ *Perform regular blood work to measure inflammation levels in the entire body*—Labs that can monitor inflammation in the body include CRP, ESR and homocysteine.

- ✓ *Vitamin D levels (blood test)*—A low vitamin D level can increase your autoimmune disease risk. I prefer to see vitamin D level around 70 to 100 on lab work.

- ✓ *Consider testing for celiac disease, gluten sensitivity, and food allergies*— These can be autoimmune disease triggers.

- ✓ *Cyrex Lab's Panel 5 (blood test)*—This test can help you determine if you have developed an autoimmune disease. Cyrex Panel 5 analyses your blood to determine if you are creating antibodies against your own body, which is indicative of an autoimmune disease.

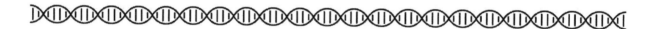

CTLA4 gene

Cytotoxic T-lymphocyte-associated protein 4

Names of CTLA4 gene genetic variants (SNP identification)	rsnumber	Risk allele
CTLA4	rs231775	Risk allele is G

What does the CTLA4 gene do?

The CTLA4 gene makes a protein called CTLA4 that is located on the surface of a white blood cell called a T-cell. The CTLA4 protein functions as an immune checkpoint that inhibits the immune system, and therefore, is important in preventing autoimmune diseases. CTLA4 is a critical regulator of the part of the immune system that controls T-cell responses.

What health problems are associated with having a CTLA4 risk allele?

Multiple autoimmune diseases, including:

- Hashimoto's thyroiditis
- Celiac disease
- Multiple sclerosis
- Lupus

- Type 1 diabetes
- Grave's disease
- Primary biliary cirrhosis

I have one or more risk allele(s) in the CTLA4 gene. What should I talk to my doctor about doing so that I can reduce my health risks?

- *Remove environmental triggers that can lead to chronic inflammation and autoimmune diseases*—Environmental triggers of inflammation include infections, processed foods, gluten, chemical toxicities, heavy metal toxicities, chronic stress and food allergies.

- *Consider supporting a tolerant immune system to decrease autoimmune disease risk*—Some simple things have been shown to improve immune tolerance and potentially decrease your autoimmune disease risk include:

  - Vitamins C and D
  - Probiotics
  - Antioxidants, such as glutathione
  - Rule out food allergies and celiac disease—These can be common autoimmune disease triggers

- *Monitor and control inflammation*—Natural ways to lower inflammation can include taking turmeric, fish oil, and following an anti-inflammatory diet low in sugar and grains and high in fruit, vegetables and fish.

I have one or more risk allele(s) in the CTLA4 gene. What labs/testing should I consider to continually monitor my health?

- ✓ *Perform regular blood work to measure inflammation levels throughout the body*—Labs that monitor inflammation in the body include CRP, ESR and homocysteine.

Christy L. Sutton D.C.

✓ **Vitamin D levels (blood test)**—A low vitamin D level can increase your autoimmune disease risk. I prefer to see vitamin D level around 70 to 100 on lab work.

✓ **Consider testing for celiac disease and food allergies**—These can be autoimmune disease triggers.

✓ **If you have digestive problems, consider a calprotectin (stool test)**—This provides a clear idea of how much inflammation exists in your digestive system. The diseases associated with having these risk alleles lead to high inflammation levels in the digestive tract.

✓ **Autoimmune blood panels**—If you're having health problems, consider autoimmune blood panels to rule out autoimmune diseases.

➢ **Cyrex Lab's Panel 5 (blood test)**—This test can help you determine if you have developed an autoimmune disease. Cyrex Panel 5 analyses your blood to determine if you are creating antibodies against your own body, which is indicative of an autoimmune disease.

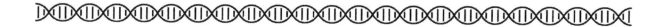

IL5 gene
Interleukin-5

Names of IL5 gene genetic variants (SNP identification)	rsnumber	Risk allele
IL5	rs2069812	Risk allele is G

What does the IL5 gene do?

The IL5 gene instructs the body to make a chemical called IL-5. IL-5 stimulates a part of the immune system called the B cells, and increases a type of white blood cell called eosinophils. The part of the immune system that IL-5 stimulates is called Th-2, which is important in fighting off bacterial and parasitic infections. It can also play a role in developing allergies and autoimmune diseases.

What health problems are associated with having an IL5 risk allele?

- *Increased risk of gastric cancer*[1]

- *Increased risk of non-Hodgkin's lymphoma (NHL)*—However, this association was only found in women with a higher body mass index[2]; women with a BMI greater than or equal to 25 kg/m2 had 50 to 90 percent increased risk of NHL.

I have one or more risk allele(s) in the IL5 gene. What should I talk to my doctor about doing so that I can reduce my health risks?

- *Manage your weight*—This is best accomplished through exercise and a diet high in fresh vegetables and healthy fats. Weight management is especially important for women with the risk allele that are both obese and have a family history of blood cancers like non-Hodgkin's lymphoma.

- *Remove environmental triggers that can lead to chronic inflammation and autoimmune diseases*—Some triggers of inflammation include infections, processed foods, gluten, chemical toxicities, heavy metal toxicities, chronic stress and food allergies.

- *Consider supporting a tolerant immune system to decrease autoimmune disease risk*—Some simple things have been shown to improve immune tolerance and potentially decrease your autoimmune disease risk include:

  - Vitamins C and D
  - Probiotics
  - Antioxidants, such as glutathione
  - Rule out food allergies and celiac disease—These can be common autoimmune disease triggers

- *Monitor and control inflammation*—Natural ways to lower inflammation can include taking turmeric, fish oil, and following an anti-inflammatory diet low in sugar and grains and high in fruit, vegetables and fish.

Christy L. Sutton D.C.

I have one or more risk allele(s) in the IL5 gene. What labs/testing should I consider to continually monitor my health?

✓ ***Regular colonoscopies and EGDs (upper endoscopy of the stomach)***— These tests are important for early detection, and possibly removal, of digestive system cancers.

✓ ***Calprotectin (stool test)***—This test provides a clear idea of how much inflammation exists in your digestive system.

✓ ***Monitor inflammation levels (blood work)***—Labs that monitor inflammation in the body include CRP, ESR and homocysteine.

✓ ***Vitamin D levels (blood test)***—A low vitamin D level can increase your autoimmune disease risk. I prefer to see vitamin D level around 70 to 100 on lab work.

✓ ***Consider testing for celiac disease, gluten sensitivity, and food allergies***— These can be autoimmune disease triggers.

✓ ***Cyrex Lab's Panel 5 (blood test)***—This test can help you determine if you have developed an autoimmune disease. Cyrex Panel 5 analyses your blood to determine if you are creating antibodies against your own body, which is indicative of an autoimmune disease.

References:

1.) Mahajan R, El-Omar EM, Lissowka J, et al. Genetic variants in T helper cell type 1, 2 and 3 pathways and gastric cancer risk in a Polish population. Jpn J Clin Oncology. 2008;9:626–633.

2.) Yantai Chen,1,2 Tong hang Zheng,2 Qing Lan,3 Francine Foss. Cytokine polymorphisms in Th1/Th2 pathway genes, body mass index, and risk of non-Hodgkin lymphoma. Blood First Edition paper, October 15, 2010.

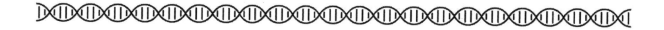

IL6 gene
Interleukin-6

Names of IL6 gene genetic variants (SNP identification)	rsnumber	Risk allele
IL6	rs2069837	Risk allele is G
IL6	rs1524107	Risk allele is T
IL6	rs2066992	Risk allele is T
IL6	rs2069840	Risk allele is G
IL6	rs1554606	Risk allele is G
IL6	rs2069849	Risk allele is T

What does the IL6 gene do?

The IL6 gene makes a chemical called IL-6 (interleukin-6), which is both an inflammatory and anti-inflammatory chemical that the body uses to communicate between cells. The IL-6 cytokine sends a signal to other cells that can both initiate or inhibit an inflammatory response in the body. IL-6 can promote chronic inflammation and progression of autoimmune diseases.

What health problems are associated with having an IL6 risk allele?

Having the IL6 risk allele can lead to higher levels of IL-6 and inflammation. Most disease processes will be exacerbated by high levels of IL-6, causing high levels of inflammation. Some health problems associated with higher levels of IL-6 include:

- *Cancer*—There is an increased cancer risk associated with having risk alleles in the IL6 genes. Specific types of cancer associated with the IL6 gene risk alleles include:

  - Multiple myeloma [5]
  - Prostate cancer [6]

- *Autoimmune disease*—Crohn's disease, lupus and rheumatoid arthritis[4,7]

- *Atherosclerosis*[1]

- *Depression*[2]

Christy L. Sutton D.C.

- *Alzheimer's disease*[3]

- *Mental illness*—High IL-6 levels contribute to schizophrenia by inhibiting the GAD67 gene, which is important for the calming neurotransmitter GABA to function properly. This leads to a decreased calming effect from GABA and an increased chance of mental illness.

I have one or more risk allele(s) in the IL6 gene. What should I talk to my doctor about doing so that I can reduce my health risks?

Ways to naturally decrease IL-6 and inflammation levels include:

- *Remove triggers that can lead to chronic inflammation and autoimmune diseases*—Some inflammation triggers include infections, processed foods, gluten, chemical toxicities, heavy metal toxicities, chronic stress and food allergies.

- *Regular aerobic exercise (at least 30 minutes every day)*—The IL-6 the body produces during exercise has an anti-inflammatory effect. However, extreme exercise can have the opposite effect and increase inflammation by increasing IL-6 levels. IL-6 can be anti-inflammatory because it inhibits a highly inflammatory chemical called tumor necrosis factor-alpha (TNF-alpha). That is why it's so important to engage in regular exercise.

- *Maintain a stable blood sugar level*—This is best accomplished by avoiding refined sugar and processed foods and eating a diet high in protein good fats and fiber.

- *Reduce stress*—Use stress-relieving techniques such as prayer, meditation, walking, talk therapy, vacations and living below your means, etc.

- *Weight management*—This is best accomplished through exercise and a healthy diet high in fresh vegetables and healthy fats.

- *Consider increasing nutrients that decrease inflammation:*

  ➤ Trace minerals—Trace minerals should include boron and magnesium, among others. Boron has shown to significantly reduce inflammation and the inflammatory marker called CRP[9].
  ➤ Turmeric
  ➤ Fish oil
  ➤ Zinc
  ➤ Vitamin D
  ➤ Probiotics
  ➤ Antioxidants (vitamin C and glutathione)

- *Avoid things that increase inflammation by increasing IL-6, including:*

  ➤ Obesity—The inflammatory chemical IL-6 is secreted by fat cells. It's thought that obese people have higher inflammation levels because they're secreting more IL-6 from fat cells.
  ➤ Stress
  ➤ Lack of sleep
  ➤ Consuming too much sugar and having an unstable blood sugar level
  ➤ Smoking
  ➤ Excess alcohol consumption
  ➤ Drinking coffee
  ➤ High blood sugar
  ➤ Viral infections
  ➤ Extreme exercise

I have one or more risk allele(s) in the IL6 gene. What labs/testing should I consider to continually monitor my health?

✓ *Perform regular blood work to measure inflammation levels throughout the body*—Labs that can monitor inflammation in the body include *CRP*, ESR and homocysteine. IL-6 is the most potent inducer of the inflammatory marker CRP. Therefore, it's important for anyone with a risk allele in the IL6 gene to monitor their CRP levels through routine blood work.

✓ *Vitamin D levels (blood test)*—A low vitamin D levels can increase your autoimmune disease risk. I prefer to see vitamin D level around 70 to 100 on lab work.

✓ *Consider testing for celiac disease, gluten sensitivity, and food allergies*—These can be autoimmune disease triggers.

✓ *Calprotectin (stool test)*—This provides a clear idea as to how much inflammation exists in your digestive system.

Christy L. Sutton D.C.

✓ **Cyrex Lab's Panel 5 (blood test)**—This test can help you determine if you have developed an autoimmune disease. Cyrex Panel 5 analyses your blood to determine if you are creating antibodies against your own body, which is indicative of an autoimmune disease.

References:

1.) Dubiński A, Zdrojewicz Z (April 2007). "The role of interleukin-6 in development and progression of atherosclerosis". Pol. Merkur. Lekarski(in Polish) 22 (130): 291–4.

2.) Dowlati Y, Herrmann N, Swardfager W, EK et al. (March 2010). "A meta-analysis of cytokines in major depression". Biol. Psychiatry 67 (5): 446–57.

3.) Swardfager W, Lanctôt K, Rothenburg L, (November 2010). "A meta-analysis of cytokines in Alzheimer's disease". Biol. Psychiatry 68 (10): 930–41.

4.) Tackey E, Lipsky PE, Illei GG (2004). "Rationale for interleukin-6 blockade in systemic lupus erythematosus". Lupus 13 (5): 339–43.

5.) Gadó K, Domján G, Hegyesi H, Falus A (2000). "Role of INTERLEUKIN-6 in the pathogenesis of multiple myeloma". Cell Biol. Int. 24 (4): 195–209.

6.) Smith PC, Hobisch A, Lin DL, (March 2001). "Interleukin-6 and prostate cancer progression". Cytokine Growth Factor Rev. 12 (1): 33–40.

7.) Nishimoto N (May 2006). "Interleukin-6 in rheumatoid arthritis". Curr Opin Rheumatol 18 (3): 277–81.

8.) Naghii MR, Mofid M, Asgari AR,. Comparative effects of daily and weekly boron supplementation on plasma steroid hormones and proinflammatory cytokines. J. Trace. Elem. Med. Bio. 2011;25:54–58.

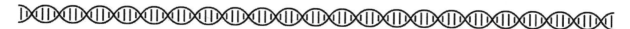

IL-13 gene
Interleukin 13 gene

Names of IL-13 gene genetic variants (SNP identification)	rsnumber	Risk allele
IL-13 C1112T	rs1800925	Risk allele is T
IL-13	rs20541	Risk allele is G

What does the IL-13 gene do?

The IL-13 gene increases inflammation and allergies[1] and provides body's instructions to make the inflammatory chemical IL-13.

What health problems are associated with having an IL-13 risk allele?

- *Asthma*—Having risk alleles in the IL-13 gene have been shown to confer an enhanced risk of inflammatory diseases such as asthma[1].

- *Lung fibrosis*—Having the risk allele for IL-13 C1112T (rs1800925) is associated with decreased lung function and idiopathic lung fibrosis[2].

- *Allergic rhinitis, psoriasis, and asthma*—Having the risk allele for IL-13 (rs20541) is associated with allergic rhinitis, psoriasis and asthma.

I have one or more risk allele(s) in the IL-13 gene. What should I talk to my doctor about doing so that I can reduce my health risks?

- *Ensure you're breathing clean air*—Avoid air pollution, don't smoke, open windows when the air outside is clean, and have house plants to produce oxygen and purify the air. Change air filters regularly in your home and car and have clean air ducts.

- *Consider increasing glutathione levels*—Having low glutathione levels can increase your asthma risk and overall inflammation levels. Read more about glutathione on pages 57.

- *Remove chronic inflammation and autoimmune disease triggers*—Some inflammation triggers include infections, processed foods, gluten, chemical toxicities, heavy metal toxicities, chronic stress and food allergies.

- *Exercise regularly*—At least 30 minutes of aerobic exercise every day.

- *Maintain a stable blood sugar level*—Avoid refined sugar and processed foods and eat a diet high in protein good fats and fiber.

- *Reduce stress*—Use stress-relieving techniques such as (prayer, meditation, walking, talk therapy, vacations, adequate sleep and living below your means.

- *Consider increasing nutrients that decrease inflammation:*

> Trace minerals—Trace minerals should include boron and magnesium, among others. Boron has shown to significantly reduce inflammation and the inflammatory marker called CRP[9].
> Turmeric
> Fish oil
> Zinc
> Vitamin D
> Probiotics
> Antioxidants (vitamin C and glutathione)

I have one or more risk allele(s) in the IL-13 gene. What labs/testing should I consider to continually monitor my health?

✓ **Monitor glutathione levels (blood test)**—Low glutathione levels can increase your asthma risk.

✓ **Perform regular blood work to measure inflammation levels throughout the body**—Labs that can monitor inflammation in the body include CRP, ESR and homocysteine.

✓ **Vitamin D levels (blood test)**—A low vitamin D level can increase your autoimmune disease risk. I prefer to see vitamin D level around 70 to 100 on lab work.

✓ **Consider testing for celiac disease, gluten sensitivity, and food allergies**—These can be autoimmune disease triggers.

References:

1.) Wikipedia. Interleukin 13. Retrieved from: https://en.wikipedia.org/wiki/Interleukin_13

2.) Ding M, Sheng H, Shen W, et al...fibrosis. Cell Biochem Biophys. 2013;67(3):905-9.

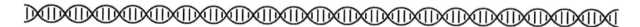

KLC1 gene
Kinesin light-chain 1 gene

Names of KLC1 gene genetic variants (SNP identification)	rsnumber	Risk allele
KLC1	rs8702	Risk allele is G

What health problems are associated with having a KLC1 risk allele?
Increased MS risk:

- The GG genotype appears to be associated with an increased risk of developing MS[1].
- The CC genotype may provide a significant protective effect from developing MS[1].
- The exact effect of the CG genotype is unclear.

I have one or more risk allele(s) in the KLC1 gene. What should I talk to my doctor about doing so that I can reduce my health risks?

- *Remove chronic inflammation and autoimmune disease triggers*—Some inflammation triggers include infections, processed foods, gluten, chemical toxicities, heavy metal toxicities, chronic stress and food allergies.

- *Consider supporting a tolerant immune system to decrease autoimmune disease risk*—Some simple things have been shown to improve immune tolerance and potentially decrease your autoimmune disease risk include:

  - Vitamins C and D
  - Probiotics
  - Antioxidants, such as glutathione
  - Rule out food allergies and celiac disease—These can be common autoimmune disease triggers

- *Monitor and control inflammation*—Natural ways to lower inflammation can include taking turmeric, fish oil, and following an anti-inflammatory diet low in sugar and grains and high in fruit, vegetables and fish.

Christy L. Sutton D.C.

I have one or more risk allele(s) in the KLC1 gene. What labs/testing should I consider to continually monitor my health?

✓ *Perform regular blood work to measure inflammation levels throughout the body*—Labs that monitor inflammation in the body include CRP, ESR and homocysteine.

✓ *Vitamin D levels (blood test)*—A low vitamin D level can increase your autoimmune disease risk. Correcting vitamin D deficiencies can help improve MS[3] symptoms. One study found that children born to mothers who were vitamin D-deficient while pregnant had a 90 percent higher risk of developing MS when compared to those whose mothers had adequate vitamin D[2]. I prefer to see vitamin D level around 70 to 100 on lab work.

✓ *Consider testing for celiac disease and food allergies, as they can be triggers for autoimmune diseases*—Many people with MS have problems with gluten; therefore, it might be worthwhile to do celiac testing and/or a trial gluten-elimination diet.

✓ *If having neurological symptoms that do not improve (i.e. headaches, numbness, tingling, dizziness), consider a MRI of the head to rule out MS.*

✓ *Cyrex Lab's Panel 5 (blood test)*—This test can help you determine if you have developed an autoimmune disease. Cyrex Panel 5 analyses your blood to determine if you are creating antibodies against your own body, which is indicative of an autoimmune disease.

References:

1.) Szolnoki Z, Kondacs A, Mandi Y, Somogyvari F. A cytoskeleton motor protein genetic variant may exert a protective effect on the occurrence of multiple sclerosis: the janus face of the kinesin light-chain 1 56836CC genetic variant. Neuromol Med. 2007;9:335–339.

2.) Brazier, Yvette. (2016, March 7th). Could low vitamin D levels in pregnancy mean a risk for MS in offspring? Retrieved from URL: http://www.medicalnewstoday.com/articles/307516.php

3.) Correale J, Ysrraelit MC, Gaitan MI.. Immunomodulatory effects of vitamin D in multiple sclerosis. Brain (2009) 132(Pt 5):1146–60.

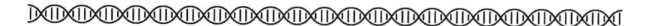

LRP6 gene
Low-density lipoprotein receptor- related protein 6 gene

Names of LRP6 gene genetic variants (SNP identification)	rsnumber	Risk allele
LRP6 Cys1270	rs1012672	Risk allele is A
LRP6 T154522C	rs2160525	Risk allele is G
LRP6	rs2302685	Risk allele is T

What health problems are associated with having a LRP6 risk allele?

- *LRP6 (rs2302685) risk alleles associated with an increased risk of developing:*

  - Crohn's disease—Genotype (G, G) is associated with early-onset Crohn's disease[1]
  - Myocardial infarction (heart attack)[2]
  - Alzheimer's disease[3]

- *LRP6 T154522C (rs2160525) risk alleles are associated with an increased risk of developing Alzheimer's disease.*

- *LRP6 (rs2302685) risk alleles are associated an increased risk of developing Alzheimer's disease.*

I have one or more risk allele(s) in the LRP6 gene. What should I talk to my doctor about doing so that I can reduce my health risks?

- *Decrease inflammation*—Increase consumption of fish or fish oil and turmeric, and eat a low-sugar diet with a lot of vegetables.

- *Avoid inflammatory triggers*—Things that can increase inflammation include stress, allergens, toxins, sugar and infections.

- *Promote a healthy immune system*—Vitamin D, turmeric, fish oil, probiotics and glutathione all help the immune system to be more tolerant and less likely to initiate an autoimmune process.

Read the section titled "How can you reduce your risk of developing Alzheimer's disease?" (pg 157).

Christy L. Sutton D.C.

I have one or more risk allele(s) in the LRP6 gene. What labs/testing should I consider to continually monitor my health?

✓ ***Blood work to monitor cholesterol, triglycerides, inflammation and blood sugar***—These labs are important for heart health and include LDL, HDL, VLDL, triglycerides, hemoglobin A1C, fasting blood glucose, homocysteine and CRP.

✓ ***Smell test***—The sense of smell is often the first sign of cognitive decline and Alzheimer's disease. Therefore, testing your sense of smell is a great way to monitor your brain health.

✓ ***Memory recall testing***

✓ ***Vitamin D level (blood test)***—Vitamin D is important for both brain and bone health. I prefer to see vitamin D level around 70 to 100 on lab work.

✓ ***Calprotectin (stool test)***—If your digestive system is a concern, you should monitor inflammation in your intestines by measuring calprotectin levels.

✓ ***Calcium score test***—This test is used to check for heart disease in an early stage and to determine how severe it is. It monitors for buildup of calcium in plaque on the walls of the arteries in the heart. This test does emit a low level of radiation, so antioxidants should be greatly increased before and after this test is performed.

✓ ***Cyrex Lab's Panel 5 (blood test)***—This test can help you determine if you have developed an autoimmune disease. Cyrex Panel 5 analyses your blood to determine if you are creating antibodies against your own body, which is indicative of an autoimmune disease.

References:

1.)Koslowski MJ, Teltschik Z, Beisner J, et al. Association of a functional variant in the Wnt co-receptorLRP6 with early onset ileal Crohn's disease. PLoS Genet. Published online 23 February 2012.

2.) Shung Xu, et al. The LRP6 rs2302685 polymorphism is associated with increased risk of myocardial infarction. Lipids in Health and Disease. 2014; 13()94.

3.)De Ferrari GV1, Papassotiropoulos A, et al,. Common genetic variation within the low-density lipoprotein receptor-related protein 6 and late-onset Alzheimer's disease. Proc Natl Acad Sci U S A. 2007 May 29;104(22):9434-9. Epub 2007 May 21.

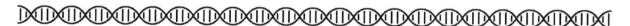

Personalized genetic report found at http://geneticdetoxification.com

FUT2 gene
Fucosyltransferase 2 gene

Names of FUT2 gene genetic variants (SNP identification)	rsnumber	Risk allele
FUT2 A12190G	rs492602	Risk allele is G
FUT2 A12404T	rs1047781	Risk allele is T
FUT2 C12376T	rs281377	Risk allele is T
FUT2 G12447A	rs601338	Risk allele is A
FUT2 G12758A	rs602662	Risk allele is A

What does the FUT2 gene do?

The FUT2 gene plays a role in intestinal health by increasing the number of intestinal binding sites available for bacteria to bind to. The more binding sites there are, the greater the risk for gastrointestinal (G.I.) infections. Because people with the FUT2 risk allele have more binding sites, they're more likely to have G.I. infections.

What health problems are associated with having an FUT2 risk allele?

- *Increased risk of developing intestinal infections, celiac disease, IBS (irritable bowel syndrome) and Crohn's disease*

    - *Celiac, inflammatory bowel disorders, and norovirus intestinal infections*—Having the risk allele for FUT2 G12447A (rs601338) is associated with an increased risk of norovirus (cruise ship stomach bug)[4] infection. This genotype is also associated with an increased risk of celiac disease and inflammatory bowel disorders[3].

    - *Crohn's disease*—Having the risk allele for FUT2 G12758A (rs602662) is possibly associated with an increased risk of developing Crohn's disease[2]. This increased risk could be a result of an infection that triggers Crohn's disease.

    - *H. pylori stomach infection*

Christy L. Sutton D.C.

- ***Vitamin B-12 deficiencies secondary to an intestinal infection, causing vitamin B-12 malabsorption***—Having an FUT2 risk allele can lead to a vitamin B-12 deficiency resulting from a gastrointestinal infection that deceases vitamin B-12 absorption. Without a G.I. infection, these FUT2 genotypes shouldn't increase the risk of a vitamin B-12 deficiency.

I have one or more risk allele(s) in the FUT2 gene. What should I talk to my doctor about doing so that I can reduce my health risks?

- ***Wash hands before eating, and avoid eating questionable food to prevent G.I. infections***—The main problem with having an FUT2 risk allele is the increased G.I. infection risk.

- ***Consider supplementing with probiotics***—High-quality probiotics are very important for anyone with an FUT2 genetic variations. Probiotics prevent G.I. infections by binding up sites in the gut that bad bacteria could potentially bind to.

- ***Monitor and prevent vitamin B-12 deficiencies***—This is especially important for anyone with a known history of H. pylori infections, Crohn's or celiac disease, as those conditions greatly increase the risk of vitamin B-12 deficiency.

- ***Consider a gluten-free diet if you're having digestive problems***—Having the FUT2 risk allele is associated with an increased risk of developing celiac disease.

I have one or more risk allele(s) in the FUT2 gene. What labs/testing should I consider to continually monitor my health?

- ✓ ***Consider the H. pylori breath test if experiencing digestive issues***—H. pylori is a bacterium that can cause stomach inflammation and pain that is normally worse when the stomach is empty. Having an FUT2 risk allele can lead to an increased risk for an H. pylori infection. The most accurate way to test for an H. pylori infection is with an H. pylori breath test.

- ✓ ***Monitor for vitamin B-12 deficiency (blood test)***—Tests to consider include methylmalonic acid, CBC and serum B12. Methylmalonic acid is the most accurate test for diagnosing a vitamin B-12 deficiency. Just testing serum B-12 levels isn't very accurate, as the vitamin B-12 deficiency has to be dangerously severe before the test flags the B-12 level as too low.

- ✓ *If having digestive issues, consider a comprehensive stool test through Genova Diagnostics or Viome*—This tests for parasite and bacterial infections and will provide a detailed understating of the health of the intestinal ecosystem, intestines, and level of inflammation in the intestines.

- ✓ *Celiac testing*—There is an increased risk of developing celiac disease associated with having a FUT2 risk allele. There is more about celiac disease and testing for celiac disease on pages 269.

References:

1.) Ikehara Y., Nishihara S., Yasutomi H., et al. Polymorphisms of two fucosyltransferase genes (Lewis and Secretor genes) involving type I Lewis antigens are associated with the presence of anti-Helicobacter pylori IgG antibody. Cancer Epidemiol. Biomarkers Prev. 2001;10:971–977.

2.) McGovern DP, Jones MR, et al.: Fucosyltransferase 2 (FUT2) non-secretor status is associated with Crohn's disease. Hum Mol Genet. 2010;19(17):3468–3476.

3.) Parmar AS1, Alakulppi N, Paavola-Sakki P, Tissue Antigens. Association study of FUT2 (rs601338) with celiac disease and inflammatory bowel disease in the Finnish population 2012 Dec;80(6):488-93.

4.) Thorven M1, Grahn A, et al. A homozygous nonsense mutation (428G-->A) in the human secretor (FUT2) gene provides resistance to symptomatic norovirus (GGII) infections. J Virol. 2005 Dec;79(24):15351-5

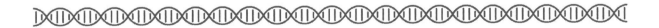

Christy L. Sutton D.C.

TLR4 gene
Toll-like receptors gene

Names of TLR4 gene genetic variants (SNP identification)	rsnumber	Risk allele
TLR4	rs4986790	Risk allele is G

What does the TLR4 gene do?

The TLR4 gene is instrumental in the immune system's ability to detect and remove pathogenic bacteria and parasites by activating an inflammatory cascade in the body. The increased level of inflammation that the TLR4 gene helps to produce can help clear infections, but long-term exposure to high inflammation levels can increase your risk of developing chronic degenerative disease, including cardiovascular disease.

What health problems are associated with having a TLR4 risk allele?

- *Increased risk of intestinal infections*—Having a risk allele for the TLR4 gene is associated with an increased risk of intestinal infections, particularly gram-negative bacterial infections[2].

- *Crohn's disease*—The TLR4 risk allele is associated with an increased risk of developing Crohn's disease and ulcerative colitis[1]. It's possible that the TLR4 risk allele is also involved in other inflammatory autoimmune diseases.

- *Type 2 diabetes and metabolic syndrome in Caucasians*[4]—There is an increased risk for developing blood sugar problems associated with having the TLR4 risk allele. In addition, type 2 diabetes patients carrying AG/GG genotypes have an increased risk of developing an eye problem called retinopathy[5].

- *Alzheimer's disease*[6]—The increased risk of developing Alzheimer's may be due to an increased amount of inflammation that can result from having a TLR4 risk allele. This inflammation is very bad for the brain[6].

- *Vascular disease*—Including heart attack, stroke and retinopathy[3].

I have one or more risk allele(s) in the TLR4 gene. What should I talk to my doctor about doing so that I can reduce my health risks?

- ***Prevent gastrointestinal infections***—Avoid intestinal infections by washing your hands and avoiding high-risk situations like eating questionable foods. Also consider supplementing with probiotics.

- ***Decrease inflammation***—Eat a diet low in sugar and inflammatory foods and high in fruits, vegetables, turmeric and healthy omega-3 fatty acids.

Read the section titled "How can you reduce your risk of developing Alzheimer's disease?" (pg 157).

I have one or more risk allele(s) in the TLR4 gene. What labs/testing should I consider to continually monitor my health?

- ✓ ***Blood work to monitor cholesterol, triglycerides, inflammation and blood sugar***—These labs are important for heart health, and include LDL, HDL, VLDL, triglycerides, hemoglobin A1C, fasting blood glucose, homocysteine and CRP. It's important to monitor inflammation with these tests because high inflammation levels increase your chance of developing Alzheimer's disease and cardiovascular disease.

- ✓ ***Memory recall testing and sense of smell***—These measures for cognitive decline are associated with Alzheimer's disease. One of the first signs of Alzheimer's is a decreased sense of smell so testing your sense of smell is a great way to monitor your brain health.

- ✓ ***Calprotectin (stool test)***—If your digestive system is a concern, you should monitor inflammation in the intestines by measuring your calprotectin levels.

- ✓ ***Cardiac stress test***—This is particularly important for men with the (G/G) genotype, as they are at an increased heart attack risk.

- ✓ ***Routine eye exams***—This is particularly important if you're diabetic.

- ✓ ***Calcium score test***—This test is used to check for heart disease in an early stage and to determine how severe it is. It monitors for buildup of calcium in plaque on the walls of the arteries in the heart. This test does emit a low level of radiation, so antioxidants should be greatly increased before and after this test is performed.

✓ **Cyrex Lab's Panel 5 (blood test)**—This test can help you determine if you have developed an autoimmune disease. Cyrex Panel 5 analyses your blood to determine if you are creating antibodies against your own body, which is indicative of an autoimmune disease.

References:

1.) Ouburg S, Mallant-Hent R, Crusius JB, , et al. The toll-like receptor 4 (TLR4) Asp299Gly polymorphism is associated with colonic localisation of Crohn's disease without a major role for the Saccharomyces cerevisiae mannan-LBP-CD14-TLR4 pathway. Gut. 2005;54(3):439–40.

2.) Agnese D. M., Calvano J. E., Hahm S. J., et al. Human toll-like receptor 4 mutations but not CD14 polymorphisms are associated with an increased risk of gram-negative infections. Journal of Infectious Diseases. 2002;186(10):1522–1525.

3.) Garcia-Bermudez M., Lopez-Mejías R., et al. Lack of association between TLR4 rs4986790 polymorphism and risk of cardiovascular disease in patients with rheumatoid arthritis. DNA Cell Biol. 2012;31:1214–1220

4.) F. S. Belforte, F. Coluccio Leskow, E. Poskus, and A. Penas Steinhardt, "Toll-like receptor 4 D299G polymorphism in metabolic disorders: a meta-analysis," Molecular Biology Reports, vol. 40, pp. 3015–3020, 2013.

5.) M. Buraczynska, I. Baranowicz-Gaszczyk, J. Tarach, and A. Ksiazek, "Toll-like receptor 4 gene polymorphism and early onset of diabetic retinopathy in patients with type 2 diabetes," Human Immunology, vol. 70, no. 2, pp. 121–124, 2009.

6.) Balistreri C. R., Grimaldi M. P., Chiappelli M., et al. (2008). Association between the polymorphisms of TLR4 and CD14 genes and Alzheimer's disease. Curr. Pharm. Des. 14, 2672–2677.

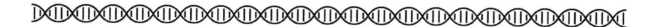

Personalized genetic report found at http://geneticdetoxification.com

TNF gene
Tumor Necrosis Factor-alpha gene

Names of TNF gene genetic variants (SNP identification)	rsnumber	Risk allele
TNF- 238	rs361525	Risk allele is A
TNF- 308.2 (TNF2)	rs1800629	Risk allele is A

What does the TNF gene do?

The TNF gene provides the body's instructions to make a protein called TNF (tumor necrosis factor-alpha), a highly inflammatory chemical messenger. When TNF is high, inflammation levels will also be high.

What health problems are associated with having a TNF risk allele?

Having a risk allele in the TNF gene can result in high TNF levels, which leads to increased inflammation levels. Health problems associated with high TNF levels include:

- *Cancer*
- *Autoimmune diseases*
- *Inflammation*

I have one or more risk allele(s) in the TNF gene. What should I talk to my doctor about doing so that I can reduce my health risks?

- *Remove chronic inflammation and autoimmune disease triggers*—Some inflammation triggers include infections, processed foods, gluten, chemical toxicities, heavy metal toxicities, chronic stress and food allergies.

- *Consider supporting a tolerant immune system to decrease autoimmune disease risk*—Some simple things have been shown to improve immune tolerance and potentially decrease your autoimmune disease risk include:

    ➢ Vitamins C and D
    ➢ Probiotics

Christy L. Sutton D.C.

> ➤ Antioxidants, such as glutathione
> ➤ Rule out food allergies and celiac disease—These can be common autoimmune disease triggers

- ***Monitor and control inflammation***—Natural ways to lower inflammation can include taking turmeric, fish oil, and following an anti-inflammatory diet low in sugar and grains and high in fruit, vegetables and fish.

- ***Ensure adequate levels of trace minerals***—Trace minerals include boron and magnesium. Boron has been shown to significantly reduce inflammation and the inflammatory marker CRP[1].

I have one or more risk allele(s) in the TNF gene. What labs/testing should I consider to continually monitor my health?

- ✓ ***Perform regular blood work to measure inflammation levels throughout the body***—Labs that monitor inflammation include CRP, ESR and homocysteine.

- ✓ ***Monitor vitamin D level (blood test)***—A low vitamin D level can increase your risk for autoimmune disease and cancer. I prefer to see vitamin D level around 70 to 100 on lab work.

- ✓ ***Calcium score test***—This test is used to check for heart disease in an early stage and to determine how severe it is. It monitors for buildup of calcium in plaque on the walls of the arteries in the heart. This test does emit a low level of radiation, so antioxidants should be greatly increased before and after this test is performed. This test is relevant due to fact that high levels of inflammation can lead to increased plaquing of the arteries.

- ✓ ***Cyrex Lab's Panel 5 (blood test)***—This test can help you determine if you have developed an autoimmune disease. Cyrex Panel 5 analyses your blood to determine if you are creating antibodies against your own body, which is indicative of an autoimmune disease.

References:

1.) Naghii MR, Mofid M, Asgari AR, Hedayati M, Daneshpour M–S. Comparative effects of daily and weekly boron supplementation on plasma steroid hormones and proinflammatory cytokines. J. Trace. Elem. Med. Bio. 2011;25:54–58.

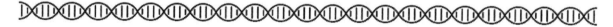

Personalized genetic report found at http://geneticdetoxification.com

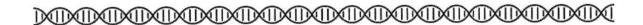

<u>Chapter 10</u>
Allergies and Hypersensitivities

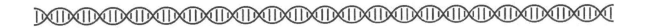

ABP1/DAO genes
Actin binding protein 1/D-amino acid oxidase gene

Names of ABP1/DAO gene genetic variants (SNP identification)	rsnumber	Risk allele
ABP1/DAO C1933G	rs1049793	Risk allele is G
ABP1/DAO C47T	rs10156191	Risk allele is T
DAO/ABP1 C995T	rs1049742	Risk allele is T

What does the ABPl/DAO gene do?

The ABP1/DAO gene provides instructions for the body to make the ABP1/DAO enzyme, which is important for histamine to be degraded and ultimately for histamine levels to be decreased. This enzyme's role in degrading histamines is why it's so important for allergies and hypersensitivities.

What health problems are associated with having an ABPl/DAO risk allele?

- *Increased risk of allergic and hypersensitivity reactions due to high histamine levels*—If you have the (T/T) genotype for ABP1/DAO C47T (rs10156191), you're more likely to have an abnormally large histamine response, which may manifest in allergies and hypersensitivity reactions. Some symptoms of an abnormal histamine response include:

  - Itching
  - Hives
  - Headaches
  - Nausea
  - Stomach aches/ Indigestion / Diarrhea
  - Drop in blood pressure
  - Increased pulse rate
  - Nasal congestion
  - Asthma
  - Runny nose
  - Irritated eyes
  - Heartburn
  - Increased risk of anaphylactic-type reaction

- *Potential increase in allergic reactions when taking NSAIDs and other drugs*—Having the T allele for the ABP1/DAO C47T (rs10156191) gene is strongly associated with a negative hypersensitivity/allergic reaction to NSAIDs. NSAIDs reduce the DAO enzyme's ability to break down the histamine. Drugs that reduce the body's ability to break down histamine include[2]:

  - Common pain killers such as aspirin and NSAIDS
  - Some diuretics ("water pills")
  - Antibiotics
  - Antidepressants

Always contact your prescribing doctor before changing or stopping any medications.

I have one or more risk allele(s) in the ABPI/DAO gene. What should I talk to my doctor about doing so that I can reduce my health risks?

Natural ways to lower histamine levels:

- *Avoid foods that increase histamine levels*—Some people may only need to adhere to a histamine-lowering diet while they're having a high-histamine response (i.e., while ovulating, menstruating, having seasonal allergies). Some foods that are known to increase histamine levels include:

  - Fermented and aged foods
  - Shellfish
  - Eggs
  - Aged or processed meat
  - Leftovers
  - Milk/cheese
  - Artificial food coloring
  - Preservatives (especially benzoates and sulphites)
  - Fermented soy
  - Chocolate
  - Alcohol

- *Ensure you're breathing clean air*—Avoid air pollution, don't smoke, open windows when the air outside is clean, and have house plants to produce oxygen and purify the air. Change air filters regularly in your home and car and have clean air ducts.

- *Heal the gut*—Leaky gut will increase histamine levels and allergic reactions. Low levels of DAO correlate with poor gut function. Intestinal damage will lead to less DAO production.

Christy L. Sutton D.C.

- ***Consider supplementing with nutrients that can help reduce histamine levels, including:***

  - ***Quercetin***—Helps prevent allergies and hypersensitivities by stabilizing the mast cells that release histamine.

  - ***Bromelain***—This enzyme is naturally found in raw pineapple and has been shown to reduce the number of circulating allergenic proteins in the blood. Bromelain has also been shown to enhance absorption of quercetin.

  - ***N-acetylcysteine (NAC)***—This can help the body make more glutathione, which is the most important antioxidant in the body. Both glutathione and NAC can help reduce the thickness of mucus.

  - ***Vitamin C***—This helps deactivates histamine.

  - ***DAO (diamine oxidase)***—This enzyme breaks down histamine and is less efficient in people with these risk alleles. It's possible to take a supplemental form of the DAO enzyme to assist in reducing histamine levels.

  - ***Vitamin D***—This is very important for maintaining a healthy immune system that doesn't overreact by producing too much histamine. I prefer to see vitamin D level around 70 to 100 on lab work.

Are your allergies better during pregnancy, but worse during certain menstrual cycle phases?

Histamine-intolerant women often suffer from headaches and menstrual pain during certain phases of their menstrual cycle—such as ovulation and right before menstruation. These women often experience other symptoms such as hives and headaches. However, these women often experience a marked decrease in symptoms during pregnancy.

This decrease in allergies and headaches during pregnancy can be a result of the placenta producing a large amount of the enzyme diamine oxidase (DAO), which is responsible for degrading excess histamine. Unfortunately, allergic symptoms tend to reoccur after pregnancy because the placenta is no longer producing extra DAO enzyme.

It is possible to increase DAO through supplementation.

I have one or more risk allele(s) in the ABPI/DAO gene. What labs/testing should I consider to continually monitor my health?

- ✓ *Consider allergy testing*—This especially includes IgE allergy testing.

- ✓ *Dunwoody labs Advanced IBA*—This measures DAO and histamine levels.

- ✓ *Monitor vitamin D level*—Having a high vitamin D level is important to maintain a healthy, properly functioning immune system. I prefer to see vitamin D level around 70 to 100 on lab work.

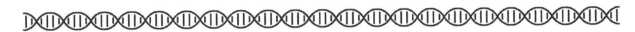

FCER1A gene
Fc fragment of IgE receptor la gene

Names of FCER1A gene genetic variants (SNP identification)	rsnumber	Risk allele
FCER1A	rs2251746	Risk allele is C

What does the FCER1A gene do?

The FCER1A gene provides the body's instructions to make the FCER1A receptor, which quickly and easily binds to allergy-inducing IgE antibodies. In doing so it plays a central role in triggering a histamine response and allergic diseases such as hay fever and asthma.

What health problems are associated with having a FCER1A risk allele?

Allergies, atopic dermatitis, hay fever and asthma—Having the risk allele for FCER1A (rs2251746) can lead to high IgE antibody levels, which are commonly found in people with allergies such as atopic dermatitis and asthma[1,2].

I have one or more risk allele(s) in the FCER1A gene. What should I talk to my doctor about doing so that I can reduce my health risks?

- • *Ensure you're breathing clean air*—Avoid air pollution, don't smoke, open windows when the air outside is clean, and have house plants to produce oxygen

Christy L. Sutton D.C.

and purify the air. Change air filters regularly in your home and car and have clean air ducts.

- **_Consider supplementing with nutrients that can help reduce histamine levels, including_:**

  ➤ **_Quercetin_**—This helps prevent allergies and hypersensitivities by stabilizing the mast cells that release histamine.

  ➤ **_Bromelain_**—This enzyme is naturally found in raw pineapple and has been shown to reduce the number of circulating allergenic proteins in the blood. Bromelain has also been shown to enhance absorption of quercetin.

  ➤ **_N-acetylcysteine (NAC)_**—This can help the body make more glutathione, which is the most important antioxidant in the body. Both glutathione and NAC can help reduce the thickness of mucus.

  ➤ **_Vitamin C_**—This helps deactivates histamine, which decreases allergic responses.

  ➤ **_Vitamin D_**—This is very important for maintaining a healthy immune system that doesn't overreact by producing too much histamine.

I have one or more risk allele(s) in the FCER1A gene. What labs/testing should I consider to continually monitor my health?

- ✓ **_Consider allergy testing_**—This especially includes IgE allergy testing.

- ✓ **_Monitor vitamin D level_**— I prefer to see vitamin D level around 70 to 100 on lab work.

References:

1.)Weidinger S1, Gieger C, Rodriguez E, et al. Genome-wide scan on total serum IgE levels identifies FCER1A as novel susceptibility locus. PLoS Genet. 2008 Aug;4(8):e1000166. Epub 2008 Aug 22.

2.) Zhou J, Zhou Y, et al. Association of polymorphisms in the promoter region of FCER1A gene with atopic dermatitis, chronic uticaria, asthma, and serum immunoglobulin E levels in a Han Chinese population. Hum Immunol. 2012 Mar;73(3):301-5.

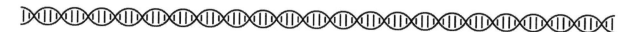

CD14 gene
Cluster of differentiation 14 gene

Names of CD14 gene genetic variants (SNP identification)	rsnumber	Risk allele
CD14	rs2569191	Risk allele is C

What does the CD14 gene do?

The CD14 gene plays a role in the immune system's ability to recognize pathogenic bacteria[1].

What health problems are associated with having a CD14 risk allele?

Having the (C, C) genotype is associated with having fewer IgE antibodies and a decreased risk of an allergic response in children exposed to pets[2].

I have one or more risk allele(s) in the CD14 gene. What should I talk to my doctor about doing so that I can reduce my health risks?

If you have a (C, C) genotype, being exposed to pets as a child might prevent allergies and immune problems as an adult.

I have one or more risk allele(s) in the CD14 gene. What labs/testing should I consider to continually monitor my health?

Monitor vitamin D level— I prefer to see vitamin D level around 70 to 100 on lab work. Vitamin D is important for maintaining a healthy immune system and preventing allergies.

References:

1.)T D LeVan1, S Guerra2, et al. The impact of CD14 polymorphisms on the development of soluble CD14 levels during infancy. Genes and Immunity (2006) 7, 77–80.

2. Bottema RW1, Reijmerink NE, et al. Interleukin 13, CD14, pet and tobacco smoke influence atopy in three Dutch cohorts: the allergenic study. 2008 Sep;32(3):593-602.

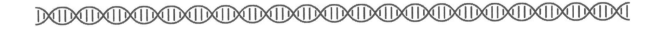

Christy L. Sutton D.C.

IL4R gene

IL-4 receptor alpha single-nucleotide gene

Names of IL4R gene genetic variants (SNP identification)	rsnumber	Risk allele
IL4R Q576R	rs1801275	Risk allele is G
IL4R	rs1859308	Risk allele is A
IL4R	rs8832	Risk allele is A

What does the IL4R gene do?

The IL4R gene plays a role in making IgE antibodies from a part of the immune system called Th-2. IgE antibodies play a central role in allergic responses such as seasonal allergies, asthma, hives and anaphylactic responses.

What health problems are associated with having an IL4R risk allele?

- **High levels of IgE antibodies**—Having the risk allele for the IL4R gene is associated with having high levels of IgE antibodies. Some health problems associated with having a high number IgE antibodies include:

  - Hypersensitivities
  - Asthma[2]

- **High cholesterol**—The (G, G) or (G, A) genotypes are associated with high cholesterol levels, but *not* with cardiovascular disease[1].

I have one or more risk allele(s) in the IL4R gene. What should I talk to my doctor about doing so that I can reduce my health risks?

- *Considers supporting a tolerant immune system to decrease the risk for developing hypersensitivities and asthma:*

  - Vitamins C and D
  - Probiotics
  - Antioxidants, such as glutathione
  - Fish oil
  - Rule out food allergies and celiac disease—These can be common autoimmune disease triggers.

- *Monitor and control inflammation*—Natural ways to lower inflammation can include taking turmeric, fish oil, and following an anti-inflammatory diet low in sugar and grains and high in fruit, vegetables and fish.

- *Remove chronic inflammation triggers*—Some triggers of inflammation can include infections, processed foods, gluten, chemical toxicities, heavy metal toxicities, chronic stress and food allergies.

- *Ensure you're breathing clean air*—Avoid air pollution, don't smoke, open windows when the air outside is clean, and have house plants to produce oxygen and purify the air. Change air filters regularly in your home and car and have clean air ducts.

I have one or more risk allele(s) in the IL4R gene. What labs/testing should I consider to continually monitor my health?

✓ *Consider allergy testing*—This especially includes IgE allergy testing.

✓ *Monitor vitamin D level*—Having an adequate vitamin D level is important to maintain a healthy, properly functioning immune system. I prefer to see vitamin D level around 70 to 100 on lab work.

✓ *Perform regular blood work to measure inflammation levels throughout the body*—Labs that monitor inflammation include CRP, ESR and homocysteine.

✓ *Monitor cholesterol levels and heart health*.

✓ *Calcium score test*—This test is used to check for heart disease in an early stage and to determine how severe it is. It monitors for buildup of calcium in plaque on the walls of the arteries in the heart. This test does emit a low level of radiation, so antioxidants should be greatly increased before and after this test is performed. This test is relevant due to fact that high levels of inflammation can lead to increased plaquing of the arteries.

References:

1.) Sánchez Muñoz-Torrero JF, et al. rs1801275 Interleukin-4 receptor alpha polymorphism in familial hypercholesterolemia. J Clin Lipidol. 2014 Jul-Aug;8(4):418-22.

2.) Al-Muhsen S., Vazquez-Tello A, et al. IL-4 receptor alpha single-nucleotide polymorphisms rs1805010 and rs1801275 are associated with increased risk of asthma in a Saudi Arabian population. Annals of Thoracic Medicine. 2014;9(2):81–86.

Christy L. Sutton D.C.

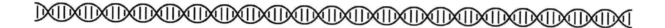

For more information on genes related to immune health, consult the following pages:

Cancer-associated genes
- ADA gene Pg. 244
- CAT gene Pg. 251

Detox genes
- NR1I2 gene Pg. 129
- Phase II detox genes
  - Glutathione genes Pg. 57
  - Methylation genes
    - MTHFR gene Pg. 87
    - MTR gene Pg. 99
    - Methylation and Autoimmune Diseases Pg. 83

Brain health genes
- MAO-B gene Pg. 187

Vitamin and mineral genes
- SLC30A8 gene Pg. 374
- VDR gene Pg. 368

Cardiovascular health genes
- NOS1, NOS2, and NOS3 gene Pg 358

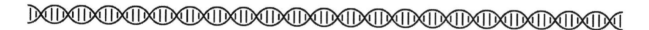

Part 5
Cardiovascular Health Genes

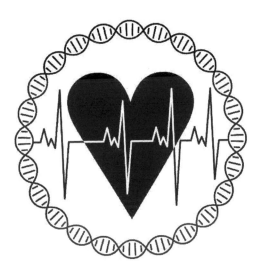

Did you know that certain genes are associated with a higher risk of having a stroke or heart attack? While you can't change your genes, you can change your environment to minimize the risk of having a cardiovascular event.

Because cardiovascular disease can often be a silent killer, it's important for everyone to have routine testing to monitor their heart health, regardless of their genotype. It's commonly accepted that the environment plays a pivotal role in developing cardiovascular disease. That's why eating a healthy diet and exercising regularly can dramatically reduce your risk for developing cardiovascular disease.

Knowing that you might have inherited certain genes that increase your risk for cardiovascular disease will enable you work with your doctor to establish a treatment plan to minimize your risk.

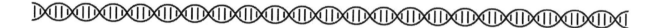

Chapter 11
Blood-Clotting Genes

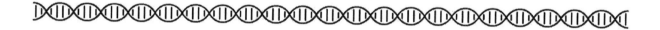

Personalized genetic report found at http://geneticdetoxification.com

<u>Factor 5 (F5) gene</u>
Coagulation factor V gene

Names of Factor 5 (F5) gene genetic variants (SNP identification)	rsnumber	Risk allele
Factor 5 (F5)	rs6025	Risk allele is T

What does the Factor 5 (F5) gene do?

The Factor 5 (F5) gene is involved in the body's ability to clot. If you have this risk allele, you are said to have the Factor V Leiden genetic mutation, and you have a significantly increased risk for forming abnormal and life-threatening blood clots.

What health problems might be associated with having a Factor 5 (F5) risk allele?

- *Increased risk for clotting disorders*—There is a very strong link between having a Factor 5 risk allele and being at an increased risk of thrombosis, abnormal clotting, and a subsequent heart attack or stroke. However, vitamin E has been shown to significantly decrease risks associated with having this high-risk allele (300 iu/ day of Vitamin E)[1]. Having this risk allele in the F5 gene is dangerous for men and women, but carries additional concerns for women. About 5 percent of women have this Factor 5 risk allele.

  ➢ *Women need to know if they have a F5 risk allele because they're at an increased risk for:*

    o *Pregnancy problems*—There is a slightly increased risk of pregnancy loss for women who have a F5 risk allele. Women with the risk allele are two to three times more likely to have multiple miscarriages or pregnancy loss during the second or third trimester[3]. There is also an increased risk for pregnancy-induced high blood pressure (preeclampsia), slow fetal growth, and early separation of the placenta from the uterine wall (placenta abruption)[3].

    o *Increased risk for clotting during pregnancy*—Having this risk allele leads to an increased risk for developing DVT (deep vein thrombosis) and pulmonary embolism by *three-fold*[1].

o *Increased risk of clotting if taking tamoxifen*—Although preliminary, a 2010 study on women taking tamoxifen as part of their treatment for early-stage breast cancer found that those women who had a clotting event were nearly *five times* more likely to have Factor 5 (F5) risk allele compared to those who did not have a thromboembolic event.

I have one or more risk allele(s) in the Factor 5 (F5) gene. What should I talk to my doctor about doing so that I can reduce my health risks?

- *Consider increasing vitamin E intake*—If you have the Factor 5 (F5) risk allele, taking 300 IU per day of vitamin E has shown to decrease health risks, including clotting[1]. Make sure you're taking the natural form of vitamin E rather than the synthetic form of vitamin E.

- *Additional ways to prevent excessive clotting:*

  - *Avoid being sedentary*— Being sedentary increases your risk for clotting. Exercise regularly and avoid prolonged periods of being sedentary if you have this risk allele. If you're limited in your level of activity, wear leg sleeves or use leg compressors.

  - *Maintain low levels of inflammation*—Inflammation can increase the risk for clotting. Increased consumption of antioxidants, fish oil and turmeric can help decrease inflammation, which can decrease the risk of clotting. Fish oil can also act as a blood thinner.

  - *Maintain a healthy weight, blood pressure and blood sugar.*

  - *Exercising caution about taking oral contraceptives.*

  - *Abstaining from smoking.*

  - *Increase garlic consumption.*

  - *Consider supplementing with an enzyme called Nattokinase, which may help prevent excessive clotting.*

I have one or more risk allele(s) in the Factor 5 (F5) gene. What labs/testing should I consider to continually monitor my health?

- ✓ ***Monitor for clotting***—It is important for anyone with the Factor 5 risk allele to be under the care of a medical doctor that can monitor their clotting levels, and help ensure that they are not clotting too fast. Clotting too fast can increase the chance of a stroke, embolism, or vascular event. Some labs to monitor clotting include:

    - ➢ ***Prothrombin Time (PT) and PTT (Partial Thromboplastin Time)***— These tests are used to determine if someone has a coagulation problem.
    - ➢ ***Fibrinogen activity test***
    - ➢ ***D-dimer***—The D-dimer test is designed to measure body's ability to break clots apart when they are no longer needed.

- ✓ ***Monitor inflammation (blood test)***—High levels of inflammation increase the risk of having a vascular event such a stroke. The best labs for monitoring inflammation in someone with an F5 risk allele include:

    - ➢ ***CRP***
    - ➢ ***Homocysteine***
    - ➢ ***Lp-PLA2 (Lipoprotein-Associated Phospholipase A2)***
    - ➢ ***Hemoglobin A1***—Because high blood sugar is very inflammatory, I also recommend testing blood sugar levels by ordering a hemoglobin A1C.

- ✓ ***Monitor blood pressure***—High blood pressure will add an increased risk to having a heart attack or stroke.

References:

1.) Glynn RJ, Ridker PM, Goldhaber SZ. Effects of Random Allocation to Vitamin E Supplementation on the Occurrence of Venous Thromboembolism. Women's Health Study. Circulation 2007;116(13):1497-503.

2.) Retrieved from: SNPedia. Rs6025. Retrieved from: http://www.snpedia.com/index.php/Rs6025

3.) NIH. Genetic Home Reference. Factor V Leiden thrombophilia. Retrieved from: https://ghr.nlm.nih.gov/condition/factor-v-leiden-thrombophilia

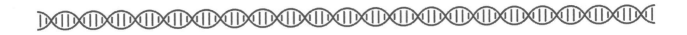

Christy L. Sutton D.C.

Factor 2 (F2) gene
Coagulation factor II (prothrombin) gene

Names of F2 gene genetic variants (SNP identification)	rsnumber	Risk allele
Factor 2 (F2)	i3002432	Risk allele is A

What does the F2 gene do?

The F2 gene is involved in the body's ability to clot.

What health problems might be associated with having an F2 risk allele?

- *Increased risk of clotting problems*—Having the (A, A) genotype can increase the risk of developing a venous thromboembolism (clot in the vein) by more than *three-fold* over having the (G, G) genotype[1]. Venous thromboembolisms are very dangerous because they are clots that form in the vein (normally in the leg) and then travel to another area of the body. If the clot travels to the brain or heart, it can cause a stroke or heart attack.

I have one or more risk allele(s) in the F2 gene. What should I talk to my doctor about doing so that I can reduce my health risks?

- *Consider supplementing with vitamin E*—In one study the group of people that supplemented with an additional 300 IU per day of vitamin E had a 67 percent lower risk of developing a deep vein thrombosis or pulmonary embolism than the group that only relied on vitamin E from food [2]. While adding vitamin E was helpful for people with one or more A alleles, vitamin E did little for women with the low risk (G, G) genotype[2]. If you supplement with vitamin E, ensure that you're supplementing with the natural form rather than the synthetic form.

- *Exercise caution if using oral contraceptives*—Taking oral contraceptives while having an F2 risk allele can significantly increase your risk for developing an unprovoked venous thrombosis (clot in the vein)[3].

- **Additional ways to prevent excessive clotting**:

  - ➤ **Avoid being sedentary**—Being sedentary increases your risk for clotting. Exercise regularly and avoid prolonged periods of being sedentary if you have this risk allele. If you're limited in your level of activity, wear leg sleeves or use leg compressors.

  - ➤ **Maintain low levels of inflammation**—Inflammation can increase the risk for clotting. Increased consumption of antioxidants, fish oil and turmeric can help decrease inflammation, which can decrease the risk of clotting. Fish oil can also act as a blood thinner.

  - ➤ **Maintain a healthy weight, blood pressure and blood sugar.**

  - ➤ **Exercising caution with taking oral contraceptives.**

  - ➤ **Abstaining from smoking.**

  - ➤ **Increase garlic consumption.**

  - ➤ **Consider supplementing with an enzyme called Nattokinase, which may help prevent excessive clotting.**

I have one or more risk allele(s) in the F2 gene. What labs/testing should I consider to continually monitor my health?

- ✓ **Monitor for clotting**—It's important for anyone with the F2 risk allele to be under the care of a medical doctor who can monitor their clotting levels and help ensure that they're not clotting too fast. Clotting too fast can increase the chance of a stroke, embolism or vascular event. Some labs to monitor clotting include:

  - ➤ **Prothrombin Time (PT) and PTT (Partial Thromboplastin Time)**— These tests are used to determine if someone has a coagulation problem.
  - ➤ **Fibrinogen activity test**
  - ➤ **D-dimer**—The D-dimer test is designed to measure the body's ability to break clots apart when they are no longer needed.

Christy L. Sutton D.C.

✓ *Monitor inflammation (blood test)*—High levels of inflammation increase the risk of having a vascular event such as a stroke. The best labs for monitoring inflammation in someone with an F2 risk allele include:

> ➢ *CRP*
> ➢ *Homocysteine*
> ➢ *Lp-PLA2 (Lipoprotein-Associated Phospholipase A2)*
> ➢ *Hemoglobin A1*— Because high blood sugar is very inflammatory, I also recommend testing blood sugar levels by ordering a hemoglobin A1C.

✓ *Monitor blood pressure*—High blood pressure will add an increased risk to having a heart attack or stroke.

References:

1.) Zee RY, Glynn RJ, Cheng S, Steiner L, et al. An evaluation of candidate genes of inflammation and thrombosis in relation to the risk of venous thromboembolism: the women's genome health study. Circ Cardiovasc Genet. 2009; 2:57-62

2.) Glynn RJ, Ridker PM, Goldhaber SZ, et al. Effects of random allocation to vitamin E supplementation on the occurrence of venous thromboembolism: report from the Women's Health Study.Circulation. 2007;116:1497–1503.

3.) Rosendaal FR (2005). "Venous thrombosis: the role of genes, environment, and behavior". Hematology Am. Soc. Hematol. Educ. Program 2005 (1): 1–12.

Factor 3 (F3) gene
Coagulation factor III gene

Names of F3 gene genetic variants (SNP identification)	rsnumber	Risk allele
Factor 3 (F3)	rs3917643	Risk allele is C

What does the F3 gene do?

The F3 gene is involved in the body's ability to clot.

What health problems might be associated with having a F3 risk allele?

- Associated with pregnancy-related venous thrombosis[1].

I have one or more risk allele(s) in the F3 gene. What should I talk to my doctor about doing so that I can reduce my health risks?

- *Pregnant women with one or more F3 risk alleles should make smart diet and lifestyle choices to help prevent clotting while pregnant*—It's important for pregnant women to talk to their doctor about what they can do to prevent clotting.

- *Additional ways to prevent excessive clotting:*

  - *Avoid being sedentary*—Being sedentary increases your risk for clotting. Exercise regularly and avoid prolonged periods of being sedentary if you have this risk allele. If you're limited in your level of activity, wear leg sleeves or use leg compressors.

  - *Maintain low levels of inflammation*—Inflammation can increase the risk for clotting. Increased consumption of antioxidants, fish oil and turmeric can help decrease inflammation, which can decrease the risk of clotting. Fish oil can also act as a blood thinner.

  - *Maintain a healthy weight, blood pressure and blood sugar.*

  - *Exercising caution about taking oral contraceptives.*

  - *Abstaining from smoking.*

  - *Increase garlic consumption.*

  - *Consider supplementing with an enzyme called Nattokinase, which may help prevent excessive clotting.*

Christy L. Sutton D.C.

I have one or more risk allele(s) in the F3 gene. What labs/testing should I consider to continually monitor my health?

✓ ***Monitor for clotting***—It's important for anyone with the F3 risk allele to be under the care of a medical doctor who can monitor their clotting levels and help ensure that they're not clotting too fast. Clotting too fast can increase the chance of a stroke, embolism or vascular event. Some labs to monitor clotting include:

  ➤ ***Prothrombin Time (PT) and PTT (Partial Thromboplastin Time)***— These tests are used to determine if someone has a coagulation problem.
  ➤ ***Fibrinogen activity test***
  ➤ ***D-dimer***—The D-dimer test is designed to measure the body's ability to break clots apart when they're no longer needed.

✓ ***Monitor inflammation (blood test)***—High levels of inflammation increase the risk of having a vascular event such as a stroke. The best labs for monitoring inflammation in someone with an F3 risk allele include:

  ➤ ***CRP***
  ➤ ***Homocysteine***
  ➤ ***Lp-PLA2 (Lipoprotein-Associated Phospholipase A2)***
  ➤ ***Hemoglobin A1***—Because high blood sugar is very inflammatory, I also recommend testing blood sugar levels by ordering a hemoglobin A1C.

✓ ***Monitor blood pressure***—High blood pressure will add an increased risk for heart attack or stroke.

References:

1.) Dahm AE1, Bezemer ID, Bergrem A, et al.Candidate gene polymorphisms and the risk for pregnancy-related venous thrombosis. Br J Haematol. 2012 Jun;157(6):753-61.

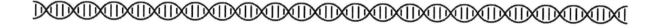

Personalized genetic report found at http://geneticdetoxification.com

Factor 11 (F11) gene
Coagulation factor X1 gene

Names of F11 gene genetic variants (SNP identification)	rsnumber	Risk allele
Factor 11 (F11)	rs2289252	Risk allele is T

What does the F11 gene do?

The F11 gene is involved in the body's ability to clot.

What health problems might be associated with having a F11 risk allele?

An increased risk for deep vein thrombosis (DVT). This F11 risk allele is associated with pregnancy-related venous thrombosis[1].

I have one or more risk allele(s) in the F11 gene. What should I talk to my doctor about doing so that I can reduce my health risks?

- *Pregnant women with one or more F11 risk alleles should make smart diet and lifestyle choices to help prevent clotting while pregnant*—It's important for pregnant women to talk to their doctor about what they can do to prevent clotting.

- *Additional ways to prevent excessive clotting:*

    - *Avoid being sedentary*—Being sedentary increases your risk for clotting. Exercise regularly and avoid prolonged periods of being sedentary if you have this risk allele. If you're limited in your level of activity, wear leg sleeves or use leg compressors.

    - *Maintain low levels of inflammation*—Inflammation can increase the risk for clotting. Increased consumption of antioxidants, fish oil and turmeric can help decrease inflammation, which can decrease the risk of clotting. Fish oil can also act as a blood thinner.
    - *Maintain a healthy weight, blood pressure and blood sugar.*

    - *Exercising caution about taking oral contraceptives.*

Christy L. Sutton D.C.

> *Abstaining from smoking.*

> *Increase garlic consumption.*

> *Consider supplementing with an enzyme called Nattokinase, which may help prevent excessive clotting.*

I have one or more risk allele(s) in the F11 gene. What labs/testing should I consider to continually monitor my health?

✓ *Monitor for clotting*—It's important for anyone with the F11 risk allele to be under the care of a medical doctor who can monitor their clotting levels and help ensure that they're not clotting too fast. Clotting too fast can increase the chance of a stroke, embolism or vascular event. Some labs to monitor clotting include:

> *Prothrombin Time (PT) and PTT (Partial Thromboplastin Time)*— These tests are used to determine if someone has a coagulation problem.
> *Fibrinogen activity test.*
> *D-dimer*—The D-dimer test is designed to measure body's ability to break clots apart when they're no longer needed.

✓ *Monitor inflammation (blood test)*—High levels of inflammation increase the risk of having vascular events such as a stroke. The best labs for monitoring inflammation in someone with an F11 risk allele include:

> *CRP*
> *Homocysteine*
> *Lp-PLA2 (Lipoprotein-Associated Phospholipase A2)*
> *Hemoglobin A1*— Because high blood sugar is very inflammatory, I also recommend testing blood sugar levels by ordering a hemoglobin A1C.

✓ *Monitor blood pressure*—High blood pressure will add an increased risk for heart attack or stroke.

References:

1.) Dahm AE1, Bezemer ID, Bergrem A, et al. Candidate gene polymorphisms and the risk for pregnancy-related venous thrombosis. 2012 Jun;157(6):753-61.

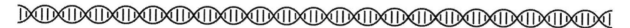

Personalized genetic report found at http://geneticdetoxification.com

CYP2C19 gene

Cytochrome P450 Phase I detoxification gene

Names of **CYP2C19** genetic variants (SNP identification)	**rsnumber**	**Risk allele**
CYP2C19	rs4244285	Risk allele is A

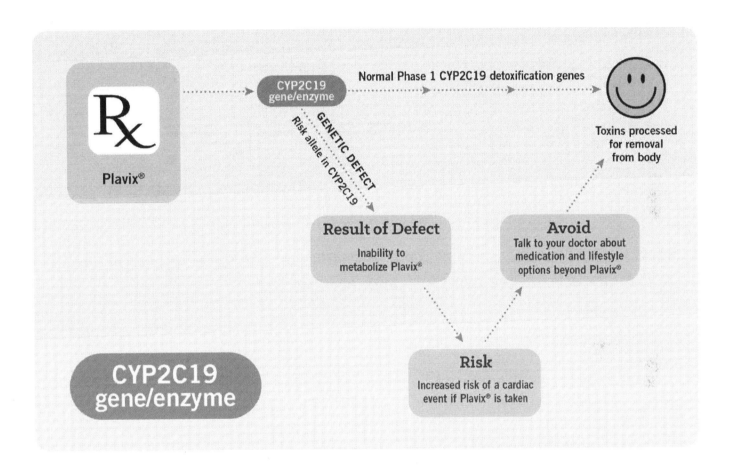

Patients with the T risk allele for CYP2C19 (rs424485) may notice less benefit from taking Plavix®, and may also have a higher risk for developing a cardiac event while on Plavix.

Make sure to contact your prescribing doctor before changing or stopping any medication.

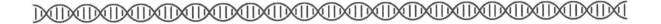

Christy L. Sutton D.C.

GP6 gene
Glycoprotein VI gene

Names of GP6 gene genetic variants (SNP identification)	rsnumber	Risk allele
GP6	rs1613662	Risk allele is G

What does the GP6 gene do?

The GP6 gene plays a role in platelet aggregation, and thus in clotting.

What health problems are associated with this GP6 genetic variant?

If you have a GP6 risk allele, then you are at an increased risk for your blood platelets getting too sticky, which can and lead to an increased risk of clotting.

I have one or more risk allele(s) in the GP6 gene. What should I talk to my doctor about doing so that I can reduce my health risks?

Some things that may help prevent excessive clotting include:

- *Consider supplementing with vitamin E*—If you supplement with vitamin E, ensure you're supplementing with the natural form rather than the synthetic form.

- *Avoid being sedentary*—Being sedentary increases your risk for clotting. Exercise regularly and avoid prolonged periods of being sedentary if you have this risk allele. If you're limited in your level of activity, wear leg sleeves or use leg compressors.

- *Maintain low levels of inflammation*—Inflammation can increase the risk for clotting. Increased consumption of antioxidants, fish oil and turmeric can help decrease inflammation, which can decrease the risk of clotting. Fish oil can also act as a blood thinner.

- *Maintain a healthy weight, blood pressure and blood sugar.*

- *Exercising caution about taking oral contraceptives.*

- *Abstaining from smoking.*

- *Increase garlic consumption.*

- *Consider supplementing with an enzyme called Nattokinase, which may help prevent excessive clotting.*

I have one or more risk allele(s) in the GP6 gene. What labs/testing should I consider to continually monitor my health?

✓ *Monitor the stickiness of your platelets with the platelet function test (blood test)*—This test will monitor and evaluate platelet function to determine if the platelets are too sticky.

✓ *Monitor inflammation (blood test)*—High levels of inflammation increase the risk of having vascular events such as a stroke. The best labs for monitoring inflammation in someone with a GP6 risk allele include:

  ➢ *CRP*
  ➢ *Homocysteine*
  ➢ *Lp-PLA2 (Lipoprotein-Associated Phospholipase A2)*
  ➢ *Hemoglobin A1*—Because high blood sugar is very inflammatory, I also recommend testing blood sugar levels by ordering a hemoglobin A1C.

✓ *Monitor and control blood pressure*—High blood pressure increases the risk of heart attack or stroke.

✓ *Calcium score test*— This test is used to check for heart disease in an early stage and to determine how severe it is. It monitors for buildup of calcium in plaque on the walls of the arteries in the heart. This test does emit a low level of radiation, so antioxidants should be greatly increased before and after this test is performed.

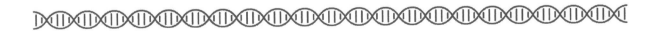

Christy L. Sutton D.C.

KNG1 gene

Kininogen 1 gene

Names of KNG1 gene genetic variants (SNP identification)	rsnumber	Risk allele
KNG1	rs710446	Risk allele is C

What does the KNG1 gene do?

The KNG1 gene plays a role in blood coagulation, and therefore in clotting.

What health problems are associated with this KNG1 genetic variant?

Increased clotting risk—The risk allele is associated with an increased risk of venous thrombosis (clotting) because it's associated with causing clots to form faster, which is known as a decreased partial thromboplastin time (PTT)[1].

I have one or more risk allele(s) in the KNG1 gene. What should I talk to my doctor about doing so that I can reduce my health risks?

Prevent clotting. Natural ways to prevent clotting include:

- *Consider supplementing with vitamin E*—If you supplement with vitamin E, ensure you're supplementing with the natural form rather than the synthetic form.

- *Avoid being sedentary*—Being sedentary increases your risk for clotting. Exercise regularly and avoid prolonged periods of being sedentary if you have this risk allele. If you're limited in your level of activity, wear leg sleeves or use leg compressors.

- *Maintain low levels of inflammation*—Inflammation can increase the risk for clotting. Increased consumption of antioxidants, fish oil and turmeric can help decrease inflammation, which can decrease the risk of clotting. Fish oil can also act as a blood thinner.

- *Maintain a healthy weight, blood pressure and blood sugar.*

- *Exercising caution if taking oral contraceptives.*

- *Abstaining from smoking.*

- *Increase garlic consumption.*

- *Consider supplementing with an enzyme called nattokinase, which may help prevent excessive clotting.*

I have one or more risk allele(s) in the KNG1 gene. What labs/testing should I consider to continually monitor my health?

✓ *Monitor the speed of clotting with Prothrombin Time (PT) and PTT (Partial Thromboplastin Time)*—These tests are used to determine if your blood is clotting too fast or slowly.

✓ *Monitor inflammation (blood test)*—High levels of inflammation increase the risk of having a vascular event such as a stroke. The best labs for monitoring inflammation in someone with a KNG1 risk allele include:

  ➢ *CRP*
  ➢ *Homocysteine*
  ➢ *Lp-PLA2 (Lipoprotein-Associated Phospholipase A2)*
  ➢ *Hemoglobin A1*— Because high blood sugar is very inflammatory, I also recommend testing blood sugar levels by ordering a hemoglobin A1C.

✓ *Monitor blood pressure*—High blood pressure increases the risk of a heart attack or stroke.

References:

1.) Morange PE, Oudot-Mellakh T, Cohen W, Germain M, Saut N, Antoni G, Alessi MC, Bertrand M, Dupuy AM, Letenneur L, Lathrop M, Lopez LM, Lambert JC, Emmerich J, Amouyel P, trégoüet DA.KNG1 ile581Thr and susceptibility to venous thrombosis. Blood. 2011; 117:3692-3694

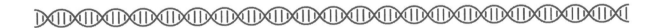

Christy L. Sutton D.C.

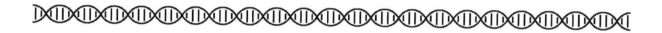

Chapter 12
Blood Pressure Genes

Did you know that high blood pressure is called the silent killer because people often have no obvious symptoms, but are at a significantly higher risk of having a stroke or vascular event?

If you have high blood pressure, then do not hesitate to go to the doctor in case you need blood pressure-lowering drugs. A healthy diet and lifestyle can go a long way toward lowering blood pressure, but it often takes a long time to naturally lower blood pressure. If you have uncontrolled high blood pressure, then taking a drug to lower blood pressure while simultaneously trying to naturally lower blood pressure is the best option for avoiding a serious health problem.

Having a heart attack or stroke while trying to correct your high blood pressure naturally will do far more harm than getting on a medication to lower blood pressure.

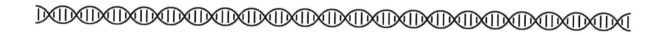

ACE gene
Angiotensin converting enzyme

Names of ACE gene genetic variants (SNP identification)	rsnumber	Risk allele
ACE G2328A	rs4343	Risk allele is G

What does the ACE gene do?

Angiotensin converting enzyme (ACE) plays an essential role in increasing blood pressure by causing the blood vessels to constrict and by increasing salt absorption[1,2].

What health problems might be associated with having an ACE risk allele?

- *Autism*[4]—Having the ACE risk allele is associated with an increased chance of developing autism.

- *Diabetic neuropathy*[1]

- *Alzheimer's*[1]

- *Hypertension (high blood pressure) and its associated health problems*— The increased risk for developing hypertension largely depends on your ethnicity. Some ethnicities are at an increased risk while others are at a decreased risk[3]. Because hypertension is so easy to diagnose through a simple blood pressure test, and because there are inconsistencies about the genotype with the ACE gene, I do not put much emphasis on the ACE gene with regard to hypertension.

  ➢ *Health problems associated with hypertension*

    ○ *Kidney disease*
    ○ *Stroke*[2]
    ○ *Cardiovascular disease*[2]

I have one or more risk allele(s) in the ACE gene. What should I talk to my doctor about doing so that I can reduce my health risks?

- *Support normal blood pressure. Some natural ways to lower blood pressure can include:*

  - *Exercise regularly.*

  - *Decrease sodium intake.*

  - *Increase garlic intake*—Fresh garlic or in supplemental form can help lower blood pressure. Supplemental form must be high in the active ingredient allicin and be enterically coated to prevent allicin from being destroyed in stomach acid.

  - *Increase fiber intake.*

  - *Increase potassium*—This should be done under the guidance of an experienced doctor. Too much potassium can lead to cardiac arrest.

  - *Increase magnesium intake.*

  - *Avoid caffeine.*

  - *Avoid and prevent psychological stress.*

  - *Correct underlying causes of pain*—Pain can lead to high blood pressure.

- *Support kidney health:*

  - *Avoid things that add extra stress on the kidneys*—Conditions that are the hardest on the kidneys include dehydration, diabetes, caffeinated beverages, teas, coffee, alcohol, high salt intake and certain nutritional deficiencies. Being deficient in CoQ10 and vitamin D can be hard on the kidneys (taking statins leads to CoQ10 and vitamin D deficiencies).

- *Consider ACE inhibitor drugs*—If you have both the risk allele for the ACE gene and high blood pressure, you may respond well to ACE inhibitor drugs to reduce blood pressure.

- *Consider autism risk*—If you're concerned about the increased risk of developing autism, then work to lower blood pressure, especially while pregnant. Also consider increasing glutathione, vitamin D and antioxidant levels, and support the methylation pathways. Also, ruling out celiac disease, gluten sensitivity or other food intolerances may be helpful.

I have one or more risk allele(s) in the ACE gene. What labs/testing should I consider to continually monitor my health?

- ✓ *Monitor blood pressure regularly.*

- ✓ *Consider autism risk*—If you're concerned about the increased risk of autism, consider lab testing to monitor glutathione and vitamin D levels, as well as homocysteine, food allergies and celiac disease.

- ✓ *Calcium score test*— This test is used to check for heart disease in an early stage and to determine how severe it is. It monitors for buildup of calcium in plaque on the walls of the arteries in the heart. This test does emit a low level of radiation, so antioxidants should be greatly increased before and after this test is performed.

References:

1.) Sayed-Tabatabaei FA, Oostra BA, et al. ACE polymorphisms. Circ Res. 2006;98:1123–1133.

2) NIH. Genetic Home References. Retrieved from: http://ghr.nlm.nih.gov/gene/ACE

3.) Wenquan N, Yue Q, Pingjin G, Dingliang Z. Review: association between angiotensin converting enzyme G2350A polymorphism and hypertension risk: a meta-analysis. J Renin Angiotensin Aldosterone Syst. 2011;12:8–14.

4.) Firouzabadi N, Ghazanfari N, et al. Genetic Variants of Angiotensin-Converting Enzyme Are Linked to Autism: A Case-Control Study.. PLoS One. 2016 Apr 15;11(4):e0153667.

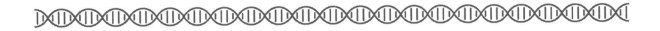

Christy L. Sutton D.C.

ADD1 gene
Adducin 1 gene

Names of ADD1 gene genetic variants (SNP identification)	rsnumber	Risk allele
ADD1 G460W	rs4961	Risk allele is T

What health problems might be associated with having an ADD1 risk allele?

High blood pressure (hypertension)—If you have the (T; G) or (T; T) genotype, you're at increased risk of developing hypertension.

I have one or more risk allele(s) in the ADD1 gene. What should I talk to my doctor about doing so that I can reduce my health risks?

- *Support normal blood pressure. Some natural ways to lower blood pressure can include:*

  - *Exercise regularly.*

  - *Decrease sodium intake.*

  - *Increase garlic intake*—Fresh or the supplemental form of garlic can help lower blood pressure. The supplemental form must be high in the active ingredient, allicin, and be enterically coated to prevent the allicin from being destroyed in stomach acid.

  - *Increase fiber intake.*

  - *Increase potassium*—This should be done under the guidance of an experienced doctor. Too much potassium can lead to cardiac arrest.

  - *Increase magnesium intake.*

  - *Avoid caffeine.*

  - *Avoid and prevent psychological stress.*

> ➤ **Correct underlying causes of pain**—Pain can lead to high blood pressure.

I have one or more risk allele(s) in the ADD1 gene. What labs/testing should I consider to continually monitor my health?

✓ **Monitor blood pressure regularly.**

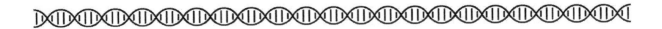

AGT gene
Angiotensin gene

Names of AGT gene genetic variants (SNP identification)	rsnumber	Risk allele
AGT M235T/C4072	rs699	Risk allele is G

What does the AGT gene do?

The AGT gene provides the body's instructions for making a protein called angiotensin (AGT). AGT causes a dramatic increase in blood pressure by causing blood vessels to constrict and by stimulating the body to absorb more salt and minerals by increasing an adrenal hormone called aldosterone.

What health problems might be associated with having an AGT risk allele?

Having a risk allele in the AGT gene can lead to higher levels of angiotensin, which has shown to lead to:

✓ **High blood pressure**[1,2]

✓ **Pregnancy-related problems, such as preeclapmsia**[3]

Christy L. Sutton D.C.

I have one or more risk allele(s) in the AGT gene. What should I talk to my doctor about doing so that I can reduce my health risks?

- *Support normal blood pressure. Some natural ways to lower blood pressure can include:*

  - ➤ *Exercise regularly.*

  - ➤ *Decrease sodium intake.*

  - ➤ *Increase garlic intake*—Fresh or the supplemental form of garlic can help lower blood pressure. The supplemental form must be high in the active ingredient, allicin, and be enterically coated to prevent the allicin from being destroyed in stomach acid.

  - ➤ *Increase fiber intake.*

  - ➤ *Increase potassium*—This should be done under the guidance of an experienced doctor. Too much potassium can lead to cardiac arrest.

  - ➤ *Increase magnesium intake.*

  - ➤ *Avoid caffeine.*

  - ➤ *Avoid and prevent psychological stress.*

  - ➤ *Correct underlying causes of pain*—Pain can lead to high blood pressure.

I have one or more risk allele(s) in the AGT gene. What labs/testing should I consider to continually monitor my health?

- ✓ *Monitor blood pressure regularly*—It's very important that pregnant women with this AGT risk allele have a doctor keep a close eye on their blood pressure.

References:

1.) Jeunemaitre X, Soubrier F, Kotelevtsev YV, et al. Molecular basis of human hypertension: role of angiotensinogen. Cell. 1992 Oct 2;71(1):169-80.

2.) Nakajima T, Jorde LB, Ishigami T, et al. Nucleotide diversity and haplotype structure of the human angiotensinogen gene in two populations. Am J Hum Genet. 2002 Jan;70(1):108-23. Epub 2001 Nov 30.

3.) Ward K, Hata A, Jeunemaitre X, et al. A molecular variant of angiotensinogen associated with preeclampsia.Nat Genet. 1993 May;4(1):59-61.

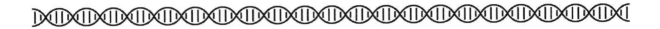

TH gene
Tyrosine hydroxylase gene

Names of TH gene genetic variants (SNP identification)	rsnumber	Risk allele
TH	rs2070762	Risk allele is C

What does the TH gene do?

The TH gene provides the body's blueprint for making the TH enzyme, which converts the amino acid tyrosine into dopamine. The TH enzyme provides the rate-limited step in the conversion of tyrosine to dopamine, which means that it tightly controls the regulation of the reaction from tyrosine to dopamine.

What health problems might be associated with having a TH risk allele?

- *Hypertension*[1]

- *Migraines*[2]

I have one or more risk allele(s) in the TH gene. What should I talk to my doctor about doing so that I can reduce my health risks?

- *Support normal blood pressure:*

  ➢ *Exercise regularly.*

  ➢ *Decrease sodium intake.*

Christy L. Sutton D.C.

➤ *Increase garlic intake*—Fresh or the supplemental form of garlic can help lower blood pressure. The supplemental form must be high in the active ingredient, allicin, and be enterically coated to prevent the allicin from being destroyed in stomach acid.

➤ *Increase fiber intake.*

➤ *Increase potassium*—This should be done under the guidance of an experienced doctor. Too much potassium can lead to cardiac arrest.

➤ *Increase magnesium intake.*

➤ *Avoid caffeine.*

➤ *Avoid psychological stress.*

➤ *Correct underlying causes of pain*—Pain can lead to high blood pressure.

I have one or more risk allele(s) in the TH gene. What labs/testing should I consider to continually monitor my health?

✓ *Blood pressure and heart rate*—Having a risk allele in the TH gene can increase dopamine, epinephrine and norepinephrine levels, which can increase blood pressure and heart rate.

✓ *Nutreval Plasma by Genova Diagnostics (blood and urine test)*—The Nutreval test measures tyrosine levels, which can be heavily affected by a genetic variant in the TH gene. High tyrosine levels could be a result of the TH enzyme functioning at a slower rate than normal due to a TH genetic variant.

✓ *Neurotransmitter testing*—There are various ways to measure neurotransmitters, but due to the inability for most neurotransmitters to cross the blood brain barrier, there is not a good way to measure the levels of neurotransmitters that are affecting the brain. While there is value in testing neurotransmitter levels, if you don't know where to start, begin with a test called the Braverman assessment.

➤ *The Braverman assessment*—This is a simple question-and-answer test designed by psychiatrist Eric Braverman. It attempts to analyze the levels of dopamine, serotonin, GABA and acetylcholine that are actually affecting the brain. The Braverman assessment can be found in Dr. Braverman's book titled, "The Edge Effect."

References:

1.)Wang L, Li B, Lu X, Zhao Q, et al. A functional intronic variant in the tyrosine hydroxylase (TH) gene confers risk of essential hypertension in the Northern Chinese Han population. Clin Sci (Lond)2008;115:151–158.

2.)Corominas R, Ribases M, Camina M, et al. Two-stage case-control association study of dopamine-related genes and migraine. *BMC Med Genet* 2009; 10:95.

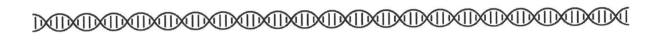

Christy L. Sutton D.C.

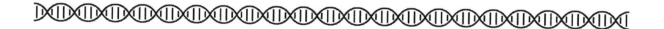

<u>Chapter 13</u>
Triglyceride and Cholesterol Genes

SLCO1B1 gene
Solute Carrier Organic Anion Transporter 1B1 gene

Names of SLCO1B1 gene genetic variants (SNP identification)	rsnumber	Risk allele
SLCO1B1	rs4149056	Risk allele is C

What does the SLCO1B1 gene do?

The SLCO1B1 gene is involved in the uptake and metabolism of cholesterol-lowering drugs called statins. If you have the C risk allele, your liver is not as good at metabolizing statins, and therefore, you will be at a higher risk of developing side effects from statins. Always talk to your prescribing doctor before stopping any medications.

What health problems might be associated with having a SLCO1B1 risk allele?

- *Muscle aches and pain from taking statins (cholesterol-lowering drugs)*—Having the C risk allele increase your risk for having muscle aches and pains from taking statins. Having the (C, C) genotype significantly increases your risk of having significant muscle pain from statin cholesterol-lowering drugs[1,2,3].

- *Less likely to have cholesterol-lowering effects from taking statin cholesterol lowering drugs.*

I have one or more risk allele(s) in the SLCO1B1 gene. What should I talk to my doctor about doing so that I can reduce my health risks?

- *Exercise caution when taking statins*—Talk to your doctor about another method to lower cholesterol, especially if you are having negative side effects while taking a statin.

  *It's important to talk to your prescribing doctor before stopping or changing any medication.

Christy L. Sutton D.C.

- *Natural ways to support lower cholesterol levels:*

  - *Exercise*
  - *Niacin*
  - *Increased fiber in diet*—Vegetables, fruits, nuts, oatmeal, or a fiber supplement)
  - *Fish oil*

I have one or more risk allele(s) in the SLCO1B1 gene. What labs/testing should I consider to continually monitor my health?

✓ *Blood work to monitor triglyceride, lipid levels, and blood sugar*—Specific blood tests include triglycerides, VLDL, LDL, HDL, hemoglobin A1C and fasting glucose.

✓ *Blood tests to monitor inflammation*—These include CRP, ESR, and homocysteine. Monitoring inflammation is essential because inflammation can be a better predictor of cardiovascular disease than cholesterol and triglyceride levels.

✓ *Calcium score test*— This test is used to check for heart disease in an early stage and to determine how severe it is. It monitors for buildup of calcium in plaque on the walls of the arteries in the heart. This test does emit a low level of radiation, so antioxidants should be greatly increased before and after this test is performed.

Statins could hurt your heart

Statins disrupt the body's ability to make CoQ10 and vitamin D, which can make you deficient in those essential nutrients.

Side effects of CoQ10 deficiencies:

- Heart disease/heart failure[1]
- Muscle pain
- Neurological problems
- Fatigue

Side effects of vitamin D deficiencies:

- Cancer
- Osteoporosis
- Immune problems

If you are taking statins, you *need* to talk to your doctor about taking CoQ10 and vitamin D to prevent unwanted side effects from the statin.

References: 1.) Mayoclinic. Retrieved from: http://www.mayoclinic.org/drugs-supplements/coenzyme-q10/evidence/hrb-20059019

References:

1.Akao H, Polisecki E, Kajinami K, et al.. Genetic Variation at the SLCO1B1 Gene Locus and Low Density Lipoprotein Cholesterol Lowering Response to Pravastatin in the Elderly. Atherosclerosis 2012;220(2):413-417.

2.) Boston Heart Diagnostics. Database of over 250,000 samples. Retrieved from: http://www.bostonheartdiagnostics.com/science_portfolio_statin.php

3.) The SEARCH Collaborative Group. SLCO1B1 variants and statin-induced myopathy – a genomewide study. N Engl J Med. 2008; 359:789–799. Retrieved from: http://www.nejm.org/doi/full/10.1056/NEJMoa0801936

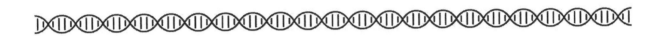

APOC3 gene
Apolipoprotein C3

Names of APOC3 gene genetic variants (SNP identification)	rsnumber	Risk allele
APOC3 3u386	rs5128	Risk allele is G

What does the APOC3 gene do?

The APOC3 modulates triglyceride metabolism through inhibition of enzymes that break down triglycerides. APOC3 is regulated by insulin, which means that APOC3 mutations could be a mechanism for glucose metabolism to affects triglyceride and other lipid levels[1].

What health problems might be associated with having an APOC3 risk allele?

The APOC3 risk allele can be associated with high triglycerides levels, high cholesterol levels, cognitive decline, blood sugar-regulating issues and cardiovascular disaease[1,2,3].

I have one or more risk allele(s) in the APOC3 gene. What should I talk to my doctor about doing so that I can reduce my health risks?

Christy L. Sutton D.C.

- ***Reduce inflammation***—Natural ways to lower inflammation include taking turmeric and/or fish oil, eating a low-sugar diet, eating raw vegetables, and increase fiber intake.

- ***Natural ways to support lower cholesterol and triglyceride levels include:***

  o ***Exercise***
  o ***Niacin***
  o ***Increased fiber in diet***
  o ***Fish oil***
  o ***Low sugar diet***

I have one or more risk allele(s) in the APOC3 gene. What labs/testing should I consider to continually monitor my health?

✓ ***Blood work to monitor triglyceride, lipid levels, and blood sugar***—Specific blood tests include triglycerides, VLDL, LDL, HDL, hemoglobin A1C, C-peptide and fasting glucose.

✓ ***Blood tests to monitor inflammation***—These include CRP and homocysteine. Monitoring inflammation is essential because inflammation can be a better predictor of cardiovascular disease than cholesterol and triglyceride levels.

✓ ***Calcium score test***— This test is used to check for heart disease in an early stage and to determine how severe it is. It monitors for buildup of calcium in plaque on the walls of the arteries in the heart. This test does emit a low level of radiation, so antioxidants should be greatly increased before and after this test is performed.

References:

1.) Smith CE, Tucker KL, Scott TM, et al. Apolipoprotein C3 polymorphisms, cognitive function and diabetes in Caribbean origin Hispanics. PLoS One. 2009;4:e5465.

2.) Singh P, Singh M, Kaur TP, Grewal SS (Nov 2008). "A novel haplotype in ApoAI-CIII-AIV gene region is detrimental to Northwest Indians with coronary heart disease". International Journal of Cardiology 130 (3): e93-5.

3.) Singh P, Singh M, Gaur S, Kaur T (Jun 2007). "The ApoAI-CIII-AIV gene cluster and its relation to lipid levels in type 2 diabetes mellitus and coronary heart disease: determination of a novel susceptible haplotype". Diabetes & Vascular Disease Research 4(2): 124–29.

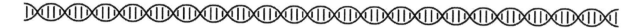

CETP gene
Cholesteryl ester transfer protein gene

Names of CETP gene genetic variants (SNP identification)	rsnumber	Risk allele
CETP C4402A	rs1800775	Risk allele is C
CETP I405V	rs5882	Risk allele is A

What does the CETP gene do?

The CETP gene is involved in the transfer and movement of cholesterol and triglycerides within the body.

What health problems might be associated with having a CETP risk allele?

- *CETP I405V (rs5882- A allele)*—This risk allele has been associated with faster aging, increased risk for dementia, less good cholesterol, increased risk of atherosclerosis and a shorter life span[1].

- *CETP C4402A (rs1800775- C allele)*—This risk allele may increase the risk of a myocardial infarction[2].

I have one or more risk allele(s) in the CETP gene. What should I talk to my doctor about doing so that I can reduce my health risks?

- *Engage in regular aerobic exercise and stress-relieving activities.*

- *Increase fiber.*

- *Increase good fats (especially omega-3 fats from fish or fish oil)*—These should be included in the routine of anyone with CETP genetic variants.

- *Limit alcohol*—It has LDL-cholesterol-raising effects.

- *Monitor sugar intake*—This can help decrease triglyceride levels and promote longevity.

Christy L. Sutton D.C.

I have one or more risk allele(s) in the CETP gene. What labs/testing should I consider to continually monitor my health?

✓ *Blood work to monitor triglyceride, lipid levels and blood sugar*—Specific blood tests include triglycerides, VLDL, LDL, HDL, hemoglobin A1C and fasting glucose.

✓ *Blood tests to monitor inflammation*—These include CRP and homocysteine. Monitoring inflammation is essential because inflammation can be a better predictor of cardiovascular disease than cholesterol and triglyceride levels.

✓ *Calcium score test*— This test is used to check for heart disease in an early stage and to determine how severe it is. It monitors for buildup of calcium in plaque on the walls of the arteries in the heart. This test does emit a low level of radiation, so antioxidants should be greatly increased before and after this test is performed.

Good news for people with the (G, G) genotype for CETP I405V (rs5882)

Having the (G, G) genotype for CETP I405V (rs5882) is associated with a longer lifespan and a decreased chance of developing high blood pressure, cardiovascular disease and metabolic syndrome[3].

References:

1.) Retrieved from: http://snpedia.com/index.php/Rs5882

2.) Wang Q, Zhou SB, Wang LJ, et al. Seven functional polymorphisms in the CETP gene and myocardial infarction risk: a meta-analysis and meta-regression. PLoS One.2014;9:e88118.

3.) Barzilai N., Atzmon G., et al. Unique lipoprotein phenotype and genotype associated with exceptional longevity. JAMA. 2003; 290:2030–2040

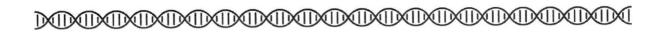

LDLR gene
Low-density lipoprotein receptor

Names of LDLR gene genetic variants (SNP identification)	rsnumber	Risk allele
LDLR	rs688	Risk allele is T

What does the LDLR gene do?

The LDLR gene plays an important role in cholesterol transportation in the brain[1]. The LDLR gene provides the body's instructions for making a protein that brings "bad" LDL cholesterol into the cell.

What health problems might be associated with having a LDLR risk allele?

Like much in life, the health problems depend on if you are a male or female.

- *For women*—This risk allele is associated with significantly higher LDL (bad cholesterol) and total cholesterol in women[1].

- *For men*—This risk allele is associated with increased Alzheimer's disease odds in males, but not in females[1].

Christy L. Sutton D.C.

I have one or more risk allele(s) in the LDLR gene. What should I talk to my doctor about doing so that I can reduce my health risks?

Support healthy cholesterol levels—Ways to naturally lower cholesterol include:

- *Limit alcohol*—It has LDL-cholesterol-raising effects[2].

- *Eat a diet high in good fats and low in bad fats*—This includes plenty of fish, olive oil, avocadoes and nuts. Minimize margarine, trans-fats, and processed and fried foods.

- *Consider supplementing with fish oil and vitamin B-3 (niacin).*

- *Follow a high-fiber diet*—This includes plenty of fruits, vegetables and nuts.

- *Exercise regularly.*

- *Exercise caution with using statins to reduce cholesterol*—Statins can lead to memory problems, muscle pain, and deficiencies in CoQ10 and vitamin D. Do not stop or change any medication without consulting your prescribing doctor.

*Read the section titled "How can you reduce your risk of developing Alzheimer's disease?" (pg 157).

I have one or more risk allele(s) in the LDLR gene. What labs/testing should I consider to continually monitor my health?

- ✓ *Blood work to monitor cholesterol, triglycerides, inflammation and blood sugar*—These labs are important for heart health and include LDL, HDL, VLDL, triglycerides, hemoglobin A1C, fasting blood glucose, homocysteine and CRP.

- ✓ *Smell test*—Loss of sense of smell is one of the first signs of Alzheimer's. Therefore, testing your smell is a great way to monitor your brain health.

- ✓ *Memory recall testing*

- ✓ *Vitamin D levels (blood test)*—Vitamin D is important for brain health. I prefer to see vitamin D level around 70 to 100 on lab work.

- ✓ *Homocysteine (blood work)*—High homocysteine is associated with an increased risk of developing Alzheimer's disease. I prefer homocysteine to be at or below 8 on blood work.

✓ *Calcium score test*— This test is used to check for heart disease in an early stage and to determine how severe it is. It monitors for buildup of calcium in plaque on the walls of the arteries in the heart. This test does emit a low level of radiation, so antioxidants should be greatly increased before and after this test is performed.

References:

1.) Zou F, Gopalraj RK, Lok J, et al. Sex-dependent association of a common low-density lipoprotein receptor polymorphism with RNA splicing efficiency in the brain and Alzheimer's disease. Hum Mol Genet.2008;17(7):929–935.

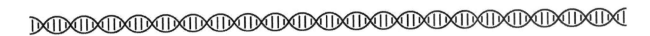

OLR1 gene
Oxidized low-density lipoprotein receptor 1

Names of OLR1 gene genetic variants (SNP identification)	rsnumber	Risk allele
OLR1	rs12316150	Risk allele is T

What does the OLR1 gene do?

The OLR1 gene helps metabolize "bad" LDL-cholesterol. The OLR1 gene encodes for the OLR1 protein, which binds, internalizes and degrades oxidized low-density lipoprotein (LDL- "bad cholesterol").

What health problems might be associated with having an OLR1 risk allele?

Having a risk allele in the OLR1 gene has been associated with atherosclerosis, myocardial infarction (heart attacks) and Alzheimer's disease[1]

I have one or more risk allele(s) in the OLR1 gene. What should I talk to my doctor about doing so that I can reduce my health risks?

Christy L. Sutton D.C.

Support health cholesterol levels naturally—Ways to naturally lower cholesterol include:

- ***Limit alcohol***—It has LDL-cholesterol-raising effects[2].

- ***Eat a diet high in good fats and low in bad fats***—This includes plenty of fish, olive oil, avocadoes and nuts. Minimize margarine, trans-fats, and processed and fried foods.

- ***Consider supplementing with fish oil and Vitamin B-3 (niacin).***

- ***Follow a high-fiber diet***—This includes plenty of fruits, vegetables and nuts.

- ***Exercise regularly.***

- ***Exercise caution with using statins to reduce cholesterol***—Statins can lead to memory problems, muscle pain, and deficiencies in CoQ10 and vitamin D. Do not stop or change any medication without consulting your prescribing doctor.

*Read the section titled "How can you reduce your risk of developing Alzheimer's disease?" (pg 157).

I have one or more risk allele(s) in the OLR1 gene. What labs/testing should I consider to continually monitor my health?

- ✓ ***Blood work to monitor cholesterol, triglycerides, inflammation and blood sugar***—These labs are important for heart health and include LDL, HDL, VLDL, triglycerides, hemoglobin A1C, fasting blood glucose, homocysteine and CRP. It's important to monitor inflammation with these tests because high levels of inflammation will increase your chance of developing Alzheimer's disease and cardiovascular disease.

- ✓ ***Smell test***—Loss of sense of smell is one of the first signs of Alzheimer's. Therefore, testing your smell is a great way to monitor your brain health.

- ✓ ***Memory recall testing.***

- ✓ ***Vitamin D levels (blood test)***—Vitamin D is important for brain health. I prefer to see vitamin D level around 70 to 100 on lab work.

- ✓ ***Homocysteine (blood work)***—High homocysteine is associated with an increased risk of developing Alzheimer's disease and cardiovascular disease. I prefer homocysteine to be at or below 8 on blood work.

✓ **Calcium score test**— This test is used to check for heart disease in an early stage and to determine how severe it is. It monitors for buildup of calcium in plaque on the walls of the arteries in the heart. This test does emit a low level of radiation, so antioxidants should be greatly increased before and after this test is performed.

References:

1.) NCBI. OLR1 oxidized low density lipoprotein receptor 1. Retrieved from: http://www.ncbi.nlm.nih.gov/gene?Db=gene&Cmd=ShowDetailView&TermToSearch=4973

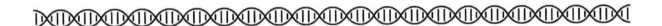

FADS1 gene
Fatty acid desaturase 1 gene

Names of FADS1 gene genetic variants (SNP identification)	rsnumber	Risk allele
FADS1	rs174546	Risk allele is T

What health problems might be associated with having a FADS1 risk allele?

This risk allele is associated with lower cholesterol levels when higher consumption of the good fats called alpha-linolenic acid (flaxseed oil and walnuts) are consumed[1]. This means that if you have the FADS1 risk allele and you also have high cholesterol, then you could benefit from increasing consumption of flaxseed oil.

I have one or more risk allele(s) in the FADS1 gene. What should I talk to my doctor about doing so that I can reduce my health risks?

Anyone with a T allele for this FADS1 genetic variant should consider increasing their intake of flaxseeds or flaxseed oil, especially if they have high cholesterol. Intake of alpha-linolenic acid (ALA) should be above 1.4 g/day[1].

References:

Christy L. Sutton D.C.

1.) Dumont J,Huybrechts I, et al. FADS1 Genetic Variability Interacts with Dietary α-Linolenic Acid Intake to Affect Serum Non-HDL–Cholesterol Concentrations in European Adolescents. J. Nutr 2011;141(7)1247-53.

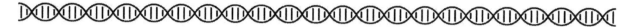

NOS1, NOS2, and NOS3 genes
Nitric oxide synthase 1, 2, and 3 genes

NOS1- Nitric Oxide Synthase 1 (Neuronal—nNOS)

Names of NOS1 gene genetic variants (SNP identification)	rsnumber	Risk allele
NOS1 A57373G	rs7298903	Risk allele is C
NOS1AP	rs12143842	Risk allele is T
NOS1AP	. rs347313	Risk allele is G

NOS2- Nitric oxide synthase 2 (Inducable NOS- iNOS)

Names of NOS2 gene genetic variants (SNP identification)	rsnumber	Risk allele
NOS2 C1823T	rs2297518	Risk allele is A
NOS2 T32235C	rs2248814	Risk allele is A
NOS2	rs944722	Risk allele is C

NOS3 – Nitric oxide synthase 3 (Endothelial NOS-eNOS)

Names of NOS3 gene genetic variants (SNP identification)	rsnumber	Risk allele
NOS3 A6251T	rs1800783	Risk allele is T
NOS3 C19635T	rs3918188	Risk allele is A
NOS3 G6797A	rs1800779	Risk allele is A
NOS3	rs891512	Risk allele is A

What do the NOS1, NOS2 and NOS3 genes do?

The NOS1, NOS2 and NOS3 genes play an essential role in the body's ability to make nitric oxide. Nitic oxide is what stimulates blood flow by opening up capillaries throughout the body. Nitric oxide has a broad impact on health and all bodily systems[12]. Nitric oxide is important for maintaining the lungs, muscles, immune system, nervous system, gastrointestinal system, sexual function and a healthy cardiovascular system. Nitric oxide can actually help the body to be more relaxed. As we age our nitric oxide production decreases dramatically.

There are three different genes that are uniquely involved in making nitric oxide. The three genes include NOS1, NOS2 and NOS3.

- **NOS1 (neuronal nitric oxide gene)**—The NOS1 gene is what makes nNOS (neuronal nitric oxide), which primarily affects the nervous system. High levels of nNOS can be a boost for the brain and nervous system.

- **NOS2 (inducible nitric oxide gene)**—The NOS2 gene is what makes iNOS (inducible nitric oxide), which is involved in increasing inflammation in the body. iNOS primarily affects the immune and cardiovascular systems. High levels of iNOS can be very inflammatory to the body.

- **NOS3 (endothelial nitric oxide)**—The NOS3 gene is what makes eNOS (endothelial nitric oxide), which is involved in increasing blood flow throughout the body by relaxing the capillaries, thus increasing blood flow.

What health problems might be associated with having an NOS1, NOS2 and/or NOS3 risk allele?

Having the risk alleles for the NOS1, NOS2 or NOS3 genes can lead to abnormal levels of nitric oxide, which can lead to a variety of health problems:

- **Health problems associated with having a risk allele in the NOS1 gene (neuronal NOS-nNOS):**

  - Asthma[2]

  - Schizophrenia[3]

  - Parkinson's disease[12]

  - Decreased cognitive function

 Christy L. Sutton D.C.

- **Health problems associated with having a risk allele in the NOS2 gene (Inducible NOS- iNOS):**

  - Coronary heart disease[10]

  - Preeclampsia[11]

  - Increased susceptibility to MS[4]

  - Leaky gut[5]

  - Autoimmune diseases[6]

  - IBS[7]

  - Migraines[8]

  - Parkinson's disease[12]

  - Bladder cancer[9]

- **Health problems associated with having a risk allele in the NOS3 gene (Endothelial NOS-eNOS):**

  - Heart attack[14]

  - Pregnancy-related hypertension[14]

  - Detachment of the placenta[14]

  - Atherosclerosis[15]

  - Erectile dysfunction or decreased libido[13]

  - Significant reduction in nitric oxide production with the (A/A) genotype for NOS3-rs1800779—Having this genotype resulted in 23 percent lower nitric oxide production[4].

  - Increased susceptibility to MS[4].

  - Hypertension

Personalized genetic report found at http://geneticdetoxification.com

Nitric oxide is a *free radical*; therefore, it can cause tissue damage at very high levels. For this reason, it's important to *increase antioxidant levels when increasing nitric oxide levels.*

I have one or more risk allele(s) in the NOS1, NOS2, and NOS3 gene. What should I talk to my doctor about doing so that I can reduce my health risks?

- *How to naturally increase nitric oxide levels if they are too low:*

  ➤ **Exercise (cardio)**—About 45 minutes of walking a day.

  ➤ **Weight control**—Lose weight if overweight.

  ➤ **Increase intake of beets and dark green vegetables.**

  ➤ **Avoid stomach acid reducers**—These can suppress nitric oxide production (antacids, Prilosec).

  ➤ **Increase intake of fruits and vegetables**[1.]

  ➤ **Ensure you aren't deficient in B vitamins or iron**—The NOS enzymes made from the NOS genes require B vitamins and iron to function properly.

  ➤ **Consider supplementing with Niacin (vitamin B-3)**—Taking niacin will cause a flush to occur that will result in an increase in nitric oxide.

- *Increase antioxidant levels*—Having an adequate nitric oxide level is essential for health. Nitric oxide is a free radical. Therefore, increasing antioxidant intake will help protect the body from damage that could occur from nitric oxide or other free radicals. Fruits and vegetables are high in antioxidants, including glutathione, vitamin C, alpha-lipoic acid, vitamin E and vitamin A.

Christy L. Sutton D.C.

- *Avoiding smoking and pesticides to prevent Parkinson's*—If you have the NOS1 or NOS2 risk alleles that are associated with an increased risk of developing Parkinson's, then some research has shown that avoiding smoking and pesticide exposure may prevent you from developing Parkinson's[12].

I have one or more risk allele(s) in the NOS1, NOS2, and NOS3 gene. What labs/testing should I consider to continually monitor my health?

✓ *Nitric oxide test (saliva)*—This is a simple, inexpensive salivary test to assess nitric oxide levels.

✓ *Nitric oxide breath test*—This test is mostly used for asthma.

✓ *Calcium score test*— This test is used to check for heart disease in an early stage and to determine how severe it is. It monitors for buildup of calcium in plaque on the walls of the arteries in the heart. This test does emit a low level of radiation, so antioxidants should be greatly increased before and after this test is performed.

References:

1.) Han X, Zheng T, Lan Q, et al. Genetic polymorphisms in nitric oxide synthase genes modify the relationship between vegetable and fruit intake and risk of non-Hodgkin lymphoma. Cancer Epidemiol Biomarkers Prev. 2009;18(5):1429–1438

2.) Wang TN1, Tseng HI, Kao CC, et al. The effects of NOS1 gene on asthma and total IgE levels in Taiwanese children, and the interactions with environmental factors.Pediatr Allergy Immunol. 2010 Nov;21(7):1064-71.

3.) Zhang Z1, Chen X1, Yu P1, et al..Evidence for the contribution of NOS1 gene polymorphism (rs3782206) to prefrontal function in schizophrenia patients and healthy controls. Neuropsychopharmacology. 2015 May;40(6):1383-94.

4.) AlFadhli S1, Mohammed EM, Al Shubaili A.Association analysis of nitric oxide synthases: NOS1, NOS2A and NOS3 genes, with multiple sclerosis. Ann Hum Biol. 2013 Jul;40(4):368-75.

5.) Tang Y1, Forsyth CB, Farhadi A, et al.Nitric oxide-mediated intestinal injury is required for alcohol-induced gut leakiness and liver damage. Alcohol Clin Exp Res. 2009 Jul;33(7):1220-30.

6.) Miljkovic D1, Trajkovic V.Cytokine Growth Factor Rev. 2004 Feb;15(1):21-32. Inducible nitric oxide synthase activation by interleukin-17.

7.) Dhillon S. S., Mastropaolo L. A.,et al. Higher activity of the inducible nitric oxide synthase contributes to very early onset inflammatory bowel disease. Clinical and Translational Gastroenterology.2014;5(1, article e46)

8.) Gonçalves F. M., Luizon M. R., et al. Interaction among nitric oxide (NO)-related genes in migraine susceptibility. Molecular and Cellular Biochemistry. 2012;370(1-2):183–189.

9.) Ryk C1, Wiklund NP, et al. .Ser608Leu polymorphisms in the nitric oxide synthase-2 gene may influence urinary bladder cancer pathogenesis. Scand J Urol Nephrol. 2011 Nov;45(5):319-25

10). Tu YC, Ding H, Wang XJ, et al. (2010) Exploring epistatic relationships of NO biosynthesis pathway genes in susceptibility to CHD. Acta Pharmacol Sin 31: 874–880.

11.) Amaral LM, Palei AC, et al. Maternal iNOS genetic polymorphisms and hypertensive disorders of pregnancy. J Hum Hypertens. 2012;26:547–552.

12.) Hancock D, Martin ER, et al. Nitric oxide synthase genes and their interactions with environmental factors in Parkinson's disease. Neurogenetics. 2008;9:249–262.

13.) Retrieved from: http://ausfp.com/nitric-oxide-deficiency/

14.) Kohlmeier, Martin Nutrigenetics, Applying the Science of Personal Nutrition. 2013. Academic Press.

15.) Dessy, C.; Ferron, O. (2004). "Pathophysiological Roles of Nitric Oxide: In the Heart and the Coronary Vasculature". Current Medical Chemistry – Anti-Inflammatory & Anti-Allergy Agents in Medicinal Chemistry 3 (3): 207–216.

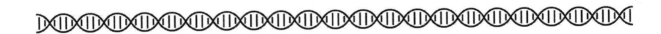

Christy L. Sutton D.C.

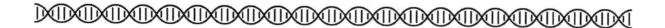

For more information on genes related to cardiovascular health, consult the following pages:

Genes associated with an increased risk for developing atherosclerosis:
- IL6 gene Pg. 291
- PON1 gene Pg. 132
- SOD2 gene Pg. 247
- TLR4 gene Pg. 304

Genes associated with an increased heart attack risk:
- CYP1A2 gene Pg. 27
- LRP6 gene Pg. 299
- ➢ UGT1A1 and UGT2A2 gene Pg. 71

Genes associated with an increased risk for high cholesterol:
- ➢ ApoE 4 gene Pg. 159
- ➢ IL4R gene Pg. 316

Genes associated with an increased risk for cardiac arrhythmia:
- ANK3 gene Pg. 219

Genes associated with an increased risk for hypertension:
- COMT gene Pg. 181

Genes associated with an increased risk for cardiovascular disease due to causing high homocysteine levels:
- MTHFR gene Pg. 87
- MTHFD1L gene Pg. 94
- MTRR gene Pg. 101
- MTR gene Pg. 99
- NBPF3 gene Pg. 366

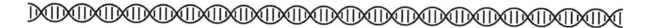

Part 6
Vitamin and Mineral Imbalances

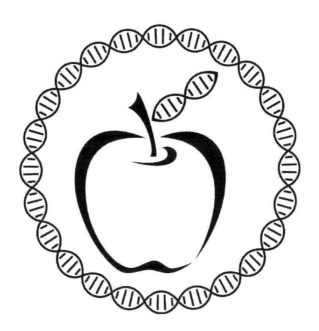

Certain genetic variants can lead to problems metabolizing specific vitamin and minerals. The side effects of this can be serious if not properly monitored and addressed.

However, genetic variants effecting vitamins and minerals can be a non-issue if properly diagnosed and resolved. In this section, you'll learn if you may have genetic predispositions that increase your risk for developing health problems from improperly metabolizing nutrients. If you do have any of these genetic predispositions, it's important to monitor your health, and talk to you doctor about making specific diet and lifestyle changes to protect yourself from developing health problems.

Christy L. Sutton D.C.

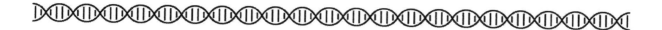

Chapter 14
Vitamin and Mineral Imbalances

Vitamin B6

NBPF3 gene
Neuroblastoma breakpoint family member 3 gene

Names of NBPF3 gene genetic variants (SNP identification)	rsnumber	Risk allele
NBPF3	rs4654748	Risk allele is C

What health problems might be associated with having a NBPF3 risk allele?

Each C allele is associated with a 15 percent lower vitamin B6 concentration[1]. This is significant when you consider that vitamin B6 is used in more metabolic pathways than all other B vitamins. Some symptoms of low vitamin B6 include:

- Muscle weakness
- Nervousness
- Irritability
- Water retention
- Depression

- Difficulty concentrating
- Memory loss (especially short-term memory)
- High homocysteine

I have one or more risk allele(s) in the NBPF3 gene. What should I talk to my doctor about doing so that I can reduce my health risks?

Consider supplementing with additional vitamin B-6—I recommend supplementing with the activated form of vitamin B-6 called pyridoxal-5-phosphate (P-5-P). Both stress and being pregnant greatly increase the body's need for vitamin B6. It's especially important for anyone with one or more NBPF3 risk alleles to consider taking extra vitamin B6 (P-5-P) while under stress or pregnant.

I have one or more risk allele(s) in the NBPF3 gene. How can I reduce my health risks?

Nutreval by Genova Diagnostics (blood and urine test)—This test will determine if you're low in vitamin B-6.

Christy L. Sutton D.C.

References:

1.) Kohlmeier, Martin Nutrigetics, Applying the Science of Personal Nutrition. 2013. Academic Press. Pg 179.

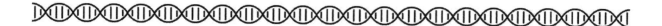

Vitamin D

VDR gene
Vitamin D receptor gene

Names of VDR gene genetic variants (SNP identification)	rsnumber	Risk allele
VDR Bsm	rs1544410	Risk allele is T
VDR Taq	rs731236	Risk allele is G

What does the VDR gene do?

The VDR gene provides the body's instructions for creating a protein called VDR, a receptor for vitamin D in the cell's nucleus. Once vitamin D has bound to the VDR receptor, then vitamin D's health-promoting effects will be initiated. If the vitamin D receptor doesn't function correctly, vitamin D won't bind as efficiently, thus diminishing its health-promoting effects.

The VDR receptor is activated by both vitamin D and lithocholic acid (LCA), a bile produced from bacteria in the colon that makes fat ingested through your diet easier to digest.

What health problems might be associated with having a VDR risk allele?

Having a risk allele in the VDR gene can lead to a decreased response to vitamin D, leading to more health problems resulting from having low Vitamin D. These health problems are far-reaching because vitamin D influences nearly 3,000 of your 20,000 genes. Some health problems that are seen more commonly in people with a VDR risk allele include:

- *Ulcerative colitis*

- *Cancer, especially breast cancer*

- *Bone loss, osteoporosis, osteopenia, impaired calcium absorption lower bone mineral density*

- *Decreased ability to detoxify*

- *Immune problems, autoimmune diseases, chronic infections[1]*

- *Type II vitamin D-resistant rickets*

- *Neurological problems*

- *Increased risk of insulin resistance*—High vitamin D levels can lead to lower rates of insulin resistance, which ultimately lead to lower blood sugar levels.

I have one or more risk allele(s) in the VDR gene. What should I talk to my doctor about doing so that I can reduce my health risks?

Consider increasing vitamin D intake—If you have a VDR risk allele, your body is less efficient at using vitamin D and requires more vitamin D to prevent symptoms of deficiency. Ask your doctor if you need to take more vitamin D.

I have one or more risk allele(s) in the VDR gene. What labs/testing should I consider to continually monitor my health?

✓ *Vitamin D (blood test)*— I prefer to see vitamin D level around 70 to 100 on lab work.

References:

1.) Kivity S, Agmon-Levin N, Zisappl M, Shapira Y, Nagy EV, Dankó K, et al. Vitamin D and autoimmune thyroid diseases. Cell Mol Immunol. 2011;8:243–7.

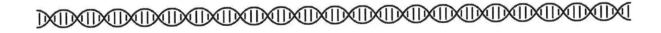

Christy L. Sutton D.C.

Vitamin D

GC gene

Group-specific component gene

Names of GC gene genetic variants (SNP identification)	rsnumber	Risk allele
GC	rs2282679	Risk allele is G
GC	rs7041	Risk allele is C

What does the GC gene do?

The GC gene transports vitamin D to the tissues.

What health problems might be associated with having a GC risk allele?

Having a risk allele in the GC gene can lead to a decreased ability for vitamin D to be transported to tissues throughout the body, which can cause those tissues to miss out on vitamin D's health-promoting effects.

Some health problems associated with having a risk allele in the GC gene include:

- *Colon cancer*—Having the risk allele for GC (rs2282679) is most strongly associated with colon cancer.

- *Ulcerative colitis*

- *Cancer*

- *Bone loss, osteoporosis, osteopenia, impaired calcium absorption and lower bone mineral density*

- *Decreased ability to detoxify*

- *Immune problems, autoimmune diseases and chronic infections*

- *Type II, vitamin D-resistant rickets*

- ***Neurological problems***

- ***Increased risk of insulin resistance***—A high vitamin D level can lead to lower rates of insulin resistance, which ultimately leads to lower blood sugar levels.

I have one or more risk allele(s) in the GC gene. What should I talk to my doctor about doing so that I can reduce my health risks?

Consider increasing vitamin D intake—If you have a GC gene risk allele, your body is less efficient at using vitamin D and requires more vitamin D to prevent symptoms of deficiency. Ask your doctor if you need to take more vitamin D.

I have one or more risk allele(s) in the GC gene. What labs/testing should I consider to continually monitor my health?

- ✓ ***Vitamin D (blood test)***— I prefer to see vitamin D level around 70 to 100 on lab work.

Vitamin D-3 and vitamin K-2 work better together

- Vitamin K-2 helps increase calcium absorption.

- Vitamin K-2 promotes calcium being deposited into the skeletal bones rather than in areas where it shouldn't be deposited, such as the organs, arteries and joint space.

- Good bacteria in the intestines will make vitamin K-2.

- Some vitamin D-3 supplements are combinations of vitamin D-3 and vitamin K-2. I have found this combination to be the most effective for bone and cardiovascular health.

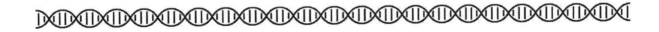

Christy L. Sutton D.C.

Vitamin A

BCMO1 gene
Beta-carotene 15, 15-prime-monooxygenase 1 gene

Names of BCMO1 gene genetic variants (SNP identification)	rsnumber	Risk allele
BCMO1	rs4889294	Risk allele is C
BCMO1 A379V	rs7501331	Risk allele is T
BCMO1 R267S	rs12934922	Risk allele is T
BCMO1 (PKD1L2) C754T	rs6420424	Risk allele is A
BCMO1	rs11645428	Risk allele is G
BCMO1	rs6564851	Risk allele is G

What does the BCMO1 gene do?

The BCMO1 gene converts vitamin A from the inactive form to the active form by metabolizing beta carotene, a precursor of vitamin A, into vitamin A (retinol). Vitamin A metabolism is important for vital processes such as vision, embryonic development, cell differentiation, and membrane and skin protection[1].

What health problems might be associated with having a BCMO1 risk allele?

Deficient in vitamin A—If you have a risk allele in the BCMO1 gene, you're significantly more likely to be deficient in vitamin A because you cannot convert beta-carotene from orange vegetables into vitamin A (retinol). Health problems related to a vitamin A deficiency are most common in people with BCMO1 risk alleles, and can lead to:

- *Eye problems*
- *Acne and eczema*
- *Infertility*

- *Immune problems*
- *Night blindness*
- *Increased cancer risk*

I have one or more risk allele(s) in the BCMO1 gene. What should I talk to my doctor about doing so that I can reduce my health risks?

If you have the high-risk alleles for the BCMO1, you may not get adequate vitamin A from only eating yellow and orange vegetables. Vitamin A is only found naturally in animal products. The precursor to vitamin A, beta carotene, is found in yellow and orange vegetables. Humans must convert beta carotene into vitamin A (retinol).
If you have risk alleles in the BCMO1 gene, then you're less efficient at converting beta carotene from vegetables into vitamin A (retinol). Therefore, you're more likely to have health problems from low vitamin A levels.

- ***Eat foods high in vitamin A***—Foods high in vitamin A include cod liver oil, dairy butter from grass-fed cows, egg yolks, fish and meat. Taking vitamin A supplements is also an option if you don't want to eat foods high in vitamin A.

- ***Consider supplementing with additional antioxidants***—This includes vitamin C, vitamin E, vitamin A, vitamin D, alpha-lipoic acid glutathione, and glucoraphanin.

- ***Consider supplementing with vitamin A***—Because vitamin A is only naturally occurring in animal products the need for vitamin A would be greatest in vegans.

I have one or more risk allele(s) in the BCMO1 gene. What labs/testing should I consider to continually monitor my health?

✓ ***Measure vitamin A (blood test)***

✓ ***Regular eye exams***

References:

1.) NCB1. BCO1 beta-carotene oxygenase 1 Retrieved from: http://www.ncbi.nlm.nih.gov/gene/53630

2.) Lietz G, Oxley A, Leung W, Hesketh J. Single nucleotide polymorphisms upstream from the β-carotene 15,15'-monoxygenase gene influence provitamin A conversion efficiency in female volunteers. J Nutr. 2012;142: 161S–5S

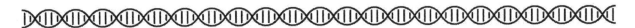

Christy L. Sutton D.C.

Zinc

SLC30A8 gene
Solute carrier family 30 gene

Names of SLC30A8 gene genetic variants (SNP identification)	rsnumber	Risk allele
SLC30A8	rs11558471	Risk allele is A

What does the SLC30A8 gene do?

The SLC30A8 gene helps the body transport zinc.

What health problems might be associated with having an SLC30A8 risk allele?

Increased risk for being zinc- deficient—Some symptoms of being deficient in zinc include:

- Skin, hair and nail problems
- Mouth ulcers or white tongue
- Smell and taste disruption
- Immune problems
- Diarrhea

- Lack of appetite
- Decline in mental health
- Delayed growth
- Pregnancy problems for mother and fetus
- Acne
- Low testosterone

I have one or more risk allele(s) in the SLC30A8 gene. What should I talk to my doctor about doing so that I can reduce my health risks?

Consider increasing zinc intake—For each A allele there is an increased need to consume an additional four to five extra mg. of zinc each day. Therefore, someone that has an AA genotype might need an extra eight to 10 mg of zinc intake daily.

Foods high in zinc include seafood, beef, lamb, wheat germ, spinach, pumpkin and squash seeds, nuts, chocolate, pork, chicken, beans, and mushrooms.

I have one or more risk allele(s) in the SLC30A8 gene. What labs/testing should I consider to continually monitor my health?

✓ **Zinc taste test**—This is a simple and fairly accurate test that consists of putting liquid zinc on your tongue. If the zinc tastes like water that indicates being low in zinc. If the liquid zinc tastes bad, that indicates adequate zinc levels.

✓ **Blood test to check zinc levels.**

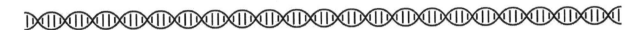

Iron

HFE gene
Hemochromatosis gene

Names of HFE gene genetic variants (SNP identification)	rsnumber	Risk allele
HFE C282Y	rs1800562	Risk allele is A
HFE H63D	rs1799945	Risk allele G

What does the HFE gene do?

The HFE gene helps the body absorb iron.

What health problems might be associated with having an HFE risk allele?

• **Hemochromatosis**—Hemochromatosis is a disorder characterized by an increased ability to absorb and retain iron, which can be problematic if iron levels get too high. Uncontrolled high iron levels can lead to cirrhosis of the liver, diabetes, hyperpigmentation of the skin, liver cancer and heart failure.

   Christy L. Sutton D.C.

> **HFE C282Y (rs1800562)**—Accounts for around 85 percent of all cases of hemochromatosis.

   o If you have the genotype (A; A), then you'll *likely* be affected by hemochromatosis due to increased absorption of iron from the intestines.

   o If you have the genotype (A; G), you're *less likely* to be affected by hemochromatosis.

> **HFE H63D (rs1799945)**

   o If you have the genotype (G; G), then you're at an *increased risk of developing a mild form* of hemochromatosis due to increased absorption of iron from the intestines.

   o If you have the genotype (C; G), then you are *unlikely* to be affected by hemochromatosis.

- *Health problems associated with hemochromatosis include:*

> Joint pain
> Abdominal pain
> Liver problems
> Fatigue/weakness
> Diabetes
> Decreased sex drive (libido)
> Alzheimer's

> Heart failure, irregular heart beat/arrhythmia
> Depression
> Gall bladder disease
> Cancer

Having a risk allele in *both* rs1049296 (TF) *and* rs1800562 (HFE) is associated with an increased risk of developing Alzheimer's, especially if you have high levels of iron on blood work[1]. Having chronically high iron levels can cause brain damage and neurodegeneration, including Alzheimer's disease[1,2,3]. If you have the risk allele for both rs1049296 (TF) and rs1800562 (HFE), you're at an increased risk of having chronically high iron levels. You can learn more about the TF gene on page 174.
Males and post-menopausal women are most likely to have hemochromatosis, as they're not losing blood every month through menstruation. Women of child-bearing

years are less likely to experience negative symptoms related to HFE genes because their iron levels are suppressed through menstruation, pregnancy and childbirth. Having a risk allele in both rs1049296 (TF) and rs1800562 (HFE) is associated with an increased risk of developing Alzheimer's[1].

I have one or more risk allele(s) in the HFE gene. What should I talk to my doctor about doing so that I can reduce my health risks?

- Donate blood regularly—Donating blood is the treatment for hemochromatosis.

- Avoid iron-rich foods such as beef.

I have one or more risk allele(s) in the HFE gene. What labs/testing should I consider to continually monitor my health?

Laboratory analysis is essential for determining if you have high iron levels due to having inherited the risk alleles in the HFE gene.

- ***Monitor for signs that the body is absorbing and storing excess iron (blood work)***—Labs should include serum iron, ferritin, transferrin, TIBC, UIBC, hemoglobin and hematocrit.

References:

1.) Kauwe J. S. K., Bertelsen S., Mayo K., et al. Suggestive synergy between genetic variants in TF and HFE as risk factors for Alzheimer's disease. The American Journal of Medical Genetics, Part B: Neuropsychiatric Genetics. 2010;153(4):955–959.

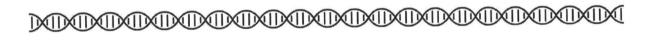

Christy L. Sutton D.C.

Vitamin B-9

DHFR gene
Dihydrofolate reductase gene

Names of DHFR genetic variants (SNP identification)	rsnumber	Risk allele
DHFR A16352G	rs1643649	Risk allele is C
DHFR A20965G	rs1643659	Risk allele is C
DHFR C19483A	rs1677693	Risk allele is T
DHFR	Rs1650697	Risk allele is A

What does the DHFR gene do?

This gene helps metabolize vitamin B-9.

What type of health problems are associated with having a DHFR risk allele?

- **Anemia**—If you have the DFHR risk allele, you're at risk for developing a specific form of anemia called megaloblastic anemia, which causes red blood cells to be too large due to low levels of B12, B9 or B6.

- **Folate (vitamin B-9) deficiency**—Folate deficiencies can cause birth defects (such as spina bifida), an increased cancer risk and a high homocysteine level (linked to a higher risk of cardiovascular problems, Alzheimer's and stroke).

I have one or more DHFR risk allele(s). What should I talk to my doctor about doing so that I can reduce my health risks?

Consider supplementing with a high-quality B-complex—Ensure that it contains the activated form of all B vitamins. Vitamin B-3 is required for DHFR to function properly.

I have one or more DHFR risk allele(s). What labs/testing should I consider to continually monitor my health?

- ✓ **CBC (blood test)**—This determines if you have megaloblastic anemia, a side effect of having the DHFR risk allele.

✓ **Homocysteine (blood test)**— I prefer homocysteine to be at or below 8 on blood work. Homocysteine is an excellent test that measures how much damage is occurring in the body due to having one or more risk allele(s) in the methylation genes.

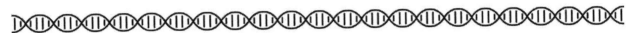

Vitamin B-9

FOLR1, FOLR2 and FOLR3 genes
Folate receptor genes

Names of folate receptor genetic variants (SNP identification)	rsnumber	Risk allele
FOLR1 G-20A	rs2071010	Risk allele is A
FOLR2 G-1316A	rs651933	Risk allele is A
FOLR2	rs7925545	Risk allele is G
FOLR3 A3771G	rs7925545	Risk allele is G

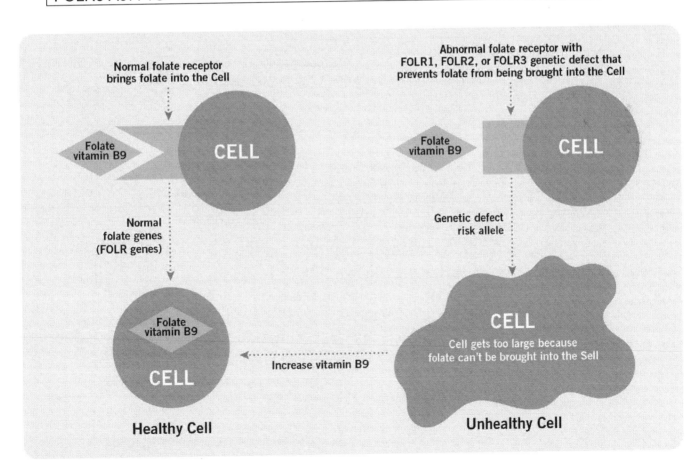

Christy L. Sutton D.C.

What do the FOLR1, FORL2 and FOLR3 genes do?

These genes help the body make receptors for vitamin B-9 (folate) to gain access to the cells. FOLR1, FOLR2 and FOLR3 receptors are like gatekeepers that allow vitamin B-9 into the cells. Vitamin B-9 (folate and folic acid) binds to the FOLR1, FOLR2 and FOLR3 receptors on the cells before being allowed to enter the cells, where it is then activated and processed by the body.

What health problems are associated with the FOLR1, FOLR2 and FOLR3 risk alleles?

- *Inability to absorb and utilize vitamin B-9 (folate) correctly*—Having the risk alleles for these folate receptor genes can decrease the body's ability to get folate to the correct locations, which can lead to a localized folate deficiency even when folate levels appear to be adequate. Therefore, it's important that anyone with a risk allele in the FOLR1, FOLR2 or FOLR3 genes take action to avoid being deficient in vitamin B-9. You should also consider supplementing with additional vitamin B-9 to help compensate for the body's decreased ability to absorb and utilize folate. Having a low vitamin B-9 level, combined with genetic variants in the FOLR1, FOLR2 and FOLR3 genes, is a dangerous combination for your health, and the health of your unborn child if you're pregnant. Being low in vitamin B-9 while pregnant will significantly increase the risk for having a child with birth defects such as spina bifida.

- *Increased risk of neural tube birth defects*—There is an increased risk of neural tube defects, such as spina bifida, and pregnancy complications due to inadequate levels of vitamin B-9 during pregnancy[1].

  - FOLR1 G-20A (rs2071010)—FOLR1 receptors play a critical role in embryonic development of a fetus. There is an increased risk of birth defects (such as spina bifida) associated with having a risk allele for FOLR1 G-20A (rs2071010). In one study done on mice that lacked the FOLR1 gene, it was found that their embryos would die in utero by day 10, whereas mice without the FOLR2 gene gave birth to embryos that developed normally. This indicated that FOLR1 genetic variations can be significant for fetal development and health.

  - FOLR2 (rs7925545)—Associated with neural tube defects such as spina bifida (birth defects)[1].

- ***Possible problems with placenta, spleen, bone marrow and thymus—*** FOLR2 receptors are located on the placenta, spleen, bone marrow and thymus; therefore, having a risk allele in the FOLR genes could lead to an abnormal response in those specific tissues.

I have one or more FOLR1, FOLR2, or FOLR3 risk allele(s). What should I talk to my doctor about doing so that I can reduce my health risks?

There is no simple way to make the folate receptors work as they would without a risk allele in the FOLR1, FOLR2 or FOLR3 genes. However, having adequate vitamin B-9 levels can minimize the risks associated with these risk alleles.

- ***Consider supplementing with vitamin B-9, especially if you're a female of child-bearing age—***If a woman has the risk alleles for these genes and waits until she is pregnant to increase her vitamin B-9 intake, then she likely missed her opportunity to prevent birth defects such as spina bifida.

- ***Eat a diet high in green, leafy vegetables—***Green, leafy vegetables are high in vitamin B-9 (folate) and help support normal folate levels.

I have a FOLR1, FOLR2 and FOLR3 risk allele. What labs/testing should I consider to continually monitor my health?

- ✓ ***CBC, homocysteine and folate (blood tests)—***These blood tests identify if you're deficient in vitamin B-9 (folate).

References:

1.) O'Byrne MR1, Au KS, Morrison AC, et al.. Birth Defects Res A Clin Mol Teratol. 2010 Aug;88(8):689-94. Association of folate receptor (FOLR1, FOLR2, FOLR3) and reduced folate carrier (SLC19A1) genes with meningomyelocele.

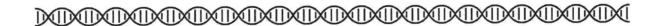

Christy L. Sutton D.C.

Vitamin B-12

TCN1 and TCN2 genes

Transcobalamin 1 and 2 genes

Names of TCN1 and TCN2 genetic variants (SNP identification)	rsnumber	Risk allele
TCN1 G4939288A	rs526934	Risk allele is G
TCN2 A8700G	rs9606756	Risk allele is G
TCN2 C766G	rs1801198	Risk allele is G

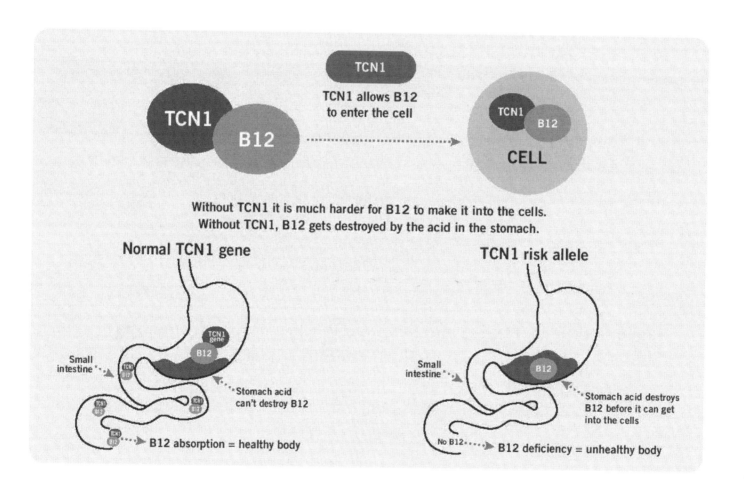

What do the TCN1 and TCN2 genes do?

The TCN1 gene helps protect vitamin B-12 from the stomach's acidic environment. The TCN2 gene helps vitamin B-12 gain access to cells so that it can be utilized by the body.

What health problems are associated with having a risk allele in the TCN1 or TCN2 genes?

- *Vitamin B-12 deficiencies*—Having the risk allele for TCN1 and TCN2 can be associated with decreased levels of vitamin B-12 because people with these risk alleles lack the ability to properly transport vitamin B-12 and keep it from being destroyed in the stomach's acidic environment[1, 2].

- *Increased cancer risk*—The increased cancer risk is largely a result of being low in vitamin B-12.

I have a risk allele for the TCN1 or TCN2 genes. What should I talk to my doctor about doing so that I can reduce my health risks?

Ensure that you're not vitamin B-12-deficient—The health problems related to TCN1 and TCN2 genes appear to be a result of low vitamin B-12 levels; therefore, it's important to prevent vitamin B-12 deficiencies. If you have these risk alleles, you may benefit from vitamin B-12 shots because the vitamin B-12 will be better absorbed as its bypassing the acidic stomach.

I have a TCN1 or TCN2 risk allele. What labs/testing should I consider to continually monitor my health?

- ✓ *Methylmalonic acid (blood test)*—This is the most accurate way to measure your vitamin B-12 level.

- ✓ *CBC (blood test)*—This shows the size of your red blood cells. Large red blood cells can be a result of low B12.

- ✓ *Serum B12 level (blood test)*—This is my least-favorite test because you have to be dangerously low in B-12 before this test flags you as having a problem.

Christy L. Sutton D.C.

References:

1.) Hazra A, Kraft P, Lazarus R, Chen C, et al. Genome-wide significant predictors of metabolites in the one-carbon metabolism pathway. Hum Mol Genet. 2009;18(23): 4677–87.

2.) Gueant JL, Chabi NW, et al. Environmental influence on the worldwide prevalence of a 776C- > G variant in the transcobalamin gene (TCN2) J Med Genet.2007;44(6):363–367.

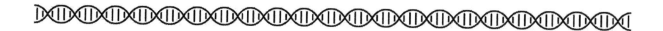

Personalized genetic report found at http://geneticdetoxification.com

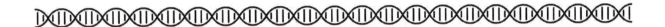

For more information on genes related to vitamins and minerals, consult the following pages:

Genes important for metabolizing *vitamin B-9*:

- MTHFR gene Pg. 87
- MTHFD1L gene Pg. 94
- MTHFS gene Pg. 96

Genes important for metabolizing *vitamin B-12*:

- MTRR gene Pg. 101
- FUT2 gene Pg. 301

Genes important for metabolizing *iron*:

- TF gene Pg. 174

Genes important for metabolizing *magnesium*:

- TRPM7 gene Pg. 237

Genes important for metabolizing *CoQ10*, even though CoQ10 is technically an antioxidant:

- NQO1 gene Pg. 255

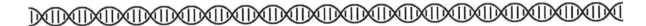

Christy L. Sutton D.C.

Part 7
Muscles/Joints and Athletic Performance

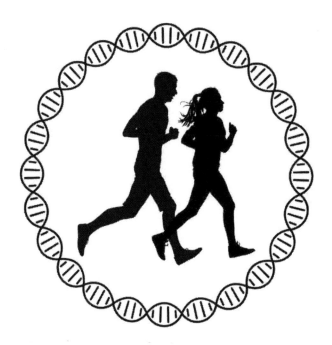

Athletic performance, muscle type, and fitness, like many other aspects of our health, is a function of much more than just genes. The genes that we inherit can influence our athletic performance, how large our muscles can become, and overall endurance.

Knowing your genetic strengths and weaknesses, energy potential, and muscle type can help guide you towards making smarter choices for your overall health.

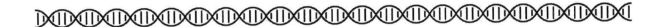

Chapter 15

Muscles/Joints and Athletic Performance

PPARGC1A gene
Peroxisome proliferator-activated receptor gamma coactivator 1-alpha

Names of PPARGC1A genetic variants (SNP identification)	rsnumber	Risk allele
PPARG1A Gly482Ser	rs8192678	Risk allele is T
PPARG1A	rs7665116	Risk allele is T
PPARG1A	rs3774923	Risk allele is T
PPARG1A	rs2970869	Risk allele is T

What does the PPARG1A gene do?

The PPARG1A gene is the blueprint for the body to make the PGC1A protein. The PGC1A protein regulates the genes involved in energy metabolism, and is the **master regulator of mitochondrial biogenesis**[1, 2, 3.] Mitochondrial biogenesis is a process that every cell undergoes to increase mitochondrial size. This is important because having larger mitochondria leads to a higher production of energy by increasing ATP (the energy molecule of the body). It is impossible to be a healthy person without healthy mitochondria.

What health conditions are associated with having a PPARG1A risk allele?

Neurodegenerative disorders— Mitochondrial dysfunctions are the prime source of neurodegenerative diseases and neurodevelopmental disorders[1]. A common hallmark of several neurodegenerative diseases is smaller and less healthy mitochondria as a result of having impaired function of PGC-1α protein and risk alleles in the PPARG1A gene. Some common neurodegenerative diseases that are associated with having unhealthy mitochondria include Huntington's, Alzheimer's, and Parkinson's Disease[1.]

Diabetes/ Insulin resistance—*The level of PGC1α mRNA in skeletal muscle was observed to be lower in individuals with insulin resistance and Type-2 diabetes*[8].It has been widely observed that improving mitochondrial function also improves *insulin sensitivity and prevents type 2 diabetes*[1]. Thus, supporting healthy mitochondria appears as a suitable strategy to treat insulin resistance[1].

PPARG1A Gly482Ser (rs8192678) risk allele (T allele) is associated with:

- Having the risk allele for PPARG1A Gly482Ser (rs8192678) is associated with having lower levels of PCG-1a protein throughout the body, including in muscles[6]. Lower levels of PCG-1a protein leads to smaller and less healthy mitochondria. Lower levels of PCG-1a protein, and the resulting decreased health of mitochondria, are likely the causes for the health conditions that are listed below. The health condition listed below are associated with having the risk allele for PPARG1A Gly482Ser (rs8192678).

  - Increased blood pressure in those under 50 years of age.
  - Earlier onset of Huntington's disease[9].
  - Increased percentage of small dense-LDL particles (bad cholesterol) [10].
  - Increased weight gain in people with diabetes that were treated with insulin[11].
  - Decreased athletic performance, especially endurance performance[12, 13].
  - Obesity and weight gain[7, 14, 18].
  - Increased risk of developing *Type-2 diabetes*[6, 8, 14,15, 16].
  - Increased risk for developing *insulin resistance*[8,16].
  - Increased risk of developing *fatty liver disease*, and having an increased level of *ALT* liver enzymes[17].
  - Increased risk for developing hypertrophic cardiomyopathy[19].
  - Increased level of cancer causing free radicals when exercise, and thus a higher need for antioxidants with exercise[21].

PPARG1A Gly482Ser (rs8192678) non-risk allele (C allele) is associated with:

- Increase in longevity[4]—The increase in longevity is likely due to an increased size and health of the mitochondria due to having a higher level of PCG-1a protein.

PPARG1A (rs7665116)—The non-risk C allele is protective against Huntington's disease[5].

PPARG1A (rs3774923 and rs2970869)—The T risk allele is associated with increased DNA damage, and therefore, an increased need for antioxidants to help prevent cancer[20].

Christy L. Sutton D.C.

I have one or more risk allele(s) in the PPARG1A gene. What should I talk to my doctor about doing so that I can reduce my health risks?

Focus on supporting your body's ability to create and maintain healthy mitochondria by increasing PCG-1a naturally:

- *Ways to naturally increase PGC-1a levels include:*

  - *Endurance exercise (Aerobic exercise)*—Exercise has been shown to activate the PGC-1α gene in human skeletal muscles, and thus increase levels of PGC-1a protein and improve mitochondrial health[22]. Aerobic exercise, such as running, has been shown to increase the size of mitochondria.

  - *A low carbohydrate diet*—Ketosis or a low carbohydrate diet has been shown to increase PGC-1a levels, which can lead to healthier mitochondria[23.]

  - *Massaging the muscles*[24.]

  - *Increase nutrition that has been shown to support healthy mitochondria*[1]:

    - ❖ **Acetyl L- carnitine**[25]

    - ❖ **Creatinine**

    - ❖ **Magnesium**

    - ❖ **CoQ10**

    - ❖ **Antioxidants**—Antioxidants are especially important to prevent free radicals that cause cancer. Some antioxidants include:

      - ○ Alpha-lipoic acid
      - ○ Vitamin C, E, and A
      - ○ Glutathione—This antioxidant is especially important to prevent neurodegenerative conditions.
      - ○ Glucoraphanin

Personalized genetic report found at http://geneticdetoxification.com

> *Increase nitric oxide levels*[26]—This has been shown to increase mitochondrial size and health by increasing PCG-1a. Ways to **naturally** increase nitric oxide levels if they are too low inlcude:

- ❖ **Exercise (cardio)**—About 45 minutes of walking a day.

- ❖ **Weight control**—Lose weight if overweight.

- ❖ **Increase intake of beets and dark green vegetables.**

- ❖ **Avoid stomach acid reducers**—These can suppress nitric oxide production (antacids, Prilosec).

- ❖ **Increase intake of fruits and vegetables**

- ❖ **Niacin (vitamin B-3)**—Niacin can cause an increase in nitric oxide, which is was causes the niacin flush

References:

1.) Valero T (2014). "Mitochondrial biogenesis: pharmacological approaches". Curr. Pharm. Des. 20 (35): 5507–9.

2.)Sanchis-Gomar F, García-Giménez JL, et al. (2014). "Mitochondrial biogenesis in health and disease. Molecular and therapeutic approaches". Curr. Pharm. Des. 20 (35): 5619–5633.

3.) Dorn GW, Vega RB, Kelly DP (2015). "Mitochondrial biogenesis and dynamics in the developing and diseased heart". Genes Dev. 29 (19): 1981–91.

4.)Clark J, Reddy S, Zheng K, Betensky RA, Simon DK. Association of PGC-1alpha polymorphisms with age of onset and risk of Parkinson's disease. BMC medical genetics. 2011;12:69.

5.)Che HV, Metzger S, et al. Localization of sequence variations in PGC-1α influence their modifying effect in Huntington disease. Mol Neurodegener. 2011 Jan 6;6(1):1.

6. Franks P.W., Ekelund U., Brage S., et al. PPARGC1A coding variation may initiate impaired NEFA clearance during glucose challenge. Diabetologia. 2007;50(3):569–573.

7.) Deeb SS, Brunzell JD. The role of the PGC1α Gly482Ser polymorphism in weight gain due to intensive diabetes therapy. PPAR Res. 2009;2009:649286.

8.) Ling C, Poulsen P, Carlsson E, et al. Multiple environmental and genetic factors influence skeletal muscle PGC-1alpha and PGC-1beta gene expression in twins.J Clin Invest. 2004 Nov; 114(10):1518-26.

9.) Weydt P1, Soyal SM, Gellera C, et al. The gene coding for PGC-1alpha modifies age at onset in Huntington's Disease. Mol Neurodegener. 2009 Jan 8;4:3.

Christy L. Sutton D.C.

10.) Sarah L. Prior, Amy R. Clark, et al. Association of the PGC-1α rs8192678 Variant with Microalbuminuria in Subjects with Type 2 Diabetes Mellitus. Volume 32 (2012), Issue 6, Pages 363-369.

11.) Deeb SS, Brunzell JD. The role of the pgc1alpha gly482ser polymorphism in weight gain due to intensive diabetes therapy. PPAR Res. 2009;2009:649286.

12.).Lucia A1, Gómez-Gallego F, et al. PPARGC1A genotype (Gly482Ser) predicts exceptional endurance capacity in European men. J Appl Physiol (1985). 2005 Jul;99(1):344-8. Epub 2005 Feb 10

13.) Eynon N1, Meckel Y, Sagiv M, Yamin C, et al. Do PPARGC1A and PPARalpha polymorphisms influence sprint or endurance phenotypes? Scand J Med Sci Sports. 2010 Feb;20(1):e145-50.

14.) Samir S. Deeb, and John D. Brunzell The Role of the PGC1α Gly482Ser Polymorphism in Weight Gain due to Intensive Diabetes Therapy. PPAR Res. 2009; 2009: 649286.

15.) Jing C , Xueyao H, Linong J. Meta-analysis of association studies between five candidate genes and type 2 diabetes in Chinese Han population. Endocrine. 2012 Oct;42(2):307-20. Epub 2012 Mar 6.

16.) Ha CD, Cho JK,et al. Relationship of PGC-1α gene polymorphism with insulin resistance syndrome in Korean children. Asia Pac J Public Health. 2015 Mar;27(2):NP544-51.

17.) Lin YC, Chang PF, et al. A common variant in the peroxisome proliferator-activated receptor-γ coactivator-1α gene is associated with nonalcoholic fatty liver disease in obese children. Am J Clin Nutr. 2013 Feb;97(2):326-31.

18.) Franks PW, Christophi CA, et al. Common variation at PPARGC1A/B and change in body composition and metabolic traits following preventive interventions: the Diabetes Prevention Program. Diabetologia. 2014;57(3):485–90

19.) Wang S, Fu C, Wang H, et al. Polymorphisms of the peroxisome proliferator-activated receptor-γcoactivator-1α gene are associated with hypertrophic cardiomyopathy and not with hypertension hypertrophy. Clinical Chemistry and Laboratory Medicine. 2007;45(8):962–967.

20.) Chao-Qiang Lai, et al. PPARGC1A Variation Associated With DNA Damage, Diabetes, and Cardiovascular Diseases: The Boston Puerto Rican Health Study. Diabetes. 2008 Apr; 57(4): 809–816.

21.) Angelique Pasquinelli, Lucia Chico. Gly482Ser PGC-1α Gene Polymorphism and Exercise-Related Oxidative Stress in Amyotrophic Lateral Sclerosis Patients. Front Cell Neurosci. 2016; 10: 102.

22.) Pilegaard H, Saltin B, Neufer PD (February 2003). "Exercise induces transient transcriptional activation of the PGC-1alpha gene in human skeletal muscle". J. Physiol. (Lond.). 546 (Pt 3): 851–8.

23.) Newman J, Verdin E. Ketone bodies as signaling metabolites. (2013). Cell Press. Vol 25. Issue 1.

24.) Crane JD, Ogborn DI, Cupido C, Melov S, Hubbard A, Bourgeois JM, Tarnopolsky MA (February 2012). "Massage therapy attenuates inflammatory signaling after exercise-induced muscle damage". Sci Transl Med. 4(119): 119ra13.

25.) Hagen, Tory M.; Wehr, et al. (1998-11-01). "Mitochondrial Decay in Aging: Reversal through Supplementation of Acetyl-l-Carnitine and N-tert-Butyl-α-phenyl-nitronea". Annals of the New York Academy of Sciences. 854 (1): 214–223.

26.) Vitor A. Lira, Dana L. Brown, et al. Nitric oxide and AMPK cooperatively regulate PGC-1α in skeletal muscle cells. J Physiol 588.18 (2010) pp 3551–3566.

Personalized genetic report found at http://geneticdetoxification.com

HIF1A gene

Hypoxia-inducible factor 1α

Names of HIF1A genetic variants (SNP identification)	rsnumber	Risk allele
HIF1A Pro582Ser	rs11549465	T allele, associated with being a **weight lifter or sprinter**. Allows for muscles to function better without oxygen. C allele- most common, associated with being an **endurance athlete**.
HIF1A	rs2301113	**Risk allele**= C allele- associated with lower levels of HIF1A, and therefore, lower levels of oxygen delivered throughout the body. A allele is associate with a decreased risk of developing obesity, hypertension, and Type-2 diabetes.

What does the HIF1A gene do?

HIF1A is important for delivering oxygen to the cells, which is imperative for athletic function and general health.

Hypoxia-inducible factor 1 (HIF-1) regulates gene expression in response to hypoxia (low oxygen) and has been associated with enhancing athletic performance[4].

What type of health characteristics are associated with having one or more risk allele(s) for HIFIA gene?

- **HIFIA Pro582Ser (rs11549465)**

  - **T allele for HIFIA Pro582Ser**—This is associated with being a **weight lifter or sprinter**[1]. *Allows* for muscles to function better without oxygen. The T allele may *increase one's ability to perform in a hypoxic (low oxygen) state*, such as what occurs with weightlifters and sprinters. The T allele may allow the HIF-1α protein to be more stable, and therefore, improve glucose metabolism, possibly lowering the risk of Type-2 Diabetes[2].

Christy L. Sutton D.C.

Having one or more T alleles for HIFIA Pro582Ser is associated with developing stable exertional angina rather than having an acute myocardial infarction[3]. Stable exertional angina is chest pain that occurs from a lack of blood flow, or oxygen, to the heart muscles. If you have the T allele for HIFIA Pro582Ser then your muscles can function better without oxygen, therefore, you may experience less damage to the heart muscles.

> **C allele HIFIA Pro582Ser**—This is the most common genotype and is associated with being an ***endurance athlete***.

- **HIF1A (rs2301113)**

  > **C allele for HIF1A (rs2301113)**—This is associated with lower levels of HIF1A, and therefore, lower levels of oxygen delivered throughout the body. *Increased* risk of developing obesity, hypertension, and Type-2 diabetes.

  > **A allele for HIF1A (rs2301113)**— This is associate with a *decreased* risk of developing obesity, hypertension, and Type-2 diabetes.

- **Genetic combo for sprinter versus endurance athlete**—Having the genetic combo of HIFIA Pro582Ser (T, T) and ACTN3 R577X (C,C) (on page 396) is highly predictive of being a ***sprinter***. Whereas having the genotype HIFIA Pro582Ser (C, C) and ACTN3 R577X (T,T,) was highly predictive of being an ***endurance*** athlete[4].

References:

1.) Gabbasov RT1, Arkhipova AA, Borisova AV, Hakimullina AM, et al. The HIF1A gene Pro582Ser polymorphism in Russian strength athletes. J Strength Cond Res. 2013 Aug;27(8):2055-8.

2.) Nagy G, Kovacs-Nagy R, et al. Association of hypoxia inducible factor-1 alpha gene polymorphism with both type 1 and type 2 diabetes in a Caucasian (Hungarian) sample. BMC Med Genet. 2009;10:79.

3.) Hlatky MA1, Quertermous T, Boothroyd DB,et al. Polymorphisms in hypoxia inducible factor 1 and the initial clinical presentation of coronary disease. Am Heart J. 2007 Dec;154(6):1035-42. Epub 2007 Sep 18.

4.) Eynon N, Alves A.J, et al. Is the interaction between HIF1A P582S and ACTN3 R577X determinant for power/ sprint performance? Metabolism. 2010;59(6):861–865.

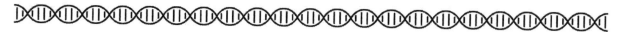

Personalized genetic report found at http://geneticdetoxification.com

Running can be good for you brain, but avoid excessive running if you have this genetic risk factor

ADAM12

Names of ADAM12 gene genetic variants (SNP identification)	rsnumber	Risk allele
ADAM12	rs3740199	Risk allele is C

If you have one or more risk allele(s) in this gene (ADAM12-rs1800562), you're at an increased risk for developing osteoarthritis in your knees[1.] The (C/C) genotype is most strongly associated with developing this issue.

How to prevent developing knee osteoarthritis if you have the risk allele for ADAM12:

- *Avoid high-impact activities*—High-impact activities, such as running and jumping (especially running downhill). These can quickly damage knee cartilage. Low-impact activities include cycling, swimming and walking.

- *Maintain a healthy weight*—For every pound of weight that you lose, you relieve four pounds of pressure from your knees.

- *Consider supplementing with collagen, glucosamine with chondroitin, and fish oil*—These can help preserve cartilage integrity in your knees.

Reference

1,) Kerna I., Kisand K., Tamm A. E., Lintrop M. Missense single nucleotide polymorphism of the ADAM12 gene is associated with radiographic knee osteoarthritis in middle-aged Estonian cohort. Osteoarthritis and Cartilage. 2009;17(8):1093–1098.

Christy L. Sutton D.C.

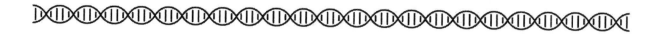

ACTN3 gene
Alpha-actinin-3

Names of ACTN3 genetic variants (SNP identification)	rsnumber	Risk allele
ACTN3 R577X The ACTN3 gene is *only* expressed in *fast twitch* muscle fibers.	rs1815739	(C, C): Better performing muscles. ***Likely a sprinter*** (C, T): ***Mix of sprinter and endurance muscle types***, but likely a sprinter. (T, T): Impaired muscle performance. Likely an ***endurance*** athlete.

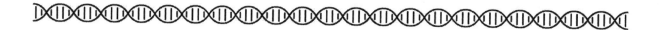

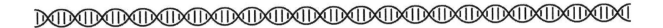

For more information on genes related to muscles/joints and athletic performance consult the following pages:

- **MTHFR gene:** Pg. 87

- **MTRR gene:** Pg. 101

- **PEMT gene:** Pg. 150

- **GCH1 gene:** Pg. 211

- For more information about genes that affect collagen, muscle, and joint recovery you can read the article titled "Genes That Can Increase Risk of Sports Injuries, and What You Can Do About It", which is found at http://geneticdetoxification.com

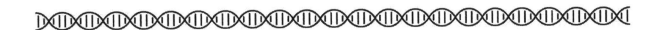

Christy L. Sutton D.C.

Glossary

Allele—An allele is a variant form of a given gene. Different form a genes are known as alleles. For example, an allele can determine if you have dark or light colored skin.

Antioxidants—A substance (such as beta-carotene, vitamin E, vitamin A, vitamin C, etc.) that inhibits oxidation or reactions promoted by oxygen, peroxides, or free radicals.

Bases—The building blocks of DNA. There are 4 bases for building DNA: Adenine (A), Cytosine (C), Guanine (G), and Thymine (T). Bases exist on each strand of the DNA double helix, and bind together in complementary pairs of A-T and C-G.

Chromosome—A tightly wound bundles of DNA strands found in the nucleus of most living cells, carrying genetic information in the form of genes. The human body has 23 chromosomes. Chromosomes structurally resemble an "X".

DNA—DNA is made up of thousands of genes. DNA is comprised of a combination of bases, which are denoted as the letters A, T, G, and C.

Epigenetics—Epigenetics is the study of biological and environmental mechanisms that will switch genes on and off. Epigenetics refers to how one's health can be influenced for the better or worse based on changes in the environment rather than changes in one's genes.

Free radical—An especially reactive atom or group of atoms that has one or more unpaired electrons. Free radicals are produced in the body by natural biological processes or introduced from an outside source (such as tobacco smoke, toxins, or pollutants) and that can damage cells, proteins, and DNA by altering their chemical structure. Free radicals can be neutralized, and thus rendered harmless, by antioxidants.

Gene— A sequence of DNA that codes for a specific protein. A unit of heredity that is transferred from a parent to offspring and is held to determine some characteristic of the offspring. Genes are located on chromosomes.

Genetic variants—Changes in one's genetic sequence that is either common, such as in a SNP, or rare, as in a mutation. Genetic variants can potentially have negative effects. See SNP and mutation.

Genotype— The genetic constitution of an individual organism.

Glutathione—An important antioxidant, detoxifier, immune modulator, and coenzyme. Glutathione is a Phase II detox pathway.

Methylation—The addition of a carbon group to a molecule or DNA strand, which alters the function. Methylation is a detoxification process that the body undergoes to remove toxins in Phase II detox.

Mutation—Uncommon changes in the genetic sequence that can potentially have negative effects.

Non-risk allele— This is the base (A, C, T, and G) that may be associated with potentially having fewer negative health effects than the risk allele. This is generally a more common genotype.

Risk allele—This is the base (A, C, T, and G) that may be associated with potentially having more negative health effects than the non-risk allele. This is generally a less common genotype.

Single nucleotide polymorphisms, SNPs—Frequently called SNPs (pronounced "snips"), are the most common type of genetic variation among people. Each SNP represents a difference in a single DNA building block, called a nucleotide. For example, a SNP may replace the nucleotide cytosine (C) with the nucleotide thymine (T) in a certain stretch of DNA. SNPs can potentially have negative effects.

Telomere—A region of repetitive nucleotide sequences at each end of a chromosome, which protects the end of the chromosome from deterioration or from fusion with

Appendix

Letter A

A2M gene, 169
AANAT gene, 7
ABCA2 gene, 167-168
Abdominal pain, 271, 376
ABP1, 310-311
ACE gene, 337-339
Acetaminophen, 28, 60, 63
Acetate, 140
Acetaldehyde, 137, 140, 141
Acetylation Detox Genes, 66-70,267
Acetylcholine, 158, 171, 187, 194, 202, 205, 210, 214, 218, 220, 222, 346
Acetyl L- carnitine, 158, 390
Acid-reducing drugs (antacids, PPI), 25, 26, 29, 34, 37, 40, 41, 43, 46, 49, 53, 362, 391
Acne, 372, 374
Actin binding protein 1- see ABPI gene
Activated B vitamins- see vitamins- B
ADA gene, 244-246, 318
ADD, Attention deficient disorder, 185, 193, 271
ADD1 gene, 340-341
Addiction, 182. Also see substance abuse.
Addison's disease, 271, 274
Adducin 1 gene-see ADD1 gene
Adenosine deaminase gene-see ADA gene
Adenosylcobalamin, 98, 104-106, 119
ADH1B gene, 137, 141
ADH1C gene, 137
ADHD, Attention deficient hyper activity
disorder, 81, 144, 182, 185, 190, 193, 200, 203, 214, 271
ADK gene, 111, 112, 113
Adrenal, 26, 34, 54, 74, 78, 80, 117, 118, 150, 180, 181, 186, 194, 201, 205, 215, 218, 220, 341
Advil, 39, 41
Aerobic exercise, 157, 184, 193, 201, 204, 209, 240, 243, 246, 265, 292, 295, 351, 390
Aflatoxin B1, 28-29
Aggressive behavior, 188-190
Aging, 13, 25, 99, 149
Agoraphobia, 208
AGT gene, 341-342.
AHCY gene, 113-114

Air pollution, 24, 29, 295, 311, 314, 317
Alcohol, 14, 16, 48, 60, 135, 136-142, 162, 167, 182, 190, 197, 198, 203, 213, 214, 217, 229, 232, 252, 293, 311, 338, 351, 354, 356
Alcohol dehydrogenase, 137
Alcoholism, 182, 190, 203, 213, 217
ALDH2 gene, 140-142
Aleve, 39, 41
Allergies and hypersensitivities, 14, 190, 212, 268, 271, 272, 273, 274, 279, 280-298, 307-317, 339
Alpha-lipoic acid, 25, 30, 34, 37, 40, 43, 46, 49, 53, 158, 230, 232, 233, 240, 242, 249, 253, 265, 361, 373, 390
Alpha-2-macroglobulin- see A2M gene
ALS, amyotrophic lateral sclerosis, 88, 248, 271
Alzheimer's disease, 15, 64, 81, 88, 92, 94, 116, 144, 148, 151, 156, 157-177, 252, 255, 257, 292, 299-306, 353-356, 376
How to potentially reduce the risk of developing Alzheimer's, 157
Ammonia, 119, 120, 121
Amphetamine, 185, 193
Amyloid beta, 170, 176
Amyloid beta A4 precursor protein-binding family B member 2 gene- see APBB2 gene, 170-171
Amyotrophic Lateral Sclerosis- see ALS
Anaphylactic, 310, 316
Androgens, 78
Anemia, 24, 29, 33, 36, 39, 42, 45, 49, 53, 101, 271, 378
Anesthesia, 103
Angiotensin gene-see AGT gene
Angiotensin converting enzyme-see ACE gene
ANKK1 gene, 216-217,
ANK3, 219-223, 364
Ankyrin repeat and kinase domain containing 1 gene- see ANKK1 gene
Ankyrin 3 gene, 219
Antibiotics, 32, 311
Anticonvulsant, 41
Antidepressant, 41, 149, 311
Antioxidant, 18, 25, 30, 34, 37, 40,43, 46, 49, 53, 57, 59, 62, 63, 70, 74, 79, 96,129, 133, 138, 148, 155, 158, 163, 184, 193, 201, 204,

Letter B

Christy L. Sutton D.C.

Drugs, 13-14, 21, 25-26, 29, 32, 34, 37, 39-49, 53, 67-69, 72, 77, 129, 162, 172, 185, 193, 197, 311, 336, 338, 347, 348
Dunwoody Labs, 63, 65, 313

Letter E

Empathy, 183, 189-190, 196
Endocrine disruptor, 85, 93
Endometriosis, 151, 153
Endothelial nitric oxide—see NOS3
Endurance, 386, 389, 390, 393, 394, 396
Epigenetics, 13, 398
Epilepsy, 41, 210, 271
Epinephrine, 181-195, 198-202, 222, 344
Erectile dysfunction, 211, 360
ESR, Erythrocyte Sedimentation Rate, 275, 278, 280, 282, 284, 286, 287, 293, 296, 298, 308, 317, 348
ESR2 gene, 262-263
Essential oil, 185, 193
Estradiol, 23, 32, 52, 229, 234, 263
Estriol, 263
Estrone, 23, 32, 52, 263
Estrogen, 22-26, 31-35, 51-54, 62, 73, 138, 153, 181-183, 185-186, 189, 229-230, 232-234, 262-264
    16-hydroxylation of estrogen, 51
    4-hydroxylation of estrogen, 31, 32
    2-hydroxylation of estrogen, 22-23
Estrogen dominance, 23, 26, 31, 32, 34, 52, 54
Estrogen receptor 2-see ESR2 gene
Ethanol, 48, 137
Excedrin, 39, 41
Exhaust, 23, 24, 28, 29
Eye problems, 373
    Macular degeneration, 59, 92

Letter F

Factor 5 (F5) gene, 321-323
Factor 2 (F2) gene (prothrombin), 324-325
Factor 3 (F3) gene, 326-327
Factor 11 (F11) gene, 329-331
FADS1 gene, 357
FADS2 gene, 154-155
Fallon, James; 187, 195-196, 199
Fast detoxifier/ metabolizer, 67-68
Fatigue, 88, 101, 200, 211, 219, 271, 276, 348, 376

Fasting, 149, 158, 232, 235, 236, 300, 305, 348, 350, 352, 354, 356
Fatty acid desaturase 1 gene-see FADS1 gene
Fatty acid desaturase 2 gene- see FADS2 gene
Fatty liver, 122, 123, 151-153, 389
Fc fragment of IgE receptor Ia gene-see FCER1A gene
FCER1A gene, 313-314
FCGR2A gene, 264, 266
Ferritin, 26, 30, 34, 38, 40, 43, 46, 50, 54, 175, 250, 254, 261, 377
Fiber, 15, 24, 33, 52, 53, 73, 117, 157, 162, 167, 237, 273, 292, 295, 338, 340, 342, 344, 348, 350-351, 354, 356, 396
Fibrinogen activity test, 323, 325, 328, 330
Fibromyalgia, 88, 109, 111, 114, 182, 190, 271
Fish oil, 24, 33, 52, 148, 154, 154, 162, 167, 184, 192, 197, 200, 204, 209, 212, 214, 217, 275, 280, 282, 284-289, 293, 296, 297, 299, 308, 316, 317, 322, 325, 327, 329, 333, 335, 348, 349, 350, 351, 354, 356, 395
Flaxseed, 357
Focus, also see concentration, 178, 182-183, 191, 197, 211
Folate, see vitamin B-9
Folic acid, see vitamin B-9,
Folinic acid, see vitamin B-9,
Food allergies, 212, 274, 279, 280-298, 308, 316, 317, 339
FOLR1, FOLR2 and FOLR3 genes, 379-381
Folate receptor genes-see FOLR1, FOLR2, and FOLR3 genes
Food dye, 78
Forkhead box protein E1 gene-see FOXE1 gene
Formic acid, 122
FOXE1 gene, 258, 259
Frontal lobe, 181, 196, 203
Frying, 69
Fucosyltransferase 2 gene-see FUT2 gene
FUT2 gene, 302-303, 385

Letter G

GABA, 120, 147, 187, 194, 202, 205, 207, 208, 210, 214, 218, 220, 222, 292, 345
GAD1, 207-210
GAD2, 207
Gall bladder disease, 72, 376
Gall stones, 72
Gamma-glutamyl hydrolase gene-see GGH gene

Letter H

Letter N

Christy L. Sutton D.C.

Christy L. Sutton D.C.

Vitamin B5, Pantothenic acid, 180, 193,
Vitamin B6; pyridoxal, P-5-P, 93, 121, 193, 218, 368
Vitamin B-9, 24, 34, 86-93, 96, 97, 100-101,
Folate, 90-93, 95, 96, 99, 122, 139, 142, 153, 379-381
    Folic acid, 90, 91, 380
    Folinic acid, 96
    Vitamin B-9 Methylation Genes, 87
Vitamin B-12, 7, 10, 24,34,86,93, 96, 99-106, 111, 113, 120, 125, 153, 279, 303, 304, 383-386
    Methylcobalamin, 34, 96, 99-106, 113, 120, 153, 279
    Adenosylcobalamin, 99, 105-107, 120
Vitamin B-12 methylation genes, 99
Vitamin C,25, 30, 35, 38, 41, 44, 47, 50, 54, 70,
Vitamin E, 25, 30, 35, 38, 41, 44, 47, 54, 159, 231, 234, 241, 243, 246, 254, 266, 322-324
Vitamin K-2, 372
Viral infections, 18, 60, 245, 246, 280, 294
Virus, 302, 304

Letter W

Warfarin, 42, 256
Warrior gene, 184, 189, 190, 192, 196, 198
Water retention, 368
Weight loss, 272
Weight gain, 272, 391, and 392
Worrier gene, 184

104, 111, 113, 120, 139, 140, 143, 153, 279, 283, 379-382, 386

159, 185, 194, 202, 205, 210, 231, 234, 241, 243, 246, 247, 250, 254, 266, 294, 297, 313, 362, 374, 391, 399
Vitamin D, 25, 27, 30, 31, 34, 35, 37, 38, 40, 41, 43, 44, 46-47, 50, 51, 54, 55, 159, 163, 164, 167-170, 172, 173, 234, 235, 239, 241, 244, 258, 266, 276, 278, 279, 281-283, 285, 287, 289, 291, 294, 297, 299, 301, 309, 314, 318, 339, 340, 349, 355, 357, 369-372
Vitamin D receptor gene-see VDR gene

Letter X

Xenobiotics, 32, 78

Letter Y

Yeast, 74, 121, 122

Letter Z
Zinc, 103-104, 113, 118-120, 177-178, 193, 232, 236, 247, 294, 297, 375, 376

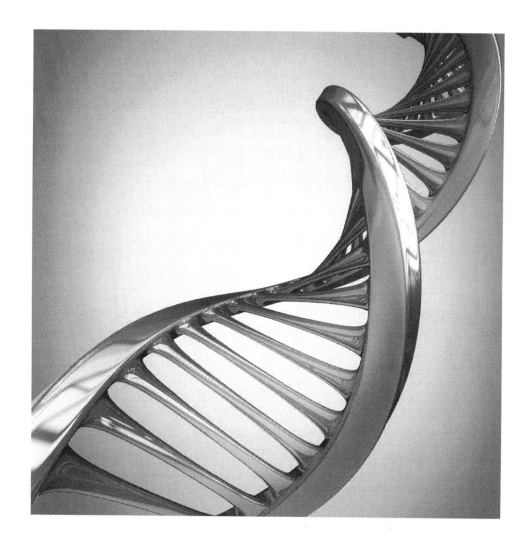

**If you have already done "23andMe", then you
can get a personalized report that follows along with this book at:
https://geneticdetoxification.com**

Made in the USA
Columbia, SC
15 May 2023

16304412R00226